CHEMOTHERAPY

Volume 1
Clinical Aspects of Infections

CHEMOTHERAPY

CHEMOTHERAPY

Volume 1
Clinical Aspects of Infections

Edited by
J.D. Williams
The London Hospital Medical College
London, U.K.

and
A.M. Geddes
East Birmingham Hospital
Birmingham, U.K.

Plenum Press · New York and London

Library of Congress Cataloging in Publication Data

International Congress of Chemotherapy, 9th, London, 1975.
  Clinical aspects of infections.

  (Chemotherapy; v. 1)
  1. Chemotherapy — Congresses. 2. Communicable diseases — Congresses. 3. Antibiotics — Congresses. I. Williams, John David, M.D. II. Geddes, Alexander McIntosh. III. Title. IV. Series.
RM260.2.C45   vol. 1   615'.58s [616.9]   76-1948
ISBN-13: 978-1-4613-4348-6   e-ISBN-13: 978-1-4613-4346-2
DOI: 10.1007/ 978-1-4613-4346-2

Proceedings of the Ninth International Congress of Chemotherapy
held in London, July, 1975 will be published in eight volumes,
of which this is volume one.

© 1976 Plenum Press, New York
Softcover reprint of the hardcover 1st edition 1976
A Division of Plenum Publishing Corporation
227 West 17th Street, New York, N.Y. 10011

United Kingdom edition published by Plenum Press, London
A Division of Plenum Publishing Company, Ltd.
Davis House (4th Floor), 8 Scrubs Lane, Harlesden, London, NW10 6SE, England

CHEMOTHERAPY

Proceedings of the
9th International Congress of Chemotherapy
held in London, July, 1975

Preface

The International Society of Chemotherapy meets every two years to review progress in chemotherapy of infections and of malignant disease. Each meeting gets larger to encompass the extension of chemotherapy into new areas. In some instances, expansion has been rapid, for example in cephalosporins, penicillins and combination chemotherapy of cancer - in others slow, as in the field of parasitology. New problems of resistance and untoward effects arise; reduction of host toxicity without loss of antitumour activity by new substances occupies wide attention. The improved results with cancer chemotherapy, especially in leukaemias, are leading to a greater prevalence of severe infection in patients so treated, pharmacokinetics of drugs in normal and diseased subjects is receiving increasing attention along with related problems of bioavailability and interactions between drugs. Meanwhile the attack on some of the major bacterial infections, such as gonorrhoea and tuberculosis, which were among the first infections to feel the impact of chemotherapy, still continue to be major world problems and are now under attack with new agents and new methods.

From this wide field and the 1,000 papers read at the Congress we have produced Proceedings which reflect the variety and vigour of research in this important field of medicine. It was not possible to include all of the papers presented at the Congress but we have attempted to include most aspects of current progress in chemotherapy.

We thank the authors of these communications for their cooperation in enabling the Proceedings to be available at the earliest possible date. The method of preparation does not allow for uniformity of typefaces and presentation of the material and we hope that the blemishes of language and typographical errors do not detract from the understanding of the reader and the importance of the Proceedings.

> K. HELLMANN, Imperial Cancer Research Fund
> A. M. GEDDES, East Birmingham Hospital
> J. D. WILLIAMS, The London Hospital Medical College

Contents

WELCOMING ADDRESS

William Brumfitt

President of the Congress

Ladies and Gentlemen,

On behalf of the Organising Committee of the 9th International Congress of Chemotherapy it is my pleasure and privilege to welcome you to London.

As in the case of previous Congresses the Organising Committee has been anxious to bring together an audience of experts actively engaged in the study of Antimicrobial and Cancer Chemotherapy. The Organising Committee was elected in order to represent the major disciplines concerned and had the difficult task of assembling a suitable programme.

Despite their importance it was necessary to exclude certain subjects because of the limited time available. The view was taken that it would be better to deal with the chosen subjects in detail rather than to discuss more subjects in less depth. The accent has been laid more on scientific and medical progress rather than technicological advances which in our view are best dealt with in communications to specialist journals. In selecting the topics for presentation we have been acutely aware of those subjects likely to lead to lively discussion.

We are pleased to see so many associate members and we must pay high tribute to Dr. David Hughes who has seen to it that an attractive and varied social programme has been arranged. I have also received great support from Dr. Jacomb, our Treasurer. Dr. Fred Wrigley, CBE, who was our business consultant, gave invaluable help over the two years of preparation and Mr. Douglas Armitage made the banking arragements which in view of the presence of delegates from 49 countries was no small task.

In spite of the many difficulties that inevitably arise in planning such a congress, a friendly atmosphere was maintained between all the members of the Organising Committee - to whom I am extremely grateful.

Finally, we must thank those members of the Pharmaceutical Industry who not only gave generous financial support but produced the compounds about which much of the discussion was based.

OPENING OF THE CONGRESS

David Owen

Minister of State

Department of Health and Social Security

My first duty is to apologise on behalf of the Secretary of State,
Mrs. Barbara Castle, that she is unable to be present owing to a
Cabinet Meeting that has been called for this morning. As a Vice
Patron of your Organisation she was looking forward very to much to
welcoming this important Congress to London and welcoming the dele-
gates on behalf of Her Majesty's Government.

It is rare in this country for a doctor to be Minister of
Health; indeed at times one suffers an identity crisis. Last night
as I was filling in my application for a new passport I had to decide what was my occupation: it could have been Minister of the
Crown, it could have been Member of Parliament but eventually I
settled for my first love and my true identity namely a Medical
Practitioner. I represent a generation of doctors that has never
known any other era than that of chemotherapy. For us it is difficult to envisage medical and surgical practice in the 1920s and
before that. We have lived all our medical lives with the knowledge
that we can use the powerful agents of chemotherapy to help our
patients and this must undoubtedly have influenced our whole attitude to medicine and science. This Congress has many distinguished
people present who have all made unique contributions to medical
science. It is in some ways invidious for me to single any of them
out but I hope you will allow me to mention three; Sir Ernst Chain,
has already been mentioned. His contribution to the discovery of
pencillin is world known. Professor Abraham, who is a Vice President
of your Congress and with me here on the platform, has made a major
contribution to the discovery not only of pencillin but also of
cephelosporin and Dr. Umezawa, from Japan, has made a major contribution in the discovery of kanamycin.

3

When I think of the advances in chemotherapy my mind goes back
to when as a young house physician, recently qualified, I admitted
straight from an ambulance into a children's ward a small child desperately ill, semi-comatose and clearly dying. That child had
bacterial meningitis, and yet, following immediate treatment, within
24 hours we had the greatest difficulty in keeping the child in bed
and from running around the ward. When one has witnessed one of
those miracles of medical science, it undoubtedly changes many of
one's basic attitudes.

It we look historically at what has happened over tuberculosis
- in the early 1940s the annual death rate from tuberculosis was
around 26,500 people in the United Kingdom, in 1971 it had dropped
to only 1,438. Notifications from tuberculosis were running at
50,000 a year in 1956, today there are less than 10,000. Improved
living standards, better hygiene, BCG vaccinations, all made their
contribution but over the last two decades no-one can doubt the
major advance has come from chemotherapy.

In cancer therapy there have too been substantial advances. In
Hodgkin's disease, chemotherapy is making a real contribution. Combination chemotherapy in many aspects of cancer therapy is showing
signs of progress and particularly in leukaemia and the leukaemia of
childhood there has been really remarkable progress in the last five
years.

If one looks at the infections that still afflict the world, the
impact of chemotherapy on syphilis, meningitis, the plague, leprosy,
has been quite dramatic.

No one individual, no one group, no one discipline has made
these advances possible, it has been the result of joint work and
multidisciplinary activity.

I am glad to pay tribute to the interest and support that the
pharmaceutical industry has given to this Congress and it would be
foolish to pretend that many of the advances that have taken place
in chemotherapy could have been done without the effort and energy
of the pharmaceutical industry. No doctor believes that advances
in chemotherapy can be undertaken in future without a genuine part-
nership developing between the pharmaceutical industry, chemists,
doctors, medical research, both in universities and institutes,

I feel I must praise the breadth and the depth of the scientific
programme which you have put on for this Congress. It shows the
range of modern chemotherapy and in particular I was interested in
the joint meetings between people facing the interesting problems
that are now arising from much of modern cancer therapy. There is an
obvious need to bring in to the discussions physicians interested in
the control of infections in view of the many people receiving strong

poisons which are given as part of the cancer chemotherapy and which
suppress the natural resistance of the body to infections. There is
a great deal that can be learnt on these difficult problems by bringing together people with experience in both fields and I am glad that
your Congress is tackling this.

It would be wrong for me as a politician, not to address myself
to some of the problems that exist over medical research. It is a
subject that has interested me personally for a number of years,
starting when I was myself involved in medical research. There are,
I believe, two fallacious but often strongly held views. On the one
hand there are those who believe that decisions on the objectives and
conduct of medical research can only be undertaken by medical scientists alone. On the other hand, there is in my view the even more
wrongly headed view held by many politicians that since the Government
is now the major funder of most medical research, the Government should
be responsible for the direction and conduct of medical research.
Both views are, in my view, wrong. I do not wish to discuss in too
great a detail the organisation of the British medical research but
many of you will know that following the recommendations of Lord
Rothschild, who was acting as a policy adviser to the then Government,
in 1972 Britain introduced a fundamental change in the management of
its research programme. Hitherto for 50 years the Medical Research
Council had been the dominant and indeed almost only vehicle for controlling medical research. There is no question but that the record
of the Medical Research Council was a very fine one and they and many
scientists understandably felt very anxious about any changes. I
believe, however, that the debate was too dominated by those who
wished to resist any Governmental influence. An influence which in my
view is wholly legitimate. The vital question is the extent of such
influence.

Since 1972 the Department of Health and Social Security has taken
over a new role of funding and commissioning research both on a broad
basis and in some detail from Medical Research Council. The amount of
research commissioned in this way is only about one-quarter of the
MRC's budget and it has been agreed that the management of biomedical
research, commissioned by the Department, should remain with the
Medical Research Council.

What we are trying to achieve, and I don't under-rate the difficulty, is a reconciliation of the natural wish of the politician and
of Government to think short-term and the essential need for long-term
thinking in medical research. We need a synthesis between the views of
the medical scientist thinking long, often pursuing ideas not orientated solely towards problem-solving research or mission orientated
research and the views of the Government which are bound to be influenced by the number of people who suffer from any particular ailment and
the distress and disruption that some illnesses can produce. I am
against a fusion of research effort, for example, I would not be in
favour of a fusion between the Medical Research Council and the Department of Health. I favour a separation, but co-ordination. I think

there is a lot to be said for the fact that there is an independence
under these new arrangements of the budget. Part of the budget lies
still solely under the control of the MRC, a smaller part lies under
the control of the Health Departments but by using the MRC as the
Departments' agent and by jointly discussing research priorities, I
think the much needed reconciliation and synthesis is achievable. It
will not be easy. No Minister of Health in any country in the world
at the moment can be unaware of the rising costs of medical research.
They are bound to constantly wish to put mass suffering, mass problems,
in the forefront of any research programme but it would be an extremely
foolish politician who thought that a Government Department could
itself alone spot the potential for new discoveries. We know from
history that many of the major medical advances have not come as a result of settling down and trying to establish an objective but have come
accidentally. I constantly stress that resources, though important,
are no-where near as important as people. It is because individuals
have been prepared to innovate, to discover, to follow a particular bent
or feeling that we have had some of the major breakthroughs in medical
research. We need to cherish the spirit of innovation and independence,
whether it's in our universities, medical research institutes, or
whether it's in research funded by voluntary bodies or through Government Departments.

I said at the outset that I come from a generation of physicians
that has always lived in the age of chemotherapy, that have accepted
the increasing role of science in medical practice. Perhaps therefore
it would be appropriate for me to finish by saying that - in welcoming
this Congress and in declaring it formally open - I think we would all
do well to remember the philosophy and the words of a generation of
physicians that came before the impact of chemotherapy. In our modern
science we would do well never to ignore the wisdom of experience,
perhaps best summed up for me in the words of the Physicians Prayer by
Sir Robert Hutchinson -

From inability to let well alone;
From too much zeal for the new and comtempt for what is old;
From putting knowledge before wisdom, science before art
and cleverness before common-sense;
From treating patients as cases and from making the cure of the
disease more grevious than the endurance of the same;
Good Lord deliver us.

REFLECTIONS ON RESEARCH IN CHEMOTHERAPY

Sir Ernst Chain

Professor of Biochemistry

Imperial College, London

I am greatly honoured by the invitation to give the opening address at this 9th International Congress of Chemotherapy, and am carrying out my assignment with greatest pleasure. The popularity of the subject can be gauged from the massive number of people who are gathered today in this largest hall in London.

Thirty-five years have passed since my colleagues and I published in 1940, in the Lancet, our first paper on the curative properties of one of the penicillins in experimental infections in mice, and a year later, in 1941, we published our second paper reporting the curative effect of this material in severe infection in man.

This discovery and its subsequent development which led to the production of benzylpenicillin on an industrial scale, and to the discovery and industrial production of a wide range of antibacterial substances of microbial origin, now known as antibiotics, with chemotherapeutic action against a wide range of bacterial infections, including some in which benzylpenicillin was not effective, marks a new era in antibacterial chemotherapy. The production technique for the antibiotics, with one exception, is based on fermentation technology which before the penicillin development was almost entirely unknown to the pharmaceutical industry, but since then has become one of the main pillars. Their use has revolutionised the treatment and brought under control the large majority of bacterial infections. The antibiotics development, therefore, constitutes one of the major achievements of medical research, and I should like to devote this introductory talk to some comments of general interest pertinent to the whole approach to medical research in the field of chemotherapy, not

just antibacterial, but drug therapy in general, arising partly
from my own experience in the history of the penicillin discovery.
I shall also try to make some brief comment on the future of
chemotherapy, as I see it.

The history of the penicillin discovery is perfectly simple
and straightforward, but has been distorted beyond recognition
by mass media and sometimes even the professional medical press.
Even the short introductory statement in the program of this
Congress has not got the facts quite right. Yet it contains a
number of facts of considerable general interest relevant to the
basic principles of medical research in the field of chemotherapy,
and demonstrates some of the difficulties, both conceptual and
financial - administrative, which the investigator in the field
encounters, before and even after he has been successful.

The work on penicillin, which I started at the end of 1938,
was undertaken as a study of purely scientific interest, without
any idea that it could have practical application in therapeutic
medicine. It was the direct continuation of a previous investigation on the mode of action of lysozyme, which had occupied a
Ph.D. student, L.A. Epstein, and myself in the years 1936-1938.
The aim of this investigation was to establish the mode of action
of this powerful bacteriolytic substance, discovered in 1922 by
the London bacteriologist, Alexander Fleming, in tears, nasal
secretion, and egg white, and capable of dissolving thick suspensions of a non-pathogenic micro-organism, b.lysodeicticus. We
achieved our aim and were able to show that lysozyme was an
enzyme hydrolising a polysaccharide substrate in the cell wall
of b.lysodeicticus with the liberation of n-acetyl glucosamine.
The full structure of the substrate of lysozyme was established
later; it contained another sugar, n-acetyl-muramic acid, as part
of the basic disaccharide unit.

When our work on the mode of action of lysozyme neared its
end, we undertook a literature survey to find out whether other
bacteriolytic substances, similar to lysozyme, had been described.
This literature survey led me to the discovery of quite a large
number of descriptions of the phenomenon of microbial antagonism,
i.e. the capability of some micro-organisms, bacteria, moulds, and
yeasts to produce substances inhibiting the growth of other microorganisms, but to very few description of bacteriolytic substances,
similar to lysozyme. However, I came across a paper published in
1929 by the same Alexander Fleming, in which he reported a striking
lytic action of a mould metabolite against the staphylococcus, and
the growth inhibitory action, without actual lysis, against many
gram-positive and a few gram-negative pathogenic cocci of the
culture fluid on which the mould was grown.

Fleming gave the name penicillin as an abbreviation for his mould culture fluid containing an antibacterial principle. Looking at the photograph of Fleming's paper, familiar to all of you, in which a large zone of lysis of staphylococci had appeared around a mould contaminant, later identified as Penicillium notatum, I thought that Fleming had discovered a sort of lysozyme attacking a substance common in the cell wall of pathogenic cocci, and decided immediately to isolate the supposed enzyme and its substrate. I obtained the mould culture from one of the collaborators of Professor Florey's predecessor, the late Danish bacteri-logist Professor Dreyer, and started to work on penicillin around the end of 1938. I was strengthened in my belief that penicillin was anenzyme by the great instability of this substance, described by Fleming in his 1929 paper as well as by a group of chemists who had studied this substance a few years later. I discussed the results of my literature survey towards its terminal stages with the late Professor H.W. Florey and we decided to undertake jointly a systematic study of antibacterial substances produced by micro-organisms which were known to exist, but whose biological and biochemical properties were entirely unknown. We decided to continue with the work on penicillin which I had already started several months earlier.

The point I wish to make, and the reason why I gave these few historic facts, is that penicillin, at the time I started to work on it, looked anything but promising from the point of view of practical application. A substance described as extremely unstable, and possibly of protein nature, giving in all probability rise to anaphylactic phenomena, does not hold out any promise as a drug useful in medicine. Our work was anything but mission oriented. In fact, I am quite certain that had I worked in a mission oriented atmosphere, say in the laboratory of a pharmaceutical firm, I would never have been allowed to work on penicillin; it would have been considered a waste of time. Actually, I cannot think of a single case in the field of therapeutics, where a basically new drug treatment was discovered for a cure of a disease just by setting out with the aim of finding a curative drug. Fortunately, penicillin turned out <u>not</u> to be an enzyme, but a substance of low molecular weight, and was not nearly as unstable as it appeared at first sight. It retained its non-toxicity even when highly purified, and became one of the least toxic and most powerful clinically effective antibacterial agents known.

Progress in the field of chemotherapy, and therapy in general, is invariably made by following up a novel biological observation which can be explained in terms of the action of well defined chemical entities. Pasteur and Joubert's discovery of bacterial antagonism was a novel biological observation of this kind, which led to the discovery of most antibiotics. Fleming's observation was novel as the staphylococcus is known to be particularly

resistant to lysis. This novelty consisted in the fact that he
allowed his Petri dish, on the surface of which he had grown
staphylococci, to stand for at least a month on his laboratory
bench while he was away on a holiday. During this time, at the
temperature in his laboratory, his mould contaminant, which may
have settled on his Petri dish while he observed his staphylococci, taking off the lid while he made his microscopie observations, or it may have been there even before he seeded the agar
surface, grew sufficiently fast to secrete enough penicillin to
reach the staphylococcal colonies while these were still capable
of dividing, as they naturally grew only quite slowly at room
temperature. Under these conditions, but only under these conditions, the staphylococcus is susceptible to lysis by penicillin.
Through a combination of lucky circumstances, Fleming achieved the
conditions under which the lytic effect of penicillin on the
staphylococcus manifests itself and, in consequence of his experience with the lytic phenomenon of lysozyme, which he had discovered several years earlier, followed it up by subculturing the
contaminant, later identified as P.notatum, on the surface of a
conventional culture fluid, and demonstrating that the culture
fluid, after having been covered by the mould, acquired strong
anti-bacterial activity against many important pathogenic gram-
positive and gram-negative cocci; it could be diluted 800 times
before the anti-bacterial activity disappeared.

    What is surprising, is that he missed the discovery of the
chemotherapeutic properties of penicillin. He had injected as
much as 0.5 ml of his culture into a 20 gm mouse without noticing
any toxic effects, and if he had repeated the same experiment
with the same crude culture filtrate, without any chemical puri-
fication, on a mouse infected with a few streptococci, pneumococci,
or staphylococci, against which he had shown penicillin to be
active, he would undoubtedly have obtained a pronounced chemotherapeutic effect. Many chemists would have then precipitated
themselves on the problem to isolate the active principle and
certainly would have succeeded in this without much difficulty,
as we did eleven years later. I believe that the reason why
Fleming did not carry out this simple experiment, which seems
obvious to us today, is that the atmosphere in his laboratory,
under Sir Almroth Wright, and in other bacteriological laboratories,
was prejudicial and hostile to the idea of bacterial chemotherapy.
It is a good example - there must be many others - of how preju-
dice in scientific thought can inhibit progress.

    Only observations on intact organisms in normal or pathological
conditions have so far led to progress in drug therapy. Clinical
observations are of particular importance, as the majority of the
most important diseases in man cannot be reproduced in animal
models. No progress in drug therapy has so far come from the

reductionist approach of the molecular biologist, and I do not
believe this situation will change in the foreseeable future. If
we get too far away from the biological reality, we have only
ourselves to blame for lack of success in discovering new leads
to chemotherapeutic drugs.

We are told by our political leaders that it is our duty to
give first priority in our studies to socially important diseases. The fact that these diseases exist is known to us all,
and we are all aware of their importance. However, this does
not mean that we are, at the present state of knowledge, in a
position to do anything to cure them. In fact, in the degenerative
diseases - artheriosclerosis, rheumatoid arthritis, cardiovascular
disorders - our knowledge is as limited as it was with regard to
bacterial infections before the times of Pasteur. Much money will
have to be spent on basic medical research before we have a sufficient understanding of the causes of these diseases, and even if
we understand them, it does not necessarily follow that we can
find a cure for them. This will be possible only if we succeed in
finding regulatory substances bringing back to normality the disturbed metabolic functions causing the disease. This may or may
not be possible. I believe it will not be possible in the majority of genetical disorders in the foreseeable future, and this
kind of disease delineates the limits of our chemotherapeutic
possibilities. Talk about curing these disorders through so-
called genetical engineering is, at best, science fiction.

I should like to remind listeners that one of the greatest
advances in therapeutic medicine, the discovery of the cortico-
steroid hormones, was achieved by studying a disease of no social
importance at al - Addison's disease, of which there are no more
than at most 200 cases per year in this country.

Once a new lead to chemotherapy is discovered, it is the
function of industry to develop it, and industry has done us well
in this respect. The role of industry in the development of the
antibiotics was of the greatest importance. Industry developed
penicillin from a laboratory curiosity to a cheap drug, naturally
making use of important fundamental discoveries made in academic
laboratories such as, for instance, the techniques of producing
mutations through x-rays, ultraviolet rays, and mutagens. The
large majority of antibiotics of practical importance were discovered in industrial laboratories, and it is impossible to imagine
any other organisation which would have done this in an equally
efficient manner. No centralised government controlled organisation would have produced the necessary funds for such undertaking
at a time when such investments were a considerable risk. The
history of the cephalosporin development is similar to that of
the development of penicillin.

The present state of bacterial chemotherapy is, on the whole,
satisfactory. There has been no serious problem of resistance
development in the gram-positive cocci. The percentage of clinically important gram-negative bacteria resistant to antibiotic has
not significantly increased. It must be mentioned, however, that
in the case of Salmonella typhi there have been reports, not in
Europe, but in Mexico and India, of a few strains causing epidemics
which were resistant to chloramphenicol, and there have been reports
of epidemics in small children, also in non-European countries, with
strains of S.typhimurium resistant to all known antibiotics. Furthermore, there were serious outbreaks of meningococcal meningitis
in Brazil, resistant to penicillin. This resistance is due to
genetic transfer of R factors and has to be watched carefully. It
seems to me of great importance to understand better and to streng-
then the immune forces of the body, specific and non-specific, in
the fight against bacterial infections, for if they are lacking,
through immuno-suppression, in old age, and in particular pathological conditions, the best antibiotic will be ineffective. The
field of specific and non-specific immunity seems to me the most
important area of research for the immediate future to complement
chemotherapy.

I do not think that in the future much progress will be made
through the discovery of new classes of antibiotics through the
conventional screening methods, though one can never be absolutely
certain about predicting the future. In any case, screening for
new antibiotics will be continued in a few places. Penicillins
and cephalosporins with new side chains will continue to be produced, and much effort will be expended on the chemical conversion
of penicillins into cephalosporins. In view of the fact that
beta-lactams were discovered in the laboratories of Eli Lilly,
in which the sulphur of the tiazolidine ring was replaced by oxygen, chemists will make an effort to obtain compounds of this kind
and modify them, as in the case of the penicillins and cephalosporins. Chemists will attempt to modify existing aminocyclitol
antibiotics in order to obtain more active and less toxic products.
The coupling of the anti-tumour antibiotics Adriamycin and Dauno-
mycin with specific tumour antibodies deserves attention. Progress
in antibacterial chemotherapy through the study of the mode of
action of antibiotics, including studies of the cell wall structure,
seems to me to be a very long way away from reality.

In one area of chemotherapy, that of parasitical infections,
progress has been slow. These infections include trypanosomiasis
in its different forms, such as Chagas' disease and sleeping sick-
ness, malaria, schistozomiasis, hook worm disease, filariasis,
bilharzia, and many others, and affecting millions of people, particularly in developing African, South American and Asian countries.
The lack of progress in this important field is due to the fact
that very little work is being done on the biochemistry of the

extremely complex life cycle of parasites and the interaction
of the different stages with the metabolism of the host; it is not
a fashionable subject. It needs painstaking and difficult work on
the whole intact animal, as it is not possible to grow most parasites outside the animal body. Yet biochemical parasitology seems
to me a gold mine for the biochemist interested in making basically
new biological discoveries in the host-parasite metabolic relationship which could give new leads towards chemotherapy. Whether we
shall be able to cope with a population increase of the order that
would result if an effective chemotherapy or immunotherapy for
these diseases would be found, is outside the scope of this
Congress, but is a matter of great importance, well worth while
bearing in mind and giving it careful thought. Biological equili-
bria cannot be disturbed without consequences which have to be paid
for. We have already seen a change in our hospital population
through the extension of the life spans by about 10 years through
the introduction of the antibiotics, and face now very many more
geriatric problems than we did at the time when many patients were
carried off through pneumonia at the age of 55-65.

    Iam not competent to talk in detail of tumour chemotherapy,
but it seems that slowly, but surely, considerable progress has
been made by the use of a combination of cytostatic agents of synthetic and microbial origin coupled with irradiation.

    The program of the Congress looks interesting. We have a large
number of leading specialists with us, and we can look forward to
fruitful discussions and personal contracts between the partici-
pants. I hope that this 9th International Congress of Chemotherapy
will be a notable success and will be remembered as such, and I wish
it the fullest success.

THE PROPHYLACTIC USE OF ANTI-MICROBIAL AGENTS IN THE SURGERY OF THE INTESTINE

Douglas Roy

Professor of Surgery

The Queen's University of Belfast

SUMMARY

The purpose of bowel preparation before surgery is first defined. In order to achieve the objectives of avoiding both tissue sepsis as a result of bacterial invasion from the intestine and interference with healing processes as a result of anti-bacterial therapy it is necessary to reduce the bacterial content of the intestine, and contamination of tissues, without damaging the defence mechanisms of the body.

Mechanical cleansing of the intestine is the first essential process, but may not be possible where partial or complete obstruction is present. Cleansing can be carried out both by reducing the residue of the diet and by washing out the contents of the intestine. Having achieved mechanical cleansing the merits and drawbacks of various anti-bacterial agents are then discussed, both in relation to pre-operative administration of drugs, active within the alimentary canal, and the prophylactic use of antibiotic powders and solutions at the time of operation. Finally, the systemic administration of antibiotics as a prophylactic measure after surgery is discussed.

It is emphasised that surgical technique is of fundamental importance in the prevention of subsequent infective complications.

INTRODUCTION

Operations on the intestinal tract were generally considered,

until the early thirties, to be dangerous. Death and morbidity
were usually the result of sepsis within the peritoneal cavity or
in the layers of the abdominal wall. Since then developments in
technique, in supportive measures for the patient during and after
operation and the development of antibiotics have reduced the
hazards to acceptable levels both for elective and emergency
procedures. Nevertheless, there are still patients who die as a
result of systemic infections following intestinal surgery (usually
of bacteraemic shock) or whose convalescence is delayed either
by intra-abdominal abscesses or infection of the operative incisions

Post-operative sepsis usually arises as a result of several
factors of which bacterial contamination is only one. They are:-
(1) Bacterial contamination at the time of operation by bacteria
from the lumen of the intestine. (2) The formation of collections
of blood or serum within the peritoneal cavity or within the layers
of the wounds which become culture media for contaminating
organisms. (3) Subsequent leakage of suture lines as a result of
relative or absolute ischaemia of the bowel wall.

The resistance of the peritoneum to infection makes intra-
peritoneal sepsis as a result of a single contamination at the time
of operation unlikely except, possibly, on rare occasions when an
organism is outstandingly virulent or the patient debilitated.
This is, to some extent, also true of wound sepsis. It, therefore,
follows that the most important prophylaxis against post-operative
sepsis is a surgical technique that avoids producing collections of
blood or serum and prevents the leakage of suture lines subsequently.

However, it is evident that if these rules are transgressed
then sepsis may still be avoided if:- (1) The contents of the
intestine are devoid of pathogenic organisms or (2) These
organisms can be killed in the tissues by (a) the body's defences
and (b) appropriate antibiotics.

THE BACTERIA

In normal people the stomach, duodenum and upper small
intestine are sterile. By far the commonest organisms elsewhere
are those called bacteroides which are present in the mouth, the
lower small intestine and the colon (Drasar and Hill 1974, Hill
and Drasar 1975). They are associated with coliforms, clostridia
and other entero-bacteria, and from time to time staphylococci
and various streptococci may be recovered while, in children,
yeasts will often be present. The degree of colonisation of
lower small bowel is much less than that of the colon and probably

fluctuates during the day depending on the times of meals. If achlorhydria is present the stomach will also become colonised with bacteroides and other organisms such as gram positive cocci. (Drasar, Shiner and MacLeod 1969 and Giannella et al 1972). The upper small bowel will only become colonised if there is some kind of blind loop present. (Drasar and Shiner 1969).

There is a variation in the faecal flora dependent on diet. Those people who take a high residue, vegetarian diet low in animal protein and fat, have far fewer anaerobic bacteria and more aerobic ones. (Hill et al 1971). This may explain the lower mortality from strangulated hernia in East Africa despite less favourable conditions for surgery and greater delays in seeking treatment (Hancock 1975, Wambwa 1974).

The bacterial pattern will also be altered by disease. If small bowel disease is accompanied by any degree of obstruction bacterial proliferation will occur. Unfortunately disease also interferes with attempts to achieve the first of our objectives, that is, to clear the gut of pathogenic organisms while emergency situations reduce the time available to achieve it. It is, therefore, necessary to depend more on measures to kill organisms that reach the tissues and are beginning to proliferate and invade.

There is increasing evidence that, of the bacteria present in the gut, bacteroides are the most important and the most dangerous (Leigh, Simmons and Norman 1974, Keighley et al 1975).

STERILISATION OF THE INTESTINAL LUMEN

It is not possible to destroy every organism but it should be possible so to reduce the level of organisms that the bowel lumen is, for practical purposes, devoid of pathogens. There are two ways of doing this.

Mechanical Cleansing

If the lumen is empty the possibility of contamination of tissues is much reduced. It is the faecal material which contaminates drapes, swabs and instruments and carries the bacteria to the tissues. A bowel that contains only small hard faecal masses is almost as good. The most undesirable situation is a bowel containing soft or fluid faeces and this is a situation often produced by inadequate bowel preparation especially when laxatives are given shortly before operation. It is also the situation in acute or sub-acute obstruction and can only be dealt with by an alteration in technique, usually involving staging of the procedure.

In order to achieve mechanical cleansing of the lower intestine three measures are taken. (1) (a) Low residue diet from the seventh day before operation. (b) Fluid diet for the last day before operation. (2) Magnesium sulphate laxative on the third and second day before operation. (3) Bowel washout on the morning and evening before the operation.

Anti-biotics Active in Lumen of the Intestine

Many surgeons believe that cleansing is sufficient in most cases but Cohn (1970) for instance, has shown that it is possible to reduce pathogens to a very low level with antibiotics and believes that the clinical results are better than with cleansing alone. He, further, has demonstrated in animals that antibiotics can protect an ischaemic anastomosis, although this requires irrigation of the bowel lumen after operation. Everitt, Brogan and Nettleton (1969), however, in a controlled trial, using neomycin in 50 patients, could not demonstrate an advantage in using antibiotic preparation of the bowel. McNaught (unpublished data 1975), on the other hand, has shown in a controlled trial a significant decrease in both coliforms and bacteroides with kanamycin and metronidazole, taking bacteriological samples from the lumen of the colon at operation. This correlated with a significant reduction in wound infection. Nevertheless, the really dangerous sepsis is that which occurs in the peritoneal cavity and failure of surgical technique is the main cause of this complication. There is no evidence in man, as opposed to animals, that antibiotics are protective if technique is poor.

There are several antibiotics or combinations that are effective (Cohn 1970), but one combination is particularly useful. Kanamycin has a broad spectrum of activity and low toxicity when given orally. It will usually kill all gram + ve cocci and coliform organisms as well as clostridia. It will not, however, deal with bacteroides. Metronidazole, being active against bacteroides although having no activity against the coliforms (Willis et al 1974) effectively compliments kanamycin and has the further advantage of being virtually without side effects. This combination given for three days before operation was used by McNaught in the trial referred to above. Yeasts are not a problem in adults but may be so in young children when the use of nystatin would be justified.

There may be disadvantages in using prophylactic combinations to sterilise the intestine. Aluwihare (1971) studied the effect of neomycin on the colonic mucosa and showed that it produced a direct toxic effect on colonic mucosal cells and a disappearance of lymphocytes from the submucosa. He postulates that these changes explain why superinfection with resistant organisms occurs so easily after preparation with neomycin to which many staphylococci are now resistant. He also suggests that they explain Cohn's (1964) observation that there was an increase in the rate of recurrence of carcinoma at the suture line in patients having colonic resection who received antibiotic bowel preparation. Clearly a balance must be struck between various therapeutic possibilities. The risk of implantation at the suture line is not great even in Cohn's series and other measures can be taken to inhibit implantation. Superinfection is less likely with kanamycin, although it probably has a similar effect on the colonic mucosa.

It seems reasonable, therefore, to suggest that preparation of the bowel with kanamycin and metronidazole is advisable for all large bowel surgery, surgery on the lower small bowel when there is any element of obstruction and the achlorhydric stomach provided that measures are taken to suppress suture line implantation in patients with malignancies. Antibiotics may well not be necessary in people who eat a high residue, low fat diet except in the presence of an obstructive lesion and, therefore, populations of developing countries may not need to use expensive antibiotics in this way.

PREVENTION OF BACTERIAL PROLIFERATION IN TISSUES AFTER OPERATION

The most important factor preventing bacterial proliferation in the tissues is the activity of the host cells. No agent should be used that will interfere, in any way, with their activity. Furthermore, it is unlikely that a systemically administered antibiotic or a local application either single or by irrigation is likely to diminish the serious effects of a leaking anastomosis.

There are two separate areas of infection to be considered, the first being intra-peritoneal sepsis and, the second, wound infection.

Intra-peritoneal Sepsis

The peritoneum may already be contaminated at the time of

operation (e.g. in the case of a penetrating wound of the colon) or contamination may occur at operation. In the first case invasion of tissues is already commencing and if peritonitis is already established, prophylaxis applies only in preventing subsequent wound infection. The condition is treated appropriately and washing out the peritoneal cavity with antiseptic solution can hardly improve the situation except by the mechanical removal of faecal matter.

If contamination has occurred only shortly before or at operation then it is conceivable that invasion of tissues can be aborted. The important question is whether any agent or procedure can do better than the defence mechanisms of the tissues themselves. Tolhurst Cleaver and his colleagues (1974) using rats as their experimental animal found that irrigation with Hartmann's solution reduced mortality from faecal peritonitis by 66% while irrigation with noxytiolin solution made no difference. This occurred even though Hartmann's solution was shown to inhibit peritoneal healing. However, clinical studies by Browne and Stoller (1970) and Pickard (1972) suggest some benefit from the use of noxytiolin although neither trial was in any way controlled and the comparisons they made with other series cannot be regarded as significant. It would seem logical to suggest that, if the tissues are invaded a systemic antibiotic is required, if not, irrigation with a fluid such as isotonic saline or Hartmann's solution before closure of the abdomen will remove faecal and other foreign matter and should be sufficient. Certain patients have an increased risk of developing sepsis, examples being those on steroids or those with cancer. In such cases post-operative treatment with lincomycin is justified as a prophylactic measure being active against bacteroides. (Keighley et al 1975).

Prevention of Wound Infection

Wounds may be exposed to antibiotics either by application to the surface before closure or by giving a systemic antibiotic. Both Polk and Lopez-Major (1969) and Evans and Pollock (1973) found that cephaloridine was effective, in controlled trials, in preventing wound infection. Leigh (1975) studying appendicectomy wounds found that careful culture methods showed that Bacteroides fragilis is present in 60% of infected wounds and recommended that lincomycin should be used to prevent wound sepsis after the removal of acutely inflamed appendices. Systemic antibiotics used routinely have, however, the disadvantage of promoting the emergence of resistant organisms making established infections more difficult to manage. Crosfil, Hall and London (1969) found no advantage in the use of chlorhexidine instilled locally in wounds, but Evans, Pollock and Rosenberg (1974) showed that cephaloridine applied locally reduced infection rates in contaminated wounds from 38.7% to 12.8%. There was no advantage in clean wounds and there was evidence of the emergence of resistant organisms in the treated group. Gilmore and Martin (1974) compared povidone iodine with a mixture of neomycin, bacitracin and polymixin applied locally and found that both reduced infection rates by half and that povidone iodine reduced infection equally in all groups and at all ages. They, therefore, concluded that povidone iodine justified its routine use.

Povidone iodine does not encourage the emergence of resistant organisms. It does not seem to delay healing and would seem to be the best local application at present available for preventing infection in contaminated wounds. Clean wounds should receive no topical therapy. Where a wound is heavily and obviously contaminated with material likely to contain virulent organisms then systemic antibiotics such as cephaloridine and lincomycin is indicated in addition to a local application but should only be used for positive indications not for routine use, and may in any case, be indicated for the treatment of the primary lesion within the abdomen.

CONCLUSION

Prophylaxis is never a routine procedure, it is always an individual decision. The use of antibiotics and other antimicrobial drugs can certainly reduce infection both within and without the abdomen but they are not nearly so important as careful and appropriate technique in the performance of operations on the gut and in closing abdominal wounds.

It is possible to reduce the pathogens in the intestinal tract by mechanical cleansing and the use of kanamycin and metronidazole. There is evidence that this reduces the chance of infective complications particularly affecting abdominal wounds but intra-peritoneal sepsis may not be much affected.

Contamination of tissues shortly before, or at operation, should be counteracted by irrigation of the peritoneal cavity with saline or Hartmann's solution and spraying of the wound with povidone iodine. Cephaloridine and lincomycin may be used for heavily contaminated wounds or peritoneal cavity in addition to local measures.

Established invasion should be treated with appropriate antibiotics reserving the expensive broad spectrum agents for fulminating cases.

REFERENCES

Aluwihare, A. P. R. (1971). Gut. 12. 341-349

Browne, M. K. and Stoller, J. L. (1970). British Journal of Surgery. 57. 525-529

Cohn, I. (1964). Maryland Medical Journal. 13. 45-48

Cohn, I. (1970). Surgery, Gynaecology and Obstetrics. 130. 1006-1014.

Crosfil, M., Hall, R. and London, D. (1969). British Journal of Surgery. 56. 906-908

Drasar, B. S. and Hill, M. J. (1974). Academic Press. London pp. 36-44

Drasar, B. S., Shiner, M. and McLeod, G. M. (1969). Gastroenterology. 56. 71-79

Drasar, B. S. and Shiner, M. (1969). Gut. 10. 812-819

Evans, C., and Pollock, A. V. (1973). British Journal of Surgery. 60. 434-437

Evans, C., Pollock, A. V. and Rosenberg, I. L. (1974). British Journal of Surgery. 61. 133-135

Everitt, M. T., Brogan, T. D. and Nettleton, J. (1969). British Journal of Surgery. 56. 679-684

Giannella, R. A., Broitman, S. A. and Zamchek, N. (1972). Gut. 13. 251-256

Gilmore, O. J. A. and Martin, T. D. M. (1974). British Journal of Surgery. 61. 281-287.

Hancock, B. D. (1975). Journal of the Royal College of Surgeons of Edinburgh. 20. 134-137

Hill, M. J., Drasar, B. S., Hawkesworth, G., Crowther, J. S., Aries, V. and Williams, R. E. O. (1971). Lancet 1. 95-100

Hill, M. J. and Drasar, B. S. (1975). Gut. 16. 318-323

Keighley, M. R. B., Burdon, D. W., Slaney, G., Cooke, W. T. and Alexander-Williams, J. (1975). Gut. 16. 408

Leigh, D. A. (1975). British Journal of Surgery. 62. 375-378.

Leigh, D. A., Simmons, K. and Norman, E. (1974). Journal of Clinical Pathology. 27. 997-1000

McNaught, W. (1975). Personal Communication.

Pickard, R. G. (1972). British Journal of Surgery. 59. 642-648

Polk, H. C. and Lopez-Major, J. E. (1969). Surgery. 66. 97-103

Tolhurst Cleaver, C. L., Hopkins, A. D., Kae Kwong, K. C. and Ng Rafteng, A. T. (1974). British Journal of Surgery. 61. 601-604

Wambwa, J. R. (1974). East African Journal of Medical Research. 1. 265-272

Willis, A. T. (1974). Lancet. 2. 1540-1543

PROPHYLAXIS WITH ANTIBIOTICS IN ORTHOPAEDIC AND TRAUMATOLOGIC

SURGICAL INTERVENTIONS

H.W. BUCHHOLZ

ALLGEMEINES KRANKENHAUS
2 HAMBURG 1
LOHMUHLENSTRASSE 5
W. GERMANY

Hopes that were pinned on the prophylactic use of antibiotics against infection in orthopaedics and traumatology have not been fulfilled. It has shown that this measure does not prevent the growth of infection as reliably as desired and with the introduction of prophylaxis with antibiotics the rate of infection after surgical interventions on bones and joints has not changed essentially.

Antibiotics given systemically normally miss to reach the endangered region around the bone or the joint in a therapeutically effective concentration. Furthermore, they are only effective for the time when they are given, which is insufficient to prevent the incipient infection. Haematoma in the fracture region and the compulsory zone of bone necrosis at the fracture hinder again and again the systemically given antibiotics to reach the region at risk in time and in an effective concentration by way of circulation. Furthermore, the range of action of the antibiotics in use with their locally low-effective concentration doesn't seem to be broad enough to destroy all the bacteria colonizing the fracture region or the operation area. This may cause the germs becoming resistant, whilst at the beginning of treatment they probably have had just about the adequate degree of sensitivity.

Furthermore, we must consider that any applied prophylactic therapy may encounter resistant germs, against which any given antibiotic agent fails to be effective. Today we may assure that many surgeons are not inclined to advocate using antibiotics prophylactically, but they agree to their being administered in cases of compound fractures, where there is high risk of infection, preferably those agents which have a close affinity to bone. Care must be taken that an adequate dose is given, and the period of

application should not be under 4-6 weeks, since before the end of
this time no revascularization of the necrotic marginal zone of bone
is to be expected. In general there is no indication for a systemically given prophylactic therapy in orthopaedic and traumatologic
surgery, only the aimed and sufficiently high dosed prophylaxis.
with antibiotics given over an appropriate period of time in cases
of increased risk of infection may inhibit the growth of bacteria to
some extent.

While the spread of implant surgery is going on, the need of
fundamental prophylactic measures has become obvious. Joint replacement surgery bears a high risk of infection due to implanted foreign
bodies and especially due to polymethymetacrylate which is used for
the fixation of the prosthesis into the bone. Dental investigations
have revealed that certain species of bacteria can survive on the
carbon which is an ingredient of polymethylmetacrylate and that
furthermore the irregular surface of the bone-cement with its dimples
and pores may be regarded as being ideal for bacterial settlement.

From the great number of patients treated with joint implants we
have noticed that the rate of infection in implant surgery seems to
be much higher than in the rest of the surgical procedures in orthopaedic and traumatology and that this rate may come up to 4 and 8
percent and even to 10 and 12 percent. Here a systemically given
prophylactic therapy is bound to fail, since the antibiotic agents
even when they reach the junction between bone and cement will not
succeed in entering the deep pores of the bone-cement.

We therefore have to walk on other ways in order to prevent or at
least limit the desastrous danger of high rates of failure in implant
surgery due to deep infection.

In early 1969 studies on the effectiveness of antibiotics added to
the bone-cement Palacos R were started which turned out to be
successful. The hardened polymethylmetacrylate has the property to
release incorporated water soluble substances into the surrounding
fluid when there is a corresponding gradient of concentration. The
water soluble incorporated substances which are to be found entirely
in the interstitial substance of the polymethylmetacrylate tend to
migrate continously from the depth of the hardened cement to its
surface, when the elution allows it. Essential for the use of
antibiotic substances is that they are not only water soluble but
also highly heat-resistant, since the temperature in the hardening
cement is likely to reach 60°C. Experimental work was done with
penicillin, streptomycin, erythromycin, lincomycin, cephaltin and
gentamycin. Tetracycline is unsuited since it has only a low-grade
heat-resistance.

Gentamycin has proved to be most suitable for antibiotic mixtures

with bone-cement. Besides good water soluble properties this
substance is extremely acid-resistant and highly heat-resistant. A
broad spectrum of effectiveness is another positive advantage.

Gentamycin mixed with polymethylmetacrylate has come into use as
Refobacin-Palacos R, but unfortunately only in Germany and Austria. A
series of bacteriological studies on the behaviour of gentamycin in
bone-cement was made. Furthermore, we initiated studies of diffusion with melachit green in bone-cement. Melachit green has a
constitutional formula similar to gentamycin, so that a similar
behaviour may be assumed. With melachit green it was possible to
prove that the water soluble chemical compound mixed with the
polymeric powder is located only in the interstitial substance formed
by monomer and constructing a network through the whole body of
cement.

The continous migration of incorporated water soluble substances
from the depth of the polymethylmetacrylate body has been demonstrated
by experiments on rabbits with chloramphenicol marked G 14, added to
the bone-cement Palacos R.

Since 1969 we have utilized this knowledge for the implant
surgery. At first we have tried to add penicillin to the bone-
cement and later on erythromycin. Since erythromycin must be
observed a series of late infections which were obviously entirely
caused by anaerobic bacteria. From 1971 on we have gradually
changed over to gentamycin and since February 1972 gentamycin is
used exclusively in the bone-cement Refobacin-Palacos R for prevention of infection in implant surgery.

Our results from then on are convincing. Since November 1972
we haven't observed any deep infections in hip joint replacement
surgery, and the infections developed in other joints have only been
sporadic. So we had three cases of deep infection in our knee joint
operations, which makes one percent and one infection in our ankle-
joint prostheses, which looks like being caused by secondary wound
healing and by the patient's indifference who was an alcohol addict.

The regional effectiveness of this prophylactic measure was so
convincing that in the same year in 1969, we started to treat
established deep infections by means of exchanging the total endoprosthesis, using the mixture gentamycin-Palacos-R. The dose of
gentamycin was risen from 0.5 gram to 1 gram and depending on the
sensitivity-test we had other antibiotic substances added. Healing
of these deep infections has been successful in 70 percent of the
cases under the maintenance of the joint implant.

The question prophylaxis with antibiotics in orthopaedic-
traumatologic operations should be answered with "no", when a
systemic general prophylaxis is intended, but we may answer with
"yes", if one thinks of the special prophylaxis with antibiotics,

which is done with water soluble antibiotic substances in polymethylmetacrylate and which exclusively has a local regional range
of action.

SUMMARY

It is shown why the systemic prophylaxis with antibiotics in orthopaedic and traumatologic injuries and operations should only be given
in special circumstances, as in cases of open fractures and other
situations with high risk of infection.

Then the causes for the high rates of infection in implant surgery
are discussed and a guide is given as to how the rate of infection
may be reduced decisively by applying a local regional prophylaxis
with antibiotics. Our own results in this procedure since 1969 are
discu-sed.

REFERENCES

1.   Barnes, J., Pace, W.G., Trump, D.S., & Ellison, E.H.
     Prophylactic postoperative antibiotics. A controlled study of
     1007 cases.
     Arch. Surg. 79 (1959), 190.

2.   Buchholz, H.W. & Engelbrecht, E.
     Uber die Depotwirkung einiger Antibiotica bei Vermischung
     mit dem Kunstharz Palacos.
     Chirurg 41, (1970), 511.

3.   Buchholz, H.W. & Gartmann, H.D.
     Infektionsprophylaxe und operative Behandlung der schleichenden
     tiefen Infektion bei der totalen Endoprothese.
     Chirurg 43 (1972), 446.

4.   Charnley, J.
     Postoperative Infection after total hip replacement with
     special reference to air contaimination in the operating room.
     Clin. orthop. 87 (1972), 373.

5.   Crasselt, C. & Thallwitz, M.
     Zur Wundheilungaströrung in der Orthopaedie.
     Beitr. Orthop. 18 (1972), 373.

6.   Fichtner, H.J.
     Kann auf den prophylaktischen Gebrauch von Antibiotica bei
     orthopaedischen Operationen verzichtet werden.
     Chirurg 39 (1968), 240.

7.   Hegemann, G., Beck, H. & Wagner, B.
     Hospitalismus in der Sicht des Chirurgen.
     Dtsch. med. Wschr. (1961), 593.

8.   Lindgren, L. & Lindberg, L.
     Orthopaedic infections during a 5-year period.
     Acta. orthop. Scand. 43, (1972) 325.

9.   Lodenkämper, H.
     Neuere bakteriologische Untersuchungsergebnisse zur Herdinfektion
     und Kariesentstehung.
     Physikalische Medizin und Rehabilitation, 13. Jahrgang
     (1972) Heft 7.

10. Lodenkämper, H. & Stienen, G.
     Importance and Therapy of Anaerobic Infections.
     Antibiotic Medicine, Vol 1, No. 12, December 1955.

11. Lodenkämper, H. & Stienen, G.
     The Treatment of Anaerobic Infections.
     Georg Thieme Verlag, Volume 1, No 8, p. 233.

12. Plane, R. & Hinz. P.
     Osteomyelitis: Erregerspektrum und Resistenzsituation.
     Arch. orthop. Unfall-Chir. 69 (1970), 83.

13. Plane, R. & Hinz, P.
     Infektionen nach orthopaedischen Operationen.
     Arch. orthop. Unfall-Chir. 70 (1971), 298.

14. Wahlig, H., Hameister, W'. & Grieben, A.
     Über die Freisentzung von Gentamycin aus Polymethylmethacrylat.
     I. Experimentelle Untersuchungen in vitro.
     Langenbecks Arch. Chir. 331 (1972) 169-192.

15. Wahlig, H., Hameister, W. & Grieben, A.
     Über die Freisetzung von Gentamycin aus Polymethylmethacrylat.
     II. Experimentelle Untersuchungen in vivo.
     Langenbecks Arch. Chir. 331 (1972), 193-212.

16. Weickenmeier, B.
     Die akute haematogens und exogene Osteomyelitis, Beitrag zur
     Pathogenese.
     Med. Inaug. Diss. Heidelberg 1972.

ANTIBIOTIC PROPHYLAXIS - YES OR NO? - ENDOCARDITIS

Quinn, E., Cox, F., Burch, K., Fisher, E., & Madhavan, T.

Division of Infectious Diseases, Henry Ford Hospital

Detroit, Michigan 48202 U.S.A.

Antibiotic prophylaxis of subacute bacterial endocarditis before dental manipulations and other surgical procedures in patients with known heart disease has been widely used for over 25 years but its effectiveness has never been proved.(1) The basis of this practice is the observation that a small proportion of patients with endocarditis have a dental procedure before onset of the heart infection. However, among susceptible heart disease patients, the actual rate of development of endocarditis in association with operative procedures likely to produce bacteremia is extremely low. Therefore, it has not been possible to determine the value of antibiotic prophylaxis by clinical observation. Indeed, the presumed success of recommended antibiotics may be more due to inherently low infection rates than prophylaxis per se. Thus, even after administration of penicillin according to an approved regimen, cases of penicillin-sensitive endocarditis after tooth extractions are reported.(2) In our own hospital three such patients were seen in the past 20 years. An alternate explanation for the failure of antibiotic prophylaxis is that the "approved regimen was inadequate. This may relate to the basis for recommended schedules, namely, in vitro sensitivities of the organisms and serum concentrations achieved by the antibiotic. Although bacteremia is reduced, the frequency of lodgment and multiplication of bacteria on the endocardium under these conditions is not known. Since clinical observation cannot answer this dilemma, it recently was proposed by Durack and Petersdorf, (3) and also by Beeson, (4) that clinical recommendations be developed based on data derived from the prevention of bacterial endocarditis in a suitable animal model.

This has become possible since 1970 when Garrison and Freedman described a method of producing endocarditis in rabbits in which the time of infection can be accurately defined and bacterial growth in the vegetation quantitatively studied. Using this model Durack and Petersdorf (3) defined certain parameters in the drug-parasite relationship necessary for successful antibiotic prophylaxis, namely: 1) The antibiotic must possess bactericidal activity. For example, penicillin and vancomycin were effective agents while tetracycline - a current recommended antibiotic in patients - always failed to protect the rabbits.(6) 2) The dose of the antibiotic to be effective must provide high initial as well as sustained serum bactericidal concentrations. 3) The duration of therapy required to prevent infection appeared to relate to the rapidity of bacterial killing by the antibiotic and varied for example from 8 hours with penicillin G combined with streptomycin to over 24 hours with penicillin alone.

In the original studies of Durack and Petersdorf (3) and the as yet unpublished findings of Pelletier, Durack and Petersdorf (6), which Dr. Petersdorf kindly provided me with for this presentation, unexpected difficulty was encountered in preventing circulating bacteria from lodging on the heart valve. The seeding of the vegetation occurred in less than 30 minutes after onset of bacteremia, sooner than any drug present could be expected to have completed its antibacterial action. Furthermore, even though the streptococcus was highly susceptible and the bacteremia was rapidly cleared, most antibiotics tested failed to eradicate the organism from the fibrin and platelet collection on the endocardium. Sterilization of the vegetation required both high initial and prolonged bactericidal serum concentrations.

To achieve killing of the entire population of streptococci in vitro as well as in the valve of the rabbit model, a combination of penicillin with streptomycin (and also vancomycin) was more effective than penicillin alone. All vegetations were sterile at 24 hours when the animal was given combined therapy or vancomycin. However, with penicillin alone, a few animals had vegetations containing a small number of viable streptococci at 24 hours, that is, the tail end of the in vivo killing curve. Several day bactericidal penicillin levels were needed to significantly alter the growth of persistors in the valve.

These findings raised the question of the value of multiple dose regimens. Again bacteriostatic drugs - tetracycline, clindamycin and erythromycin - consistantly failed, where as multiple doses of penicillin V or cefazolin were effective.

These animal studies constitute the only firm experimental evidence that antibiotics can prevent endocarditis. Translation to man poses certain problems such as difference in pharmocokenetics, etc. With these limitations the 1975 Edition of the Text Book of Medicine edited by Beeson and McDermott contains the following

choice and schedules of antibiotics as recommended by Paul Beeson.
(Table 1)

Table 1. Guidelines for Antibiotic Prophylaxis of Bacterial
          Endocarditis

For dental extractions:			
1. Penicillin G	1,000,000 Units	IM	Just
plus Streptomycin	0.5 Gm	IM	before or
or, 2. Vancomycin	1.0 Gm	IV	after
or, 3. Penicillin G	2,000,000 Units	IM	procedure
plus Propaine penicillin G	600,000 Units	IM	
For urethral or gynecologic procedures:			Just be-
1. Ampicillin	1.0 Gm	IM	fore and
plus Streptomycin	0.5 Gm	IM	6 hrs after procedure

Based on the as yet unpublished data presented at the September 1974 Interscience Conference on Antimicrobial Agents and Chemotherapy in San Francisco Dr. Pelletier suggested the following
multiple antibiotics dose schedule for prevention of streptococcal
endocarditis:

Table 2. Additional Guidelines for Oral and Multiple Dose Anti-
          biotic Prophylaxis for Penicillin-Sensitive Strepto-
          coccal Endocarditis

1. Penicillin V	2.0 Gm x 1, then 0.50 Gm Q6H x 8 doses	Oral
or, 2. Cefazolin	1.0 Gm Q6H x 6 doses	IM

In considering other aspects of antimicrobial prophylaxis of
endocarditis several areas deserve comment: prevention of endocarditis in patients receiving other antibiotics; prevention of
endocarditis following cardiac surgery; and prevention of endocarditis in heroin addicts and the compromised host.

It is well established that patients on oral penicillin develop
a relatively penicillin-resistant alpha streptococcal mouth flora
and in those at risk, endocarditis due to such organisms may occur.
(8) Again, with no proof of effectiveness from clinical observation or experimental data, larger doses of penicillin G or combinations of penicillin plus streptomycin or large doses of nonpeni-
cillin bactericidal antibiotics have been recommended.(9) It is
hoped tests of such organisms in the rabbit model may provide new
information for clinical recommendations.

The value of antibiotic prophylaxis is directed at the organisms most frequently causing postcardiotomy endocarditis (PCE),
although probably universally employed, is also unproven. Several
factors deserve comment. An effective program would require protection against many different species of organisms including
ubiquitous organisms of low pathogenicity such as Staphylococcus
epidermidis, diphtheroids, etc. Since early postcardiotomy endocarditis becomes manifest 3-8 weeks after the operation, "persistors" which are not eradicated by prophylactic antibiotics, could
account for endocarditis due to organisms fully susceptible to the
prophylactic agent employed. Another factor to be considered is
the altered pharmocokenetics of antibiotics related to cardiopulmonary bypass. Benner (10) and also Kluge and coworkers (11) showed
that antibiotic levels were rapidly reduced to ineffective levels
after beginning extracorporal circulation. Finally it is recognized that the source of bacteria causing postcardiotomy endocarditis may originate not only from perioperative contaminants in the
surgical field but also intervascular cannulae, postoperative sepsis
from other organs, blood transfusions, etc. Therefore, this multi-
factorial problem probably does not have a simple answer. It is
also recognized that prophylaxis with antibiotics often fails to
prevent infection due to multiple organisms. Thus, antibiotic
prophylaxis may not be possible. Indeed, this pessimistic attitude
should require us to study proven or potentially valuable preventive measures other than antibiotics.

If antibiotics are used during heart surgery, how should they
be chosen? A significant reduction in the incidence of postoperative wound infection can be accomplished in abdominal operations
with potential contamination by bacteria provided that a potent
level of an appropriate antibiotic is present during the operation
and immediately in the postoperative period. Furthermore, the same
principles established in the rabbit model probably should also be
followed, namely, the agent or agents should provide a high initial
bactericidal level and a prolonged lower bactericidal level and as
prompt as possible 100% killing of bacteria. However, since postcardiotomy endocarditis is caused by multiple different organisms,
it very likely would be impossible to prevent infection by all
such micro-organisms and the most one could hope for would be to
prevent infection by the most common causative organisms. Even if
an effective regimen is employed, the antibiotics themselves may
predispose to infection with unusual organisms such as fungi, etc.

Is there any rational to the use of antibiotic prophylaxis of
infective endocarditis in parenteral drug abusers? The exact source
of organisms causing endocarditis in these patients has not been
clarified. Preceding local infections are uncommon predisposing
factors in our series as well as those reported by other investi-

gators and perhaps constitute less than 10% of cases. Likewise,
street heroin and injection paraphernalia have not proved to be the
source of causative organisms. Perhaps it is significant that
Staphylococcus aureus carriage is high (35%) in actively "shooting"
drug addicts compared to a low rate (11%) in appropriately matched
controls. It is thus of interest that addicts with Staphylococcus
aureus endocarditis are always mucocutaneous carriers of the same
strain of staphylococcus.(12) If drug users are the source of their
own organism, one might consider possible preventive measures.
Elimination of parenteral drug abuse is, of course, the best solution. Another measure could be employment of bacterial interference by therapeutic colonization with a "nonpathogenic" strain
of staphylococcus. Finally, courses of antibiotics might be given,
but since this method fails to control recurrent infections from
patients carrier organism, it would seem to have little merit;
therefore, antibiotic prophylaxis of endocarditis in parenteral
drug abusers is not feasible.

Finally, in the compromised host, prevention of endocarditis
due to bacteremia from intravascular cannula, A-V shunts, etc.
requires appropriate medical and surgical techniques and prompt
therapy of infected sites rather than prophylactic antibiotics.

In summary, the value of antibiotic prophylaxis for endocarditis is not established at present. If clinical trials cannot be
arranged to answer this question and prophylactic antibiotics are
given, data derived from experimental observation should be used
to formulate clinical recommendations.

REFERENCES

1. Quinn, E. L. Bacterial Endocarditis. Postgrad. Med. 44(3):
      82-88, 1968.
2. Durack, D. T., Littler, W. A. Failure of "Adequate" Penicillin
      Therapy to Prevent Bacterial Endocarditis After Tooth Extrac-
      tion. Lancet 2:846-847, 1974.
3. Durack, D. T., Petersdorf, R. G. Chemotherapy of Experimental
      Streptococcal Endocarditis. I. Comparison of Commonly
      Recommended Prophylactic Regimens. J Clin Invest 52:592,
      1975.
4. Beeson, P. B. and McDermott, W. (Editors): Cecil-Loeb Textbook
      of Medicine. Ed 14. Philadelphia, W. B. Saunders Company,
      1975.
5. Garrison, P. K. and Freedman, L. R. Experimental Endocarditis.
      I. Staphylococcal Endocarditis in Rabbits Resulting from
      Placement of a Polyethylene Catheter in the Right Side of
      the Heart. Yale J Biol Med 42:394, 1970.

6. Southwick, F. S. and Durack, D. T. Chemotherapy of Experimental
   Streptococcal Endocarditis Part III Failure of a Bacteriostatic agent (tetracycline) in prophylaxis. J Clin Path
   27:261-264, 1974.
7. Pelletier, L. L., Jr., Durack, D. T. and Petersdorf, R. G.
   Chemotherapy of Experimental Streptococcal Endocarditis.
   In press. Presented in part at the 19th Interscience Conference on Antimicrobial Agents and Chemotherapy, San Francisco, California, September 11, 1974. Personal communication
   from Dr. Petersdorf.
8. Garrod, L. P. and Waterworth, P. M. The Risk of Dental Extraction During Penicillin Treatment. Brit Heart J 24:39, 1962.
9. Editorial: Prevention of Rheumatic Fever. Brit Med J
   1:1625, 1965.
10. Benner, E. J. Metabolism of Antibiotics During Cardiopulmonary
    Bypass for Open-Heart Surgery. Antimicrobial Agents and Chemo-
    therapy. p. 373-377, 1968.
11. Kluge, R. M., Calia, F. M., McLaughlin, J. S. and Hornick, R. B.
    Serum Antibiotic Concentrations Pre- and Postcardiopulmonary
    Bypass. Antimicrobial Agents and Chemotherapy. 4(3):270-
    276, 1973.
12. Tuazon, C. U. and Sheagren, J. N. Staphylococcal Endocarditis
    in Parenteral Drug Abusers: Source of the Organism. Ann
    Intern Med 82:788-790, 1975.

CHEMOPROPHYLAXIS OF MENINGOCOCCAL MENINGITIS

Edmund C. Tramont and Malcolm S. Artenstein

Walter Reed Army Institute of Research

Washington, D. C. 20012

There are primarily two situations where the question of prophylaxis against meningococcal disease is raised, first the community epidemic and second, for close contacts of patients with meningococcal meningitis or meningococcemia.

Recently, two countries, Brazil and Finland, have had epidemics affecting the general populations, while other countries, i.e. the United States, have encountered epidemic disease only in closed populations such as military recruit camps.

In the late 1960's meningococcal polysaccharide vaccines to serogroups A and C organisms were developed (1). These have proven effective in studies carried out in the United States, Brazil, Egypt and Finland in children over the age of two years and in young adults. Unfortunately, neither vaccine has been shown to be protective in children under the age of two years. Nor does one know how long the protective effect will last, although studies have shown protective (bactericidal) antibodies for up to five years. Adverse reactions to these purified polysaccharide vaccines have been distinctly rare.

As yet, no vaccine effective against other serogroups of meningococci has been developed, therefore, chemoprophylaxis must be considered. The ideal chemoprophylactic agent is one which would eliminate the carrier state and prevent spread to noncarriers, could be used for treatment of disease, have of low magnitude the development of resistant strains, have a low incidence of side effects, have little impact on the microbial ecology of the host and environment and be of low cost. Prior to 1963, sulfadiazine came the closest chemotherapeutic agent to fulfilling these

criteria. Both the carrier rate and the number of cases were
markedly reduced. The only significant problem was the incidence
of side effects which was minimized by giving a short course of
treatment (two grams for two days). The low magnitude at which
resistant strains developed was attested to by the fact that it
took over 20 years for significant clinical resistance to develop.
In 1963, disease of epidemic proportions caused by sulfa resistant
organisms first appeared. Since then the search for a replacement
for sulfadiazine chemoprophylaxis has been going on in earnest.
By considering antibiotic concentrations in saliva or lacrimal
duct secretions as a reflection of nasopharyngeal concentration
and finding them to be below the minimal inhibitor concentration
of meningococci, or by actually testing them in field studies,
the list of unsuccessful chemoprophylactic drugs would now include
sulfonamides, penicillin G, penicillin V, benzathine penicillin,
ampicillin, oxytetracycline, doxycyline, erythromycin,
ethoxzolamide, nalidixic acid, cephalexin, coumermycin,
trimethoprim and sulfadiazine, pyrimethamine and sulfadiazine, and
immune serum globulin (Table 1).

Three agents with some promise are sulfonamides, minocycline
and rifampin (2,3) (Table 1). Sulfonamides are listed in both
categories since data from the Center for Disease Control in the
U. S. on strains isolated in 1973 show that 80 percent of group B
case strains and 96 percent of group Y case strains were sensitive
in vitro to sulfonamides. Thus, if the index case strain is found
to be serogroup B or Y, the probability that it is sensitive to
sulfonamides is high. However, it must be emphasized that the
standard antibiotic disc sensitivity assays using Kirby-Bauer
methods are not applicable for the purpose of determining sulfonamide sensitivity to meningococci as it relates to prophylactic
efficacy. In this circumstance either an agar dilution technique
or disc method of Bennett et al. (2) must be applied. Also,
having a laboratory with the ability to serogroup strains
accurately is helpful. Seventy-five percent of group C and 57
percent of group A strains remain resistant to sulfonamides and,
therefore, prophylaxis with sulfadiazine for these serogroup
isolates remains impractical.

Several studies have shown that 100 mg minocycline given every
12 hours for five days eliminated meningococci from the nasopharynx
of 60-95 percent of treated asymptomatic adult carriers. The early
field trials revealed few serious side reactions. However, recently
minocycline given in chemoprophylactic doses was associated with
true vertigo in about one-third of the individuals (5). Whether
this discordance is unique to different lots of the antibiotic used
is not known at this time. But these results currently cause doubt
as to whether minocycline would be appropriate as a prophylactic
agent. Also, one is loathe to use a tetracycline derivative in
children.

Table 1

Possible Chemoprophylactic Agents for
Meningococcal Infection

A. Unsuccessful

    1. Sulfonamides

    2. Penicillin G, oral, intramuscular

        Penicillin V, oral

        Benzathine Penicillin, intramuscular

    3. Ampicillin

    4. Oxytetracycline

        Doxycycline

    5. Erythromycin

    6. Ethoxzolamide

    7. Nalidixic acid

    8. Cephalexin

    9. Coumermycin

    10. Trimethoprim-sulfadiazine

    11. Pyrimethamine-sulfadiazine

    12. Gamma globulin

B. Promising agents

    1. Sulfonamides

    2. Minocycline

    3. Rifampin

Rifampin has been strikingly effective (95-100 percent) in eradicating the carrier state. However, when the development of rifampin-resistant meningococci was sought their presence was regularly found (6). In addition, these strains were shown to have occurred in untreated individuals suggesting an ability for them to spread. Nevertheless, no disease due to rifampin resistant organisms has been recorded. Six hundred mg daily for four days is recommended for adults and 10-20 mg/kg for children.

On the basis of these results it was only natural that a minocycline-rifampin combination would be tried (3). The results were gratifying in that the development of rifampin resistant organisms was low, but in one of the studies the incidence of side reactions (33 percent) was disturbing.

Also, it must be emphasized that neither of these agents has proven effective in preventing meningococcal disease when used as chemoprophylaxis in a controlled field study.

Close contacts are one specific group which are at a relatively high risk of developing disease. Defining close contacts as "individuals who frequently slept and ate in the same dwelling with index cases", Kaiser et al. (7) determined a secondary attack rate of 5.9 percent. Secondary case rates were inversely proportional to age; the rate being 11.8 percent in close contacts between the ages of one and four years. Other studies have concurred with these findings. Prophylaxis for close contacts is thus warranted. However, vaccination in this setting would be unlikely to be effective since more than 50 percent of second cases in families occur less than five days after the onset in the index case, whereas vaccine-induced immunity requires five to seven days. Chemoprophylaxis, then, must be considered.

However, as has already been pointed out, minocycline and rifampin have not been shown to be effective in preventing disease and sulfa drug sensitivity determinations requires certain expertise not commonly available in routine laboratories.

Thus, at the present time the cornerstone for caring for susceptible individuals must be careful, repeated clinical surveillance, the objective being to recognize and treat infection (disease) at its earliest stages. Other contact situations such as school, bus, airplane or hospital association have not been found to be at a high risk. Day care nursery contacts should probably be considered as close contacts.

Contact with possible susceptibles must be made two-three times per day by medical personnel, preferably the primary physician, and they must be examined if any symptoms, however mild, develop. At the earliest objective signs such as fever, pharyngitis, otitis, exanthem or stiff neck the individual should be hospitalized, blood cultures and a lumbar puncture performed and treatment begun. If, after 36-48 hours, the cultures are negative and the symptoms abate, the patient may be discharged.

Whether or not to administer minocycline, rifampin, or even sulfadiazine, must be regarded as an additive measure only. The point is, no matter how the stiuation is handled and for whatever reasons, medical, social or political, the potential susceptible individual must be closely monitored.

An uncommon, although important, exception is when the chance of an immediate bacteremia is high such as after an accidental injection (laboratory accident) or mouth-to-mouth resuscitation (high inoculum effect). In such situations 500,000 units of procaine penicillin G should be administered intramuscularly three times daily for two days, followed by orally administered penicillin V, 500 mg thrice daily for eight days.

Because carrier rates are highly variable under normal conditions, positive cultures do not necessarily indicate recent acquisition (the average carrier state lasts approximately nine months) and cannot be interpreted as to whether or not that individual is at a greater risk. Thus, throat cultures for meningococci do not contribute to the management of meningococcal contacts.

In summary, when the disease occurs as an epidemic, vaccination with groups A and C meningococcal vaccines will be effective against those serogroups while the chances are that sulfadiazine would be effective against groups B and Y disease. The use of minocycline and rifampin must be weighed against the incidence of side reactions and the development of resistant strains.

With regards to close contacts, frequent observation of those at risk must be maintained and the use of chemoprophylaxis can be regarded only as an additive measure at this time. In those situations where the chance of blood stream invasion is high, emperical treatment appears warranted.

References

1. Gotschlich, E. C., Goldschneider, I. and Artenstein, M. S.:
   Human immunity to the meningococcus. IV. Immunogenicity
   of group A and group C meningococcal polysaccharides in
   human volunteers. J. Exp. Med. 129:1367-1384, 1969.

2. Guttler, R. B., Counts, G. W., Avent, C. K. and Beaty, H. N.:
   Effect of rifampin and minocycline on meningococcal carrier
   rates. J. Infect. Dis. 124(2):199-205, Aug. 1971.

3. Munford, R. S., Vasconcelos de, Z. J. S., Phillips, C. J.,
   et al.: Eradication of carriage of Neisseria meningitidis
   in families: A study in Brazil. J. Infect. Dis. 129(6):
   644-649, June 1974.

4. Bennett, J. V., Camp, H. M. and Eickhoff, T. C.: Rapid
   sulfonamide disc sensitivity test for meningococci.
   Appl. Microbiol. 16:1056-1060, 1968.

5. Center for Disease Control. Morbidity and Mortality Weekly
   Report 24(6):55-56, 8 Feb. 1975.

6. Eickhoff, T. C. In vitro and in vivo studies of resistance
   to rifampin in meningococci. J. Infect. Dis. 123:414-420,
   Apr. 1971.

7. Kaiser, A. B., Hennekans, C. H., Saslaw, M. S., et al.:
   Seroepidemiology and chemoprophylaxis of disease due to
   sulfonamide-resistant Neisseria meningitidis in a civilian
   population. J. Infect. Dis. 130:217-224, 1974.

TREATMENT OF ACUTE AND LIFE-THREATENING INFECTIONS

Klaus Jensen M.D.

Head of Dept. of Clinical Microbiology
University Clinic of Infectious Diseases
Blegdamshospitalet, Copenhagen
Denmark

Infective endocarditis has changed much during the last three decades. Before the introduction of chemotherapy a rather clearcut distinction could be made between acute bacterial endocarditis (ABE) and subacute bacterial endocarditis (SBE)

	ABE	SBE
previous endocardial damage	unnecessary	necessary
causative micro-organisms	invasive	non invasive
metastatic infections	common	uncommon
valve involved most commonly	aortic	mitral
valvular disease	ulcerative necrotizing	indolent
valve rupture	common	rare
change in murmur	rapid	slow

SBE has become less frequent, mainly due to the decrease in rheumatic heart disease; maybe also to the improved dental hygiene and the much disputed chemoprophylaxis used to protect patients with congenital or rheumatic heart disease. It occurs later in life, and recurrent attacks are seen more often as a consequence of the effective therapy.

ABE in previous healthy subjects caused by Diplococcus pneumonia and Streptococcus haemolyticus has decreased considerably and Neisseria endocarditis is now an extremely rare disease. This is a consequence of the very effective chemotherapy of the primary infections caused by these microorganisms.

ABE in patients with severe predisposing diseases as leukaemia, patients undergoing open heart surgery, patients in chronic haemodialysis, patients in immunosuppressive therapy and mainline narcotic addicts has increased. Hospital acquired endocarditis are also more frequent, 50% of the cases are related to the use of intravascular katheters.

Staphylococcus aureus is still the most common organism, but acute endocarditis caused by microorganisms of low pathogenicity or opportunistic microorganisms as Pseudomonas aeruginosa Streptococcus faecalis, Bacillus species and mycotic endocarditis caused by Candida albicans, Cryptococcus neoformans etc are encountered with an increasing frequency. Mixed infections and recurrent infection with different microorganisms are seen more often. ABE occurs in a later age, 30% of the patients being more than 60 years old.

These factors have complicated the diagnosis of ABE and made the therapy difficult and complex. In spite of more effective antimicrobial agents and an increased knowledge of how to use them; the prognosis has not improved during the last ten to fifteen years. The mortality rate is still about 20%, in patients over the age of 60 it is 72%, and the sequelae are frequent and serious.

As Dr Gorback has already focused upon the predisposing factors and the aethiology, I shall continue by discussing the diagnosis, the pathology of the lesions and the immunopathology of the complications. A study of these factors is the basis for improving the therapy.

A rapid diagnosis with identification of the causative microorganisms is the most important factor for a good prognosis. When the clinical diagnosis is obvious the damage to the heart valves is however often far progressed and the complications caused by embolic manifestations severe and irreversible.

Finding the causative microorganism in the blood of the patient is of major importance to the selection of the most effective chemotherapy, and to the guidance of this therapy; but the search for microorganisms must not delay the initial chemotherapy which should be given as soon as the suspicion of acute endocarditis has been raised. However conflicting as these two problems seem to be, it is often possible to fulfill both requirements: The bacteriaemia in ABE is often massive and constant. In 85% of the cases the blood cultures are positive. 70-90% of the cases with positive blood culture are positive in the first blood culture and none of them become positive later than the sixth blood culture. The requirements for blood cultures can thus be fulfilled by taking six blood samples with five to ten minute intervals. Venous blood samples are sufficient, arterial blood samples and bone marrow cultures do not seem to add to the positive results. In addition to the blood cultures samples should be taken from any possible focal lesions, including the tips of intravascular catheters. The samples should be cultivated in good allround media including anaerobic media. If penicillin or cephalosporin has been given the media should contain B-lactamase, and hypertonic media should be added to facilitate the growth of L-forms. In cases suspected for ABE no microorganisms should be disregarded as possible contaminants. This is also true when more than one microorganism is found. All microorganisms found should be kept in stock culture for subsequent studies of MIC and of the bactericidal levels in the blood of the patient of the antibiotics used. A blood sample should be taken for the microscopic search for intracellular microorganisms in the leucocytes in the buffy coat, and the serum should be studied with countercurrent immunoelectrophoresis for the occurrence of microbial antigens - a new method which can give reliable results within less than an hour. All these measures can be carried out within less than two hours whereafter the initial chemotherapy should be started.

Dr Gorback has already commented on the initial therapy, and I shall now focus upon the pathology of the heart lesions. The nature of the lesions in ABE is necrotic and destructive. In the centre of the lesions enormous numbers of bacteria are multiplying and producing toxins - e.g. leucocidin, coagulase, fibrinolysin and necrotoxin. In addition to this they will also in many instances produce B-lactamases and other enzymes capable of inactivating antibiotics. The bacteria are surrounded by fibrin or fibrous tissue. It is remarkable and quite characteristic for the lesions in ABE that no inflammatory cells are found in the cardiac lesions. The reason for this is most possibly the violent blood current on the surface of the lesions. It does not allow the leucocytes to adhere and immigrate from the bloodstream and it removes leucotaccines so fast that a gradient necessary for the attraction of leucocytes cannot be established.

Inside the lesions the concentration of leucocidal toxins is far
too high for the leucocytes to survive. That this type of lesion
is a consequence of the local factors on the endocardium and not
a common mode of reaction of the host organism can be seen by the
fact, that the metastatic foci in other places of the body has a
structure which is quite similar to ordinary inflammatory
reactions.

The consequences of this type of lesions are clearly
reflected by the type of complications: Necrotoxins will destroy
the valves and the cordae tendineae. Lumps of fibrin, aggregated
platelets and immunocomplexes and bacteria are torn loose and
causes embolic manifestations and metastatic infection. One
third of patients with ABE show symptoms of embolism in the
central nervous system. Of fatal cases infarction in the kidneys
were found in 56%, in the spleen in 80% and myocardial infarction
was found in 40% of the cases. The great production of bacterial
antigens directly into the circulation gives rise to immunocomplex
diseases. A high proportion of the patients develop IgM anti-
IgG, autoantibodies. 80% of the patients have haematuria and
albuminuria, and 10% develop renal failure. The well known
pathalogical picture of a "flea bitten kidney" was until recently
thought to be produced by multiple emboli, but is now showed to be
an immunocomplex glomerulonephritis as indicated by the "lumpy-
bumpy" deposits of immunocomplexes found on the glomerular
membrane.

The consequences for the chemotherapy are as follows:
Only bactericidal antibiotics will be able to erradicate the
bacteria, since the antimicrobial defence mechanism of the host
is ineffective. The penetration of antimicrobial drugs into the
lesions is only passive by diffusion and the inactivation of
antimicrobials inside the lesions can be expected to be very
pronounced if the microorganisms produce B-lactamases or other
enzymes inactivating antimicrobials. Persisters in the form of
resting bacteria and L-forms have the optimal possibility to
survive for prolonged periods. The possibilities for selection
of resistant mutuants are very favourable because of the large
number of bacteria, the low concentrations of antibiotics and
the ineffective phagocytoses.

On this basis the following recommendations for the
chemotherapy of ABE can be set up:

Staphylococcus aureus: Penicillin G or penicillinase stable
penicillins in accordance to sensitivity testing. Great care
must be used to detect even the slightest production of penicillinase as this will make therapy with penicillin G ineffective. If
the patient is allergic to penicillin a cephalosporin can be used
instead. The pencillins or cephalosporins should be given
intraveneously in doses equal to 15-20 megaunits of penicillin

G per day initially. In addition to penicillin or cephalosporin
should be given fucidic acid or rifampicin or an aminoglycocide
e.g. gentamycin. The reason for this is that these drugs will
inhibit the production of B-lactamases, kill the persisters and
stop the production of bacterial antigens. Much discussion has
dealt with the problem of antagonism between fucidic acid and
B-lactam antibiotics. However the antagonistic effect can only
be demonstrated in vitro under circumstances where the influence
of the antibiotics is of relative short duration. In our hands
the combination of methicillin and fucidic acid has given
excellent results, and we have now seen seven cases of staphylococcal endocarditis which have not responded to methicillin
alone respond on the addition of fucidic acid.

Methicillin resistant Staphylococcus aureus: Fucidic acid +
rifampicin which is bactericidal. Rifampicin can also be used
in combination with erythromycin, lincomycin or aminoglycocides
e.g. gentamycin.

Other gram positive microorganisms: Penicillin G or ampicillin
in combination with an aminoglycocide antibiotic, most often
streptomycin, but in case of Streptococcus faecalis infection,
gentamicin should be preferred for streptomycin as many Streptococcus faecalis are completely resistant to streptomycin. Even in
endocarditis caused by Diplococcus pheumonia or Streptococcus
haemolyticus a combination of penicillin and streptomycin should
be used.

Pseudomonas aeruginosa Tobramycin in combination with
Carbenicillin intraveneously in doses of 20 -30 g per day. To
block the activity of the B-lactamases produced by most strains
of Pseudomonas aeroginosa 2-4 g of carbenicillin can be
substituted by methicillin.

Other gram negative rods Aminoglycocides or polymyxins in
combination with B-lactam antibiotics in accordance to sensitivity
testing using a technique revealing the combined activity of the
drugs in question.

     In all instances the therapy should be continued for at
least two to three months. Aminoglycocides or other toxic
antibiotics should be given in full doses during the first 14
days. After that time the dosage can be reduced. The antibiotic
levels in serum should be measured regularly using the patients
own microorganism as test organism.

     Finally it should be stressed, that chemotherapy can only
kill microorganisms. It cannot heal ruptured valves or
reconstitute the function of the central nervous system after
embolism. These grave consequences can only be prevented by an
early diagnosis and immediate institution of chemotherapy.

RECENT TRENDS IN THE EPIDEMIOLOGY OF ACUTE MENINGITIS

David L. Miller

Professor of Community Medicine
The Middlesex Hospital Medical School
Central Middlesex Hospital
London N.W.10

Two recent reports from Devon carried vivid reminders of the extreme potential dangers of infections in which micro-organisms reach and multiply in the meninges or brain. In an outbreak of meningococcal disease in Devon in 1972-73 there were 31 cases with six deaths, several of which occurred within hours of onset (Easton et al, 1974). One case, for example, was in a 10-month-old infant who had refused his feeds and was observed to be lethargic with a low-grade fever; after several hours he developed an extensive petechial rash and died within an hour. In another case a boy aged 17 came home late from a dance and was found dead in bed next morning. Cases of fulminating bacterial infections such as these, usually associated with infection with the meningococcus, are familiar to clinicians, particularly those who work with infectious diseases.

The second of the two reports to which I have referred told, perhaps, a less familiar story. Two years earlier, on 23rd September, 1970, a nine-year-old Exeter girl collapsed and died in her school cloakroom. At necropsy there were signs of acute encephalitis and echovirus type 17 was grown from her brain and spinal cord (Hart and Miller, 1973). This case occurred during a nation-wide outbreak of infections due to this virus, in which 152 cases were reported to the Public Health Laboratory Service, of which just over half had encephalitis or meningitis.

These reports are cited to emphasise the fact that, despite having had in our possession antimicrobial drugs effective against most species of bacteria that cause meningitis for 30 years or more, such infections still kill and often do so very rapidly. Indeed, although case fatality rates have been greatly reduced

where appropriate drugs are given early in the course of illness,
rates have declined little in the last 10 - 15 years. Viral
infections of the central nervous system present different
problems and generally give rise to fewer anxieties. Serious
neurological involvement is rare and most patients who develop
such illnesses make a full recovery. However, no specific treatment is available and no prophylactic measures can be taken to
prevent most infections of this kind and such impotence against
potentially dangerous agents is uncomfortable.

BACTERIAL MENINGITIS

Global Epidemiology

The commonest cause of bacterial meningitis after infancy is
still meningococcal infection. This organism spreads with
particular facility in residential groups such as military recruit
camps, sometimes causing serious epidemics. In the general
population most cases arise sporadically but sometimes the infection
spreads to affect whole communities. The most severely affected
parts of the world were for many years those areas of Africa lying
between the Sahara and the equator known as the "meningitis belt".
Elsewhere the reported incidence had shown a steady decline after
the war. But there have been disturbing reports of an increased
frequency of outbreaks of the disease in many countries in the last
few years.

Starting in June 1971 there have been recurrent outbreaks of
meningococcal meningitis in Sao Paulo, Brazil, which later spread
to other parts of the country. In each of the succeeding four
winters there were increasingly severe winter epidemics, mainly at
first due to serogroup C strains, but with a change to group A
strains in 1974; in both cases a high proportion of strains were
sulphonamide resistant (W.H.O., 1974 (b) : PAHO, 1974). More
recently outbreaks have also been reported from Argentina, mainly
due to group C strains (W.H.O., 1975 (b)).

In Europe, Belgium has reported a sharp increase in cases
since 1969, affecting mainly children under ten years of age
(W.H.O., 1975 (a)). There has been a similar increase during this
period in Britain (Lambert, 1973) but in both countries the
predominant serotype belonged to group B. In Finland an outbreak
due to sulphonamide resistant group A strains began in the south·in
1973 and spread throughout the country during 1973 and 1974 (W.H.O.
1974 (a)).

Of other forms of bacterial meningitis Haemophilus influenzae
infection is reported to be the commonest cause in the United States
Canada, Australia and Sweden and there is evidence that its frequenc

has increased in the U.S.A. over the last three or four decades
(Michaels, 1971). Pneumococcal meningitis is usually the commonest cause in developing countries and is the third most common
in most developed countries.

Bacterial Meningitis in Britain

The relative frequency with which different species were
isolated from the cerebrospinal fluid of patients with bacterial
meningitis and reported to the Public Health Laboratory Service
from laboratories in the United Kingdom in 1974 is shown in
Table 1. Meningococcal infections were by far the most common,
comprising more than half the total, compared with 42% in 1962-63
(Bevan-Jones and Miller, 1967). Haemophilus influenzae and
pneumococcal infections were about equally frequent and together
comprised another one-third of the total. No other one species
was often isolated. The steep increase in the number of cases of
meningococcal infection notified since 1970 has already been
mentioned (Figure 1). In the first quarter of this year, however,
there has been a fall of about one-third both in the number of
cases notified and in the number of isolations of meningococci
reported to the PHLS (BMJ, 1975) and it is possible that the
current wave has passed its peak. The cases reported are mostly
sporadic.

The incidence of meningococcal infections shows a strong
seasonal variation, with the highest rates in the first quarter of
the year, in contrast to other forms of meningitis which are
commoner in the third quarter (Figure 2)

Table 1

BACTERIAL MENINGITIS : Infections Reported to the PHLS, 1974

	No.	%
Meningococcus	1048	53.7
Haemophilus	325	16.7
Pneumococcus	275	14.1
Coliforms	111	5.7
Staphylococcus	77	3.9
Streptococcus	69	3.5
M. Tuberculosis	29	1.5
Listeria	15	0.8
Other	2	0.1
	1951	100.0%

NOTIFICATIONS MENINGOCCAL INFECTION ENGLAND & WALES 1954-74

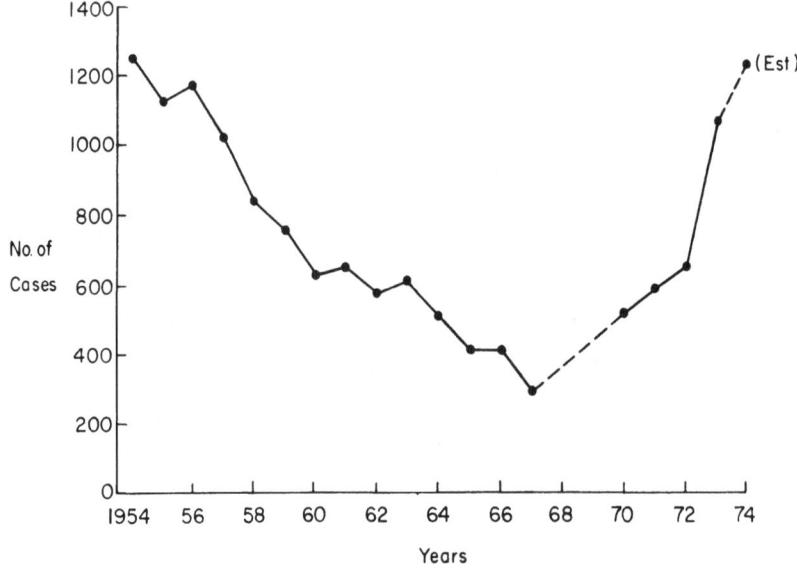

Figure 1

QUARTERLY NOTIFICATIONS MENINGITIS 1970-74

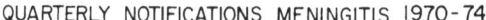

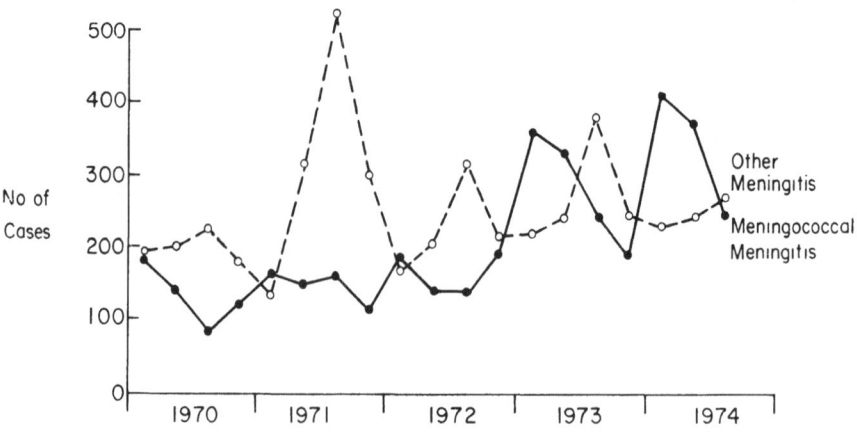

Figure 2

The age distribution of cases differs with causative organism. Only cases of meningococcal meningitis are separately identified in notifications and of these over half are in children under the age of five years (Table 2). In an analysis of isolations reported by laboratories Bevan-Jones and Miller (1967) found relatively few cases of either meningococcal or haemophilus meningitis over the age of five years but 43% of cases of pneumococcal meningitis were in adults (Table 3). Almost all cases due to gram-negative enteric organisms were in children under one year old: most of these occur in the neonatal period (Goldacre, M.J. and Miller D.L., unpublished data). For all types of infection males seem to be somewhat more vulnerable than females.

Table 2

Notifications of Meningococcal Meningitis by Age and Sex - England and Wales, 1973

Age (years)	Males	Females	Total No.	Total %
Under 1	145	95	240	22.5
1 -	89	54	143	13.4
2 -	109	112	221	20.7
5 -	128	102	230	21.6
15 -	62	53	115	10.8
25 +	47	58	105	9.8
N.K.	4	9	13	1.2
TOTAL	584 / 54.7	483 / 45.3	1067	100.0

The numbers of deaths attributed to various forms of meningitis in England and Wales in the last twenty years are shown in Figure 3. Deaths due to tubercular meningitis have declined steadily and are now rare. Those due to meningococcal infection have shown a recent increase similar to that for notifications but there has been relatively little change in the numbers due to other causes. Precise case fatality rates are hard to obtain but some indication is given by relating deaths recorded by the Registrar General to the estimated numbers of admissions to hospital recorded by the Hospital In-Patient Enquiry (HIPE) (Table 4). This assumes that most patients with meningitis are admitted. Rates are highest in young children and older adults and are higher for infections due to pneumococci and gram-negative organisms than for meningococcal and haemophilus infections (Bevan-Jones and Miller, 1967). In gram-negative infections in infants the case fatality rate may exceed 50% (Goldacre and Miller, unpublished data).

54   D.L. MILLER

Table 3

Age Distribution of Cases by Organism Isolated

Infecting Organism	No. of Cases	Percent Distribution by Age (Years)					
		0-	1-	5-	15-	30-	50+
Meningococcus	324	42	38	8	7	3	2
Pneumococcus	145	23	21	13	9	14	20
Haemophilus	121	37	55	7	0	0	2
Gram-negative organisms	54	83	11	0	0	0	6

From: Bevan-Jones and Miller (1967)

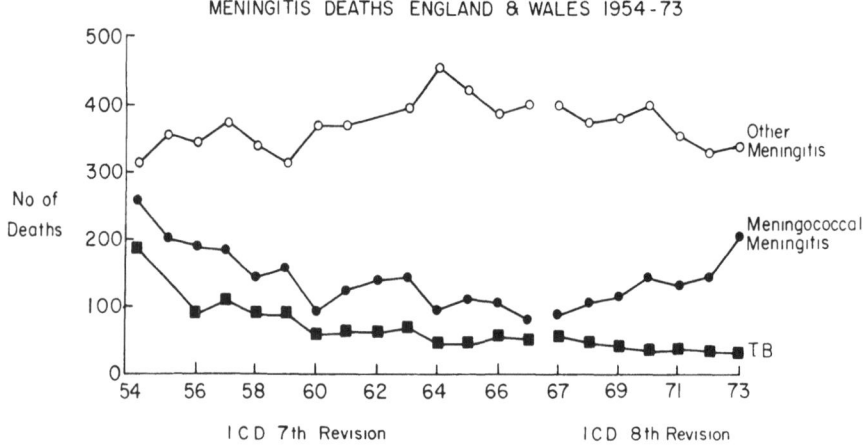

Figure 3

Table 4

Mean Case Fatality Ratios for Meningitis

(R.G. Deaths/H.I.P.E. Admissions 1962-71)

	Age (Years)					
	0-4	5-14	15-44	45-64	65+	TOTAL
	Rates per cent					
T.B. Meningitis	16	7	8	40	38	13
Meningococcal Infection (ICD Code 036)	13	7	9	27	56	13
Meningitis (ICD Code 320)	12	2	3	18	38	10
TOTAL	12	3	5	20	38	11

VIRAL MENINGITIS

A wide range of viruses may cause aseptic meningitis or encephalitis. The illnesses that result are usually less severe than those caused by bacteria and are rarely fatal, although occasionally there may be serious sequelae. Infection with some enteroviruses is occasionally associated with illnesses indistinguishable from paralytic poliomyelitis (Miller et al, 1970) and other forms of neurological damage, though Mitchell and Walker (1970) found no evidence of an increased prevalence of behavioural disorders in children after aseptic meningitis.

The relative frequency of different viruses isolated from patients with acute neurological illnesses reported to the Public Health Laboratory Service in 1974 is shown in Table 5. Enteroviruses and mumps virus are the most commonly reported agents. The predominant enterovirus type prevalent in the population varies from one year to the next. Characteristically one particular virus begins to increase in prevalence in the year prior to a major outbreak, its frequency reaches a peak in the summer months of the second year and it continues to be active, but at a diminishing rate, during the third year (Hart and Miller, 1973). In 1974 the epidemic strain happened to be echovirus type 19: the previous year it had been echovirus types 9 and 11 (BMJ 1974, (b)). Typically the virus is isolated more often from young children than from older children and adults, and neurological symptoms are reported more often in adults than in children. For instance, in the echovirus 9 outbreak in 1973 about 20% of children under 5 from whom the virus was isolated and about 70% of patients over this age had meningitis (BMJ, 1974 (a)). The virus was isolated from the cerebrospinal fluid in 60% of reported cases of meningitis, but in most of the remainder it was recovered from the nose, throat or faeces and the aetiological significance in these cases is doubtful. Also, cases selected for laboratory investigation are not necessarily representative of the usual pattern of infection.

The commonest complication of mumps infection involves the central nervous system. In a retrospective survey of 2,482 cases admitted to hospitals in England and Wales between 1958 and 1960, 25% of males and 18% of females suffered such complications, most often meningitis (Association for the Study of Infectious Diseases 1974). In five cases there was apparently permanent eighth nerve damage suggesting that serious permanent damage is probably rare.

Treatment and Prophylaxis

A worrying feature of the recent increased incidence of meningococcal infection has been the frequency with which sulphonamide resistant strains have been found. Reference has

Table 5

Virus Infections with C.N.S. Symptoms
Reported to the P.H.L.S. 1974

	No.	%	
Adenovirus	112	7.9	
Coxsackie A	31	2.2	
Coxsackie B5	66	4.7	) 11.5
Coxsackie B Other Types	96	6.8	)
Echovirus 6	97	6.8	)
Echovirus 9	62	4.4	)
Echovirus 19	316	22.3	) 42.0
Echovirus Other Types	121	8.5	)
Herpes Simplex	150	10.6	
Mumps	193	13.6	
Poliomyelitis	22	1.6	
Other Agents	153	10.8	
	1419	100.0%	

already been made to epidemics in South America in which a high
proportion of strains of both groups A and C were sulphonamide
resistant, and to an outbreak in Finland due to sulphonamide-
resistant Group A strains. In Britain, the PHLS has reported
that of 266 isolates examined so far this year 65% were group B,
18% were group C and 10% were group A (BMJ, 1975). Of the strains
whose sensitivity was reported four out of 98 group B strains (4%),
3 out of 23 group C strains (13%) and 7 out of 13 group A strains
(54%) were resistant to sulphonamides. Twelve of the resistant
strains were resistant to sulphonamide at a concentration of
50μg/ml.

Reports from Scotland suggest sulphonamide resistance is
increasing in frequency. In 1971, 72% of strains isolated in
Scotland were fully sensitive to sulphadiazine, whereas by 1974
the proportion was only 29% (Fallon, 1975). This shift, however,
was accounted for by an increase in the proportion of strains
showing only partial resistance (i.e. resistant 0.1 mg/100 ml)
rather than of fully resistant strains.

These changes, apart from their implications for treatment,
also threaten the effectiveness of the main current means of

prophylaxis. Sulphonamides have long been used successfully to control carrier states and became routine in the U.S. military camps until sulphonamide resistance began to appear (Lancet, 1970). They remain the drug of choice for this purpose (B.M.J., 1974 (c)). but with the emergence of resistance the possibility of developing vaccines has received increasing attention. Purified polysaccharide vaccines prepared from group C meningococci confer good protection against infection with this serotype (Artenstein et al, 1970). A group A vaccine is also now available and is reported to have been useful in the recent Finnish outbreak (W.H.O., 1974(a)). Unfortunately, so far no vaccine is available against group B strains, the commonest type in many countries, including Britain.

The use of vaccines in military groups is of proven value but their application to preventing the disease in civilian populations is more doubtful. Studies of the spread of infection within households in the Sao Paulo epidemic, suggest that meningococcal infection is usually introduced into families by adults, spreading subsequently to other members of the family (Munford et al, 1974). If vaccination reduced the rates of acquisition and carriage of meningococci, vaccination of older household members might prevent disease in young children and infants by reducing introductions to the family. This seems to be a practical approach that would beworth putting to the test.

SUMMARY

Acute meningitis is still sometimes rapidly lethal. In many parts of the world there has been a resurgence of meningococcal meningitis. In Britain, more than half of cases of bacterial meningitis reported are due to meningococci, with Haemophilus influenzae and pneumococci together accounting for about another one-third of cases. The incidence of meningococcal infection has increased in the last five years, with group B strains predominating. Case fatality rates have not improved in the last decade or more. Sulphonamide resistance to meningococci is increasing in frequency. Group specific polysaccharide vaccines may be a useful alternative prophylactic both for preventing meningococcal infection in vulnerable groups such as military recruits and in controlling epidemics. Viral meningitis is caused mainly by enteroviruses with a different type prevalent in most summers.

Acknowledgements: I am grateful to Dr. Michael J. Goldacre for permission to refer to some of his unpublished work. I also wish to thank the Director of the Public Health Laboratory Service for permission to include figures on cases reported by laboratories which will be incorporated in forthcoming publications from the P.H.L.S.

References

Artenstein, M.S., Gold, R., Zimmerly, J.G., Wyle, F.A., Schneider, H., and Harkins, C., (1970) New Engl. J. Med., 282, 417

Association for the Study of Infectious Disease (1974)
    J. Roy. Coll. Gen. Practit., 24, 552

Bevan-Jones, H., and Miller, D.L., (1967)
    Mon.Bull.Min.Hlth.Lab.Serv., 26, 22

British Medical Journal   (1974 (a)) 1, 652

                           (1974 (b)) 3, 123

                           (1974 (c)) 3, 295

                           (1975)   2, 625

Easton, D.M., Estcourt, P.G., Brimblecombe, F.S.W., Burgess, Winifred, Haas, L., and Kurtz J.B. (1974).
    Brit. med. J., i, 507

Fallon, R.J. (1975), Communicable Diseases Scotland 75/7 (v)

Hart, R.J.C., and Miller, D.L. (1973) Lancet, ii, 661

Lambert, P.M., (1973) Comm.Med., 1, 279

Lancet (1970), 1, 663

Michaels, R.H., (1971) New Engl.J.Med., 285, 666

Miller, D.L., Reid, D. and Diamond, Judith R. (1970) Publ.Hlth. Lond., 84, 265

Mitchell, S. and Walker, J. (1970) Medical Officer, 124, 151

Munford, R.S., Taunay, A. de. E., de Morais, J.S., Fraser, D.W. and Feldman R.A. (1974), Lancet, 1, 1275

Pan American Health Organisation (1974) Morbid. and Mortal. Wkly. Rep., 23, 349

World Health Organisation (1974, a) Wkly.Epidem.Rec., 49, 362

                          (1974, b)   Ibid.   49, 381

                          (1975, a)   Ibid.   50, 9

                          (1975, b)   Ibid.   50, 161

THE CURRENT STATUS OF OSTEOMYELITIS

William J. Holloway

Head, Section of Infectious Disease
Wilmington Medical Center
Wilmington, Delaware   USA

It appears proper to include osteomyelitis in a panel discussion on life-threatening infections in man. Although the mortality and morbidity of osteomyelitis have been greatly reduced in recent decades, if this disease is un-recognized and untreated, the mortality rate is still about 20 percent.[1] Equally important is the fact that rapid diagnosis and treatment are necessary to prevent progression to the disabling and frequently life-long chronic osteomyelitis.

One would like to assume that the decreased incidence of acute hematogenous osteomyelitis in infants and chil-dren is a result of early discrete antibiotic use by the primary physician, but there is no data to support this assumption. A better understanding of the predisposing circumstances extant in those who develop this disease is necessary before evaluating factors influencing its prev-alence.

The availability of newer antistaphylococcal agents was suggested to be the reason for the decrease in noso-comial staphylococcus infections in the past decade. How-ever, recent reports of the resurgence of the staphylococ-cus as a major cause of hospital-acquired infections put this theory to rest.[2,8]

Important changes have been noted in the clinical as-pects of osteomyelitis in children and adults. The staph-ylococcus continues to be the most common pathogen in this type of infection, and it appears to have replaced He-

mophilus influenzae as the most frequent cause of osteomyelitis in very young infants.[4] In addition, penicillin-
resistant staphylococci are by far the more common pathogen in children with hematogenous osteomyelitis, reflecting the marked increase in penicillinase-producing strains
of staphylococci present in the community.[2]

The availability of more practical anaerobic culture
techniques has increased the recovery of anaerobes from a
variety of infections, including osteomyelitis. Classic
anaerobic osteomyelitis complicating decubitus ulcers and
severe trauma have been recognized for years but current
experience may indicate that acute hematogenous osteomyelitis due to anaerobes is more common then previously recognized.

Nosocomial infections due to gram-negative bacilli
and yeast have resulted in an increased incidence of osteomyelitis due to these opportunistic organisms. These infections frequently occur in patients in whom there has
been suppression of humoral or cellular defense or those
in whom natural anatomical barriers have been breached.

Finally, an entity recently recognized is pseudomonas
osteomyelitis secondary to a puncture wound of the foot.[5,6]

OSTEOMYELITIS AT THE WILMINGTON MEDICAL CENTER

As an orientation for this discussion of osteomyelitis I have reviewed the experience with osteomyelitis at
the Wilmington Medical Center for the three-year period,
1971-1973. This clinical experience does not represent
all of the patients with osteomyelitis during this period
at this 1100-bed general hospital, but will review the patients with osteomyelitis who came to the attention of the
Infectious Disease Section of the Department of Medicine.
This designation does not indicate that members of the Infectious Disease Section were responsible for the selection of therapy in all of these patients so we do not assume credit for the many successes or blame for the few
failures.

During the three-year period 71-73, a total of sixty-
eight patients with osteomyelitis were followed at the
Wilmington Medical Center. Thirty-six of the patients had
acute osteomyelitis with twenty-three of these classified
as acute hematogenous osteomyelitis, eleven acute post-
traumatic (including surgical) osteomyelitis and in two
patients the acute osteomyelitis was secondary to paranasal sinusitis.

The thirty-one patients with chronic osteomyelitis were classified as follows: post-traumatic infection in fifteen patients, post-surgical infection in six patients, and infection secondary to vascular disease and diabetes in ten patients. One patient was suffering from tuberculous osteomyelitis.

In fifteen of the twenty-three patients with acute hematogenous osteomyelitis, the infecting organism was Staphylococcus aureus and only one strain was penicillin-susceptible. In six patients with clinically obvious acute hematogenous osteomyelitis no infecting organism was identified. One infant was infected with Hemophilus influenzae type B and one additional patient in whom leukemia was the underlying disease was infected with Pseudomonas aeruginosa.

A majority of the patients with acute hematogenous osteomyelitis gave a history of trauma prior to the onset of symptoms and in sixteen of the twenty-three patients x-ray evidence of the disease was present within ten days of the initial day of illness. The age range was three weeks to thirty-nine years with a median of nine years; male patients outnumbered female by twenty to three. In each case a single bone was involved and in the majority of patients the infected bone was in the lower extremity.

Fourteen of the patients were treated with antibiotics alone while in nine patients antibiotics were combined with surgical drainage (Table 1). Nafcillin was the single antibiotic in six patients in whom surgery was also utilized with a good response in all six. In five patients, nafcillin was used without surgical intervention with only

Table I
ACUTE HEMATOGENOUS OSTEOMYELITIS

Initial Therapy
    Antibiotic + Surgery - 9
    Antibiotic Alone   - 14

Failures on Initial Therapy
    Cephalosporin 2 ⟶ Lincomycin
    Nafcillin   1 ⟶ Surgery + Nafcillin
    Pen + Doxy   1 ⟶ Surgery + Nafcillin (chronic)

Revised Antibiotic + Surgery - 11
        Antibiotic Alone   - 12

one failure; this patient subsequently responded to surgical drainage and a continuation of nafcillin.

Lincomycin was the single antibiotic administered to five patients in this series; three patients were treated with antibiotic alone while in two patients surgery was necessary. A good outcome was experienced by all five patients. Lincomycin was used successfully in two additional patients who had failed to respond to cephalosporin antibiotics. The only clear-cut failure recorded was a patient with S. aureus osteomyelitis treated with penicillin and doxycycline who rapidly progressed to chronic osteomyelitis.

In summary then, there were four failures on initial therapy; two patients who initially received parenteral cephalosporins and were subsequently successfully treated with lincomycin without surgical drainage; one patient who failed to respond to nafcillin alone and subsequently responded when surgical drainage was added to nafcillin therapy; and a fourth patient who received penicillin and doxycycline and was subsequently treated with surgical drainage and nafcillin, but progressed to chronic osteomyelitis.

Eleven patients with acute osteomyelitis were categorized as having post-traumatic or post-surgical osteomyelitis. These patients are grouped together because most patients who experienced trauma were also subjected to operative procedures, e.g. surgical reduction of fractures. An exception was the patient with post-traumatic osteomyelitis following a puncture wound of the foot in whom the infecting organism was Pseudomonas aeruginosa.

Staphylococcus aureus was the most common pathogen in our patients with acute post-traumatic osteomyelitis, being isolated from six of eleven patients. However, in the majority of patients, other organisms such as Group A streptococcus and coliforms co-existed with the staphylococcus.

Therapy in the patients with acute post-traumatic osteomyelitis always included surgical debridement and a variety of antibiotic regimens. This approach prevented chronic osteomyelitis in ten of eleven cases and adequate surgical debridement would appear to be the keynote to success in these patients. The eleven-year old girl with acute pseudomonas osteomyelitis secondary to a puncture wound was treated with debridement and two weeks of therapy with gentamicin and carbenicillin with a good result.

One of the two patients who experienced acute osteomyelitis secondary to paranasal sinusitis was infected
with a streptococcus while in the other patient the pathogen was not identified. Both patients responded to large
doses of penicillin.

Fifteen of the thirty-one patients classified as
having chronic osteomyelitis had suffered trauma in the
recent or distant past, such as fracture of bone or penetrating wound of bone (e.g. neurosurgical tongs). Five
of the fifteen patients with chronic post-traumatic osteomyelitis had a Staphylococcus aureus isolated as the single
pathogen, while in two additional patients the culture revealed Staphylococcus aureus and a coliform. In four instances a pure or mixed coliform flora was isolated on
culture. Anaerobic organisms were responsible for infection in two of these patients while in an additional two
patients the pathogens were unidentified.

The treatment of chronic osteomyelitis is difficult
to evaluate since long-term follow-up is necessary to differentiate temporary from permanent cure. Ten of the fifteen patients in this group had improvement for the period
of time of follow-up while five failed to respond to any
therapy. Eight of the fifteen patients were treated with
antibiotics, while in seven patients surgical debridement
or drainage was combined with the antibiotic therapy.
Three of the patients with chronic staphylococcal osteomyelitis were treated with long-term (eight to twenty-four
months) therapy with lincomycin with good results in each
instance to the date of this writing. One additional patient who probably had staphylococcal osteomyelitis failed
to respond to lincomycin. In the remainder of the patients
in this category antibiotic therapy was haphazard and subject to frequent change so that no significant conclusion
can be reached. Three of these fifteen patients with post-
traumatic chronic osteomyelitis underwent amputation for
permanent cure.

Six of the patients with chronic osteomyelitis developed their infection as a direct result of a surgical procedure, four of the six occurring after a hip pinning. In
four of these six patients the infecting organism was
known to be a staphylococcus, while in one patient the
pathogen was Proteus mirabilis and in the other the organism was unidentified. Two of the post-surgical patients
with staphylococcus infection were treated with nafcillin,
with a good response in each case. The other two patients
with staphylococcal post-surgical osteomyelitis were
treated with lincomycin and clindamycin respectively,

again with adequate initial responses. Unfortunately,
these four patients have been lost to long-term follow-up.

Ten of the patients with chronic osteomyelitis in
this series suffered from vascular insufficiency associated with diabetes, obstructive vascular disease or decubitus ulcer. Multiple bacteria were isolated from the
lesions in these patients and the pathogenicity of these
isolates was difficult to assess. One exception was an
elderly patient with peripheral gangrene in whom the significance of <u>Clostridium</u> <u>perfringens</u> in the wound was confirmed by the presence of significant amounts of gas in
the soft tissue. The vascular insufficiency responsible
for this type of disease prevents the antibiotic from
reaching the site of infection in these patients, relegat-
ing systemic antimicrobial therapy to an unimportant role
in the therapy of patients. Surgical debridement is the
mainstay of treatment in this setting with amputation as
the common consequence.

DISCUSSION

Acute Osteomyelitis

It seems apparent that the rapid diagnosis of osteomyelitis is the single most important factor relating to
outcome and imperative to a favorable prognosis. A high
index of suspicion remains the most important diagnostic
tool since such parameters as x-rays, sedimentation rates,
and white blood counts are unreliable and often delayed
in reflecting the disease process. Early bone scan may
aid in rapid diagnosis of this disease; however, the logis-
tics of bone scanning will have to be drastically improved
in our institution for this procedure to play any role in
the early detection of any disease.

Since the majority of patients with acute osteomyelitis are infected with a penicillinase-producing strain of
staphylococcus, appropriate initial therapy should include
potent agents resistant to this enzyme. We prefer nafcillin because of its stability, bone and joint penetrability,
and relative effectiveness against streptococci and penicillin-sensitive strains of staphylococci. Obviously other
penicillinase-resistant semisynthetic penicillins could be
used in this role. When patients give a history of recent
penicillin allergy we prefer to use lincomycin as alternative therapy in acute osteomyelitis. Although some authors
have expressed hesitancy about using this agent alone, our
extensive experience suggests that it is a superb agent

for parenteral administration in the management of acute
staphylococcal osteomyelitis.[8,9]

We avoid the use of cephalosporin antibiotics in the
treatment of penicillin-allergic patients because of our
clinical experience with cross allergenicity between these
two antibiotic groups. In addition, experience at our institution suggests that the cephalosporins are inferior to
the penicillin antibiotics in the treatment of infections
due to staphylococci, Escherichia coli, and Proteus mirabilis. The only two patients in our series with acute osteomyelitis who were treated with cephalosporin antibiotics
failed to make a satisfactory response and were subsequently successfully treated with lincomycin.

Rapid initiation of therapy in acute osteomyelitis
should preclude the need for surgical intervention in a
great majority of patients. Unfortunately, this favorable
situation does not exist in our institution as approximately half of our patients required surgery during their course
of treatment.

Interpretation of Wound Cultures

No one questions the significance of a pathogen isolated from the blood of patients with acute hematogenous
osteomyelitis or any other type of osteomyelitis. However,
evaluation of the pathogenicity of organisms recovered from
a draining wound associated with bone infection is a difficult problem and mistakes can result from overinterpretation.
Nosocomial colonization is commonly misread as a changing
infection prompting changes in therapy; to wit, a recent
experience with a sixteen-year old boy admitted to the hospital with obvious osteomyelitis of the humerus. Three
blood cultures taken on admission grew Fusobacterium necrophorum as did the anaerobic culture taken in the operating
room at the time of surgical drainage (aerobic cultures
were sterile). Appropriate therapy was instituted with
high-dose penicillin but a delayed response (probably due
to late treatment of the initial infection) prompted re-
culturing of the draining wound. An Enterobacter sp. was
isolated from the aerobic culture and the attending surgeon
discontinued the penicillin and instituted therapy with
gentamicin. Ten days later, clinical worsening and a septic
course prompted a repeat blood culture which again grew
Fusobacterium necrophorum. Repeat surgical drainage obtained purulent material from which the Fusobacterium and
the Enterobacter were isolated. Sequential therapy with
clindamycin and carbenicillin has resulted in improvement
although an eventual sequestrectomy will be necessary.

If nosocomial organisms are repeatedly isolated from draining wounds of patients who are not improving, bone biopsy through healthy tissue may be necessary for stain and culture to identify the significant pathogen(s).

Acute Pseudomonas Osteomyelitis

While acute hematogenous pseudomonas osteomyelitis only occurs in patients with immune deficiencies, we are recognizing an increasing number of patients with acute post-traumatic osteomyelitis due to Pseudomonas aeruginosa. This clinical syndrome, first described in 1968, almost always follows a puncture wound of the foot.[5,6] Since 1973, we have seen five such patients at the Wilmington Medical Center, four children or teenagers and the fifth an adult female. All five patients required surgical drainage, debridement, and curettage, and prolonged antibiotic therapy. Three of the five patients received parenteral gentamicin and carbenicillin, while one patient was treated with gentamicin alone. A fifth patient was treated with Amikacin. While the clinical course is somewhat prolonged in all of these patients an eventual successful outcome has been realized in each instance.

Opportunistic Osteomyelitis

Medical and surgical advances in the treatment of serious diseases have resulted in a striking increase in opportunistic infections due to less common pathogens, not usually the cause of infection in healthy individuals. Numerous reports of osteomyelitis occurring alone or in association with other types of infection have been reported in the literature. The prototype of such infection is salmonella osteomyelitis occurring in patients with sickle cell anemia. Additionally, we are now seeing opportunistic osteomyelitis in nosocomial sepsis, hemodialysis, extensive surgical procedures, and intravenous heroin use, to name but a few. This type of osteomyelitis is characterized by an insidious onset, atypical clinical presentation, unusual anatomic location, and an esoteric pathogen. For example, the patient who uses heroin intravenously is particularly prone to infection of the sternoclavicular joint, the vertebra, and the intervertebral disc space. Patients with immunologic suppression as seen with leukemia, cancer chemotherapy, and steroids are particularly prone to osteomyelitis in the pelvis and other flat bones. Proper therapy in these patients is difficult and depends upon recovery of the infecting organism by aspiration or direct surgical approach. Patients with opportunistic osteomyelitis require prolonged therapy with appropriate antibiotics and control of the underlying disease.

SUMMARY

Although acute hematogenous osteomyelitis is lessening in mortality and frequency, it is still a serious affliction seen in children and immunocompromised adults. Staphylococcus aureus continues to be the most common pathogen and virtually all of the strains causing this infection in our community are penicillin-resistant. A penicillinase-resistant penicillin (nafcillin is our choice) is the treatment of choice for osteomyelitis. A lincomycin antibiotic is the preferred alternative agent in penicillin-allergic patients.

Chronic osteomyelitis requires a combination of surgical and antibiotic treatment usually including long-term antimicrobial therapy. Many of these infections are likewise due to staphylococcus and will respond to antistaphylococcal therapy; however, attempts to identify other pathogens are important.

There is a changing pattern in osteomyelitis due to the increasing incidence of this infection associated with serious nosocomial infections.

The clinical syndrome of acute post-traumatic (puncture wound) pseudomonas osteomyelitis has become more apparent and the primary physician must be prepared to recognize this entity.

REFERENCES

1. Nade, Sydney, "Acute Haematogenous Osteomyelitis",
    The Medical Journal of Australia, Vol. 2, p. 708-711,
    1974.

2. Holloway, W.J., and Clark, J.L., "Changing Patterns of
    Penicillin Susceptibility of Community Strains of
    Staphylococci", The Delaware Medical Journal, Vol. 47,
    No. 5, p. 241-243, 1975.

3. Scott, E.G., Unpublished Data.

4. Weissberg, E.D., Smith, A.L., and Smith, D.H., "Clini-
    cal Features of Neonatal Osteomyelitis", Journal of
    Pediatrics, Vol. 53, p. 505-510, 1974.

5. Johnson, P.H., "Pseudomonas Infections of the Foot Fol-
    lowing Puncture Wounds", JAMA, Vol. 204, No. 3, p. 170-
    172, 1968.

6. Miller, E.H., Semian, D.W., "Gram-Negative Osteomyeli-
    tis Following Puncture Wounds of the Foot", Jour-
    nal of Bone and Joint Surgery, Vol. 57-A, No. 4, June
    1975.

7. Nunes, H.L., Pecora, C.C., Judy, K., Rosenman, S.B.,
    Warren, G.H., and Martin, C.M., "Turnover and Distri-
    bution of Nafcillin in Tissues and Body Fluids of
    Surgical Patients", Antimicrobial Agents and Chemo-
    therapy, p. 237-249, 1964.

8. Martin, R.R., and White, A.C., "Osteomyelitis", Infec-
    tious Diseases, Paul Hoeprich, Editor, Harper and Row,
    Co., p. 1189-1199, 1972.

9. Holloway, W.J., Lincomycin, Wallace E. Herrell, Editor,
    Modern Scientific Publications, Inc. Chapter VIII,
    1969.

MANAGEMENT OF BACTERIAL INFECTIONS IN CANCER PATIENTS

Gerald P. Bodey, M.D., Victorio Rodriguez, M.D., Manuel
Valdivieso, M.D., Ronald Feld, M.D., & K. B. McCredie, M.D.

Department of Developmental Therapeutics, The University
of Texas System Cancer Center, M. D. Anderson Hospital
and Tumor Institute, Houston, Texas, U.S.A.

The prognosis for patients with hematological malignancies and
some metastatic cancers has improved substantially during recent
years. Major factors in this progress have been the discovery of
more effective antitumor agents and the introduction of combination
chemotherapy. Although these advances have been most encouraging,
they have not been accomplished without risk to the patients due to
toxicity of antitumor agents. The primary toxicities of most antitumor agents are myelosuppression and immunosuppression. The consequence of these toxicities is increased susceptibility to infection which may be further enhanced by mucosal ulceration of the
gastrointestinal tract which facilitates invasion of enteric organisms into the bloodstream.

We have recently reviewed the causes of death in a series of
patients with solid tumors, lymphoma and acute leukemia who came to
autopsy examination (7,9,10). Infection was the proximate cause
of death in 47% of the 816 patients with solid tumors, 51% of the
206 patients with lymphoma and 75% of the 315 patients with acute
leukemia. The major sites of fatal infection were pneumonia and
septicemia or other disseminated infections (Table 1). Disseminated
infection was much more common in patients with acute leukemia than
in patients with lymphoma or solid tumors.

The etiologic agent causing fatal infection was identified in
214 patients with acute leukemia, 104 patients with lymphoma and 221
patients with solid tumors (Table 2). Over half of the identified
infections in every tumor category were caused by gram-negative
bacilli. Escherichia coli was the most common single organism causing fatal infection in patients with solid tumors whereas the
Klebsiella-Enterobacter-Serratia group were most common in patients

TABLE 1. Types of Fatal Infections in Cancer Patients

	ACUTE LEUKEMIA	LYMPHOMA	SOLID TUMORS
Patients Dying of Infection	234	104	380
Pneumonia (%)	21	40	50
Disseminated (%)	75	53	39
Peritonitis (%)	1	3	7
Other* (%)	3	4	4

* Includes cases of pyelonephritis, CNS infections, viral
  hepatitis, abscesses, tetanus and enterocolitis

with acute leukemia. Gram-positive cocci were an infrequent cause
of fatal infection, especially in patients with acute leukemia.
Infections caused by multiple organisms occurred most frequently in
patients with acute leukemia.

Neutropenia is probably the most important factor responsible
for the susceptibility to infection during cancer chemotherapy.
Table 3 illustrates the median lowest neutrophil counts observed
during combination chemotherapy for bronchogenic carcinoma (12).
Between 14% and 25% of these patients had to be hospitalized for
antibiotic therapy of presumed or proven infection. Combination
chemotherapy has become accepted as routine management for patients
with advanced lymphoma. We have recently examined the frequency of
infections during this type of therapy (Table 4). During MOPP
therapy for Hodgkin's disease, 27% of patients developed infectious
complications and 25% of these infections were associated with

TABLE 2. Bacterial Organisms Causing Fatal Infection

	ACUTE LEUKEMIA		LYMPHOMA		SOLID TUMORS	
Etiologic Agent Identified†	214		104		221	
Gram-Negative Bacilli (%)	52		60		68	
E. coli (%)		13		14		23
P. aeruginosa (%)		13		13		11
K-E-S* (%)		22		13		17
Gram-Positive Cocci (%)	2		8		9	
Staph. aureus (%)		1		6		4
Multiple Organisms (%)	15		3		7	

* Klebsiella-Enterobacter-Serratia
† Includes non-bacterial infections, also

TABLE 3. Myelosuppressive Toxicity from Combination Chemotherapy
          for Bronchogenic Carcinoma

REGIMEN	MEDIAN LOWEST NEUTROPHIL COUNT/mm^3	% COURSES WITH MEDIAN LOWEST NEUTROPHIL COUNT <500/mm^3	PERCENT PATIENTS HOSPITALIZED FOR ANTIBIOTIC THERAPY
COMB #1	300	67	25
COMB #2 & #3	600	44	19
BACON #1	1000	38	17
BACON #2	1000	22	14

COMB = Combination of cyclophosphamide, vincristine, methylCCNU
       and bleomycin
BACON = Combination of bleomycin, adriamycin, CCNU, vincristine,
        and nitrogen mustard

neutropenia which was usually drug-induced. Among patients with non-
Hodgkin's lymphoma, 33% developed infectious complications during
COP therapy and 42% during regimens containing adriamycin. With
these latter regimens, 53% of the infectious complications were
associated with neutropenia. Often chemotherapeutic agents have a
more profound effect on the concentration of circulating neutrophils
than on lymphocytes.

     Profound and prolonged neutropenia is a special problem in pa-
tients receiving chemotherapy for acute leukemia. The relation between neutrophil count and infection has been studied in 52 patients
with acute leukemia who were followed from onset of remission induction therapy until death (1). During 38% of the total 17,743 patient

TABLE 4. Infectious Complications During Chemotherapy of Lymphoma

	MOPP[1]	COP[2]	CHOP & HOP[2]
Number of Patients Treated	131	135	81
Percent of Patients Infected	27	33	42
Number of Infections	51	59	58
Infections per Patient	0.4	0.4	0.7
Percent Infections Associated with Neutropenia	25	27	53

1 Patients with Hodgkin's disease only
2 Patients with non-Hodgkin's lymphoma only
MOPP = Nitrogen mustard, vincristine, prednisone and procarbazine
COP = Cyclophosphamide, vincristine and prednisone
CHOP = Cyclophosphamide, adriamycin, vincristine and prednisone
HOP = Adriamycin, vincristine and prednisone

days observed, the patients had active leukemia. The patients spent about 50% of their time with neutrophil and lymphocyte counts less than 1500/mm^3. Figure 1 illustrates the inverse correlation between the concentration of circulating neutrophils and lymphocytes and the frequency of infection. When the neutrophil count was less than 100/mm^3, 53% of the patient days were spent with identified infection. The proportion of time spent with identified infection decreased sharply as the neutrophil count increased, but there was no further reduction when the neutrophil count exceeded 1000/mm^3. There was a similar correlation between the lymphocyte count and the proportion of time spent with identified infection.

The relative importance of neutropenia and lymphopenia on the frequency of major organ or disseminated infection was investigated. There were 28 episodes of major infection per 1000 patient days when both the neutrophil and lymphocyte count were less than 1000/mm^3.

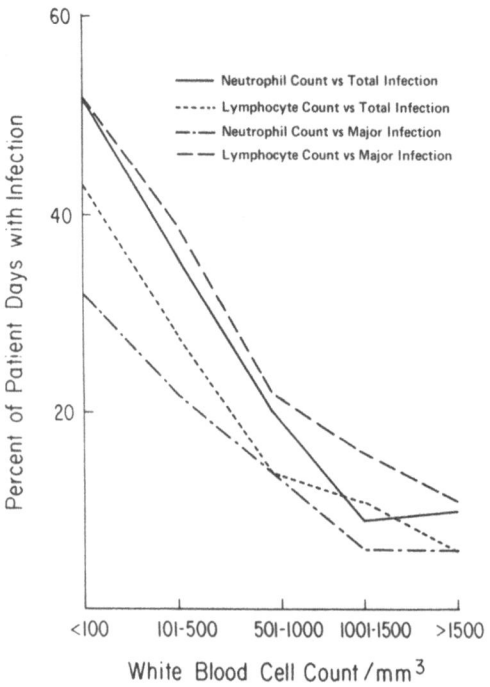

FIGURE 1.   Relation Between White Blood Cell Counts and Infection

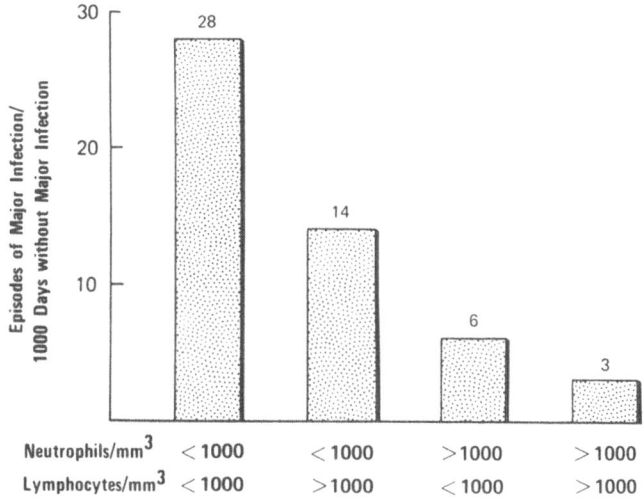

FIGURE 2.   Relation Between Neutrophil and Lymphocyte Counts and
            Episodes of Major Infection

There were 14 episodes per 1000 patient days when the neutrophil
count was less than 1000/mm^3 but the lymphocyte count was greater than
1000/mm^3. When the converse was true, there were only 6 episodes of
major infection per 1000 patient days. Hence, neutropenia was a
greater risk than lymphopenia (Figure 2).

The 52 patients experienced 331 episodes in which the neutrophil
count fell significantly during a one week period usually due to
their antileukemic chemotherapy. During 117 (36%) of these episodes,
the neutrophil count decreased by more than 500/mm^3. Any decrease in
the neutrophil count, regardless of the magnitude, was associated
with a 12% frequency of infection. If the neutrophil count was less
than 1000/mm^3 initially and there was a further reduction, there was
a 28% frequency of infection. However, the final neutrophil count
was the most important determinant of the risk of infection. Regardless of the magnitude of the decrease, the frequency of infection
inversely correlated with the final neutrophil count. Thus, the
frequency of infection was only 2% if the neutrophil count decreased
but remained above 2000/mm^3, whereas it was 28% if the neutrophil
count decreased to less than 100/mm^3. Among the total 115 major infections in these 52 patients, 36% occurred following a decrease in
the neutrophil count during the preceding week.

TABLE 5. Neutrophil Count Related to Cause of Death in Acute
          Leukemia

NEUTROPHILS/mm^3	NUMBER OF SUBJECTS	% WHO DIED OF INFECTION
<100	173	85
101 - 500	38	71
501 - 1000	36	67
>1000	68	53
TOTAL	315	74

The fatality rate from major infection was related to fluctua-
tions in the neutrophil count during the first week of infection.
The fatality rate was 80% among those patients whose initial neutrophil count was less than 100/mm^3 and persisted at that concentration.
Among those patients with an initial neutrophil count of less than
1000/mm^3, the fatality rate from major infection was 59% if their
neutrophil count remained unchanged or decreased. However, among
those patients who had the same initial neutrophil count but it increased to greater than 1000/mm^3 during their infection, the fatality
rate was only 27%. In our study of the causes of death in adults with
acute leukemia, there was a correlation between the cause of death
and the patients' neutrophil counts (Table 5). Among those patients
with less than 100 neutrophils/mm^3, 85% died of infection, whereas
among those patients with greater than 1000 neutrophils/mm^3, only
53% died of infection (7).

Although the majority of bacterial infections are caused by the
common gram-negative bacilli, the cancer patient is peculiarly susceptible to infections caused by several bacteria. About 20% of
systemic Salmonella infections occur in cancer patients. Patients
with hematological malignancies and tumors of the gastrointestinal
and genitourinary tracts are especially susceptible. S. typhimurium
seldom causes more than gastroenteritis in the general population but
is a common cause of serious Salmonella infections in cancer patients.
Salmonella spp. may cause pneumonia, peritonitis, osteomyelitis or
meningitis and 30% of infections are associated with septicemia.

Tuberculosis used to be a common complication of lymphoma and
chronic lymphocytic leukemia. During the past two decades, less than
1% of patients with any form of cancer developed tuberculosis (11).
Tuberculosis is now most prevalent in patients with bronchogenic carcinoma, head and neck cancers and lymphoma. Among patients who develop active tuberculosis during cancer therapy, as many as 30%
disseminate. Infection is most likely to be disseminated in patients
with hematological malignancies. In a recent study during a 5 year
period, we found that 50% of mycobacterial infections were caused by
atypical strains (8). Most of these infections were caused by M.
kansasii and M. fortuitum.

Listeria monocytogenes is a gram-positive bacillus which causes meningitis and septicemia in cancer patients (15). Patients with lymphoma are most susceptible to infection. Listeria infections can be rapidly fatal and the mortality rate is 20% within the first 48 hours after the onset of symptoms.

Patients with hematological malignancies and tumors of the gastrointestinal and genitourinary tracts are susceptible to infections caused by Clostridium perfringens, although these infections occur infrequently (6). This organism is a normal inhabitant of the bowel and vagina and may invade the bloodstream through mucosal defects. Over 90% of infections in cancer patients are associated with septicemia. The clinical features of Clostridial septicemia include tachycardia, hypotension, oliguria, jaundice and intravascular hemolysis. The fatality rate is about 75% within 48 hours if not treated promptly.

The cancer patient with neutropenia is susceptible to infection caused by organisms of low pathogenicity, including Corynebacterium acnes, Bacillus cereus, Aeromonas hydrophila and Staphylococcus epidermidis. Both C. acnes and S. epidermidis are part of the resident flora of the skin and it is often difficult to ascertain whether their presence in a culture respresents infection or contamination. When these organisms are isolated from blood cultures, the possibility of their causing infection should be considered very seriously and be considered as definitely causing infection if isolated from repeated cultures.

Fever is a common complication in patients with malignant disease and its cause is often difficult to ascertain. Fever in most cancer patients indicates infection. Patients with lymphoma are the main exception, since nearly 50% of febrile episodes are due to their malignant disease. In patients with acute leukemia, who frequently have granulocytopenia, over 60% of febrile episodes are due to documented infection. These patients are unable to produce an adequate inflammatory response, and may have urinary tract infection without pyuria, meningitis without cerebrospinal fluid pleocytosis, and pneumonia without physical signs or pulmonary infiltrates on chest X-ray films. In a study of 31 patients with acute leukemia and major pulmonary infection at autopsy examination, only 13 infections were recognized clinically and the etiologic agent was identified in only 7 (4). A normal chest x-ray examination was found in 30% of these patients after the onset of the infection.

Broad-spectrum antibiotic therapy should be instituted promptly when the neutropenic develops fever because infection is likely to disseminate widely and rapidly. Septicemia occurred in 35% of 40 pediatric patients with pneumonia which was confirmed by autopsy examination (2). None of the patients with neutrophil counts greater than 1000/mm^3 had septicemia, as compared with 64% of the patients with neutrophil counts less than 1000/mm^3. Eight of the

10 patients with neutrophil counts less than 100/mm^3 had septicemia in association with their pneumonia.

The aminoglycosides have gained wide acceptance because of their broad spectrum of activity. Gentamicin has been used extensively in cancer patients because it is active against most gram-negative bacilli, including P. aeruginosa. In our study in which we used an intermittent dosage schedule of 30 mg/M^2 intravenously every 6 hours, the response rate to gentamicin therapy was 51% in 122 infections in cancer patients (12). The majority of infections were cases of pneumonia, septicemia, cellulitis and urinary tract infection caused by Serratia marcescens, Pseudomonas aeruginosa and Klebsiella pneumoniae. Although, gentamicin was very effective against infections in patients with adequate neutrophils, it was suboptimal in patients with neutropenia initially and in patients whose neutrophil count fell during their infection (Table 6). The failure of gentamicin in neutropenic patients is not due to inadequate serum concentrations or to the emergence of resistant organisms. Serum from patients failing to respond inhibited their organisms in vitro at dilutions of 1:4 or greater. Furthermore, a 50% to 150% increase in the dose of gentamicin did not result in cure of the infections. Nephrotoxicity is a special concern in cancer patients because they often receive multiple courses of gentamicin therapy. In these patients, the frequency of nephrotoxicity was 4% after a single course but increased to 37% after multiple courses. Occasional patients develop acute renal failure after only a few days therapy. Nephrotoxicity is usually reversible if the patient is supported with dialysis until recovery.

Tobramycin is an aminoglycoside antibiotic with a spectrum of activity similar to gentamicin except it is more active in vitro against P. aeruginosa. Unfortunately, most organisms resistant to gentamicin are also resistant to tobramycin. We have used tobramycin in an intermittent dosage schedule of 50 mg/M^2 intravenously every 6 hours for the therapy of 82 infections in cancer patients (16). The overall response rate of 54% was similar to that obtained with gentamicin. The majority of infections were cases of pneumonia and septicemia and were caused by E. coli, P. aeruginosa and K. pneumoniae. Like gentamicin, tobramycin was quite effective in patients with adequate circulating neutrophils but was only minimally effective in patients with neutropenia (Table 6). Failure in the neutropenic patient was not related to emergence of resistant organisms or to inadequate serum concentrations, nor was it related to inadequate serum inhibitory activity. The major toxicity of tobramycin is renal but it appears to be somewhat less nephrotoxic than gentamicin.

The penicillins are bactericidal antibiotics and are the most effective group of antibiotics in patients with impaired host defenses. Even in neutropenic patients, these antibiotics cure the majority of infections caused by sensitivity organisms. This was first recognized when methicillin was introduced for the treatment of penicillin G resistant S. aureus infections. Prior to that time, these infections were treated with erythromycin and chloramphenicol, which were only minimally effective in these patients. Before the availability of methicillin, S. aureus was the leading cause of fatal infection, whereas at present, few patients die of these infections if treated promptly with one of the antistaphylococcal penicillins.

The penicillin which has been studied most extensively in cancer patients is carbenicillin, because of its activity against P. aeruginosa. It is also active against both indole positive and indole negative Proteus spp., and some Enterobacter spp. and E. coli. The total daily dose of carbenicillin is critical when it is used for the treatment of systemic infections. The total daily dose should be at least 30 grams which may be administered in a schedule of 5 grams every 4 hours. The overall response rate in a series of 59 episodes of Pseudomonas infections in cancer patients was 75% (5). Carbenicillin has been found to be effective even in patients with severe neutropenia (Table 6). Considerable concern has arisen because of the purported rapid emergence of resistant strains of P. aeruginosa during carbenicillin therapy. While resistance does occur, this problem may have been over-emphasized. In many instances, apparent resistance has been due to faulty in vitro sensitivity testing.

Ticarcillin is a new semi-synthetic penicillin which has a spectrum of activity similar to carbenicillin but is somewhat more active against P. aeruginosa in vitro. We have administered it at a dose of 3.5 grams every 4 hours to 20 patients with Pseudomonas infections. Sixteen of these 20 patients were cured of their infection (14). Like carbenicillin, ticarcillin is effective regardless of the patient's neutrophil count. Unfortunately, organisms resistant to carbenicillin are also resistant to ticarcillin.

No single antibiotic has a sufficiently broad spectrum of activity to be used alone as initial therapy of presumptive infection in cancer patients since they are susceptible to such a wide variety of organisms.

TABLE 6. Effect of Neutrophil Count on Response to Infection

NEUTROPHIL COUNT/mm^3	PERCENT CURED WITH		
	CARBENICILLIN[1]	GENTAMICIN[2]	TOBRAMYCIN[2]
<100	75	23	24
101-1000	88	53	70
>1000	56	79	79
Decreased	72	31	39
Increased	82	74	69

1 Pseudomonas infections only
2 Single organism gram-negative bacillary infections only

TABLE 7. Response to Bacterial Infection with White Blood Cell Transfusions

	INFECTIONS	RESPONSE (%)
Septicemia	38	61
Pneumonia	21	67
Septicemia + Pneumonia	9	78
Others	13	100
Total	81	70

Two regimens which have become especially popular as initial therapy for presumed infection are carbenicillin plus gentamicin and carbenicillin plus a cephalosporin. It is not clear what is the most optimum regimen, but we feel that carbenicillin should be included in initial therapy, especially of neutropenic patients because of the high frequency of Pseudomonas infections.

Even though the infection has been identified and appropriate antibiotic therapy has been instituted, the neutropenic patient may fail to respond. Leukocyte transfusions have been found to be useful in this situation. Initial studies of the efficacy of leukocyte transfusions used patients with chronic myelogneous leukemia as donors. In a series of 92 bacterial infections occurring in neutropenic patients which failed to respond to antibiotics alone, 46% responded to leukocyte transfusions from these donors (17). More recently, leukocytes have been collected from normal donors by using a continuous blood cell separator or by continuous-flow filtration (13). In a series of 81 bacterial infections in neutropenic patients, 70% responded to leukocyte transfusions from normal donors after failing to antibiotic therapy alone (Table 7).

Considerable progress has been made in our understanding of the unique problems of infection in cancer patients, the effects of antitumor agents on host defense mechanisms, and the limitations of antibiotic therapy. The introduction of other supportive measures such as leukocyte transfusions has improved our ability to control these infections. Hopefully, future studies with new antibiotics and other supportive measures such as immunotherapy, transfer factor and specific vaccines may provide us with better capabilities to cure the infectious complications of cancer patients.

REFERENCES

1. Bodey, G.P., Buckley, M., Sathe, Y.S., and Freireich, E.J: Quantitative Relationships Between Circulating Leukocytes and Infection in Patients with Acute Leukemia. Ann. Int. Med. 64:328-340, 1966.

2. Bodey, G.P., and Hersh, E.M.: The Problem of Infection in
Children with Malignant Disease. In: Neoplasia in Childhood.
Proc. 12th Annual Clinical Conference at The University of Texas
M. D. Anderson Hospital and Tumor Institute at Houston, Houston,
Texas. Chicago Year Book Medical Publishers, Inc., pp. 135-154,
1969.

3. Bodey, G.P., Middleman, E., Umsawasdi, T., and Rodriguez, V.:
Infections in Cancer Patients - Results with Gentamicin Sulfate
Therapy. Cancer 29:1697-1701, 1972.

4. Bodey, G.P., Powell, R.D. Jr., Hersh, E.M., Yeterian, A., and
Freireich, E.J: Pulmonary Complications of Acute Leukemia. Cancer
19:781-793, 1966.

5. Bodey, G.P., Whitecar, J.P. Jr., Middleman, E., and Rodriguez,
V.: Carbenicillin Therapy of Pseudomonas Infections. J.A.M.A. 218:
62-66, 1971.

6. Cabrera, A., Tsukada, Y., and Pickren, J.W.: Clostridial Gas
Gangrene and Septicemia in Malignant Disease. Cancer 18:800-809,
1965.

7. Chang ,H.Y., and Rodriguez, V.: Causes of Death in Adult Acute
Leukemia. To be Published.

8. Feld, R., Bodey, G.P., and Groschel, D.: Mycobacteriosis in
Patients with Malignant Disease. Arch. Int. Med. In Press.

9. Feld, R., Bodey, G.P., Rodriguez, V., and Luna, M.: Causes of
Death in Patients with Malignant Lymphoma. Am. J. Med. Sci. 268:97-
106, 1974.

10. Inagaki, J., Rodriguez, V., and Bodey, G.P.: Causes of Death in
Cancer Patients. Cancer 33:568-573, 1974.

11. Kaplan, M.H., Armstrong, D., and Rosen, P.: Tuberculosis Complicating Neoplastic Disease. A Review of 201 Cases. Cancer 33:850-858,
1974.

12. Livingston, R.B., Einhorn, L.H., Bodey, G.P., Burgess, M.A.,
Freireich, E.J, and Gottlieb, J.A.: COMB (Cyclophosphamide, Methyl-
CCNU and Bleomycin): A Four-Drug Combination in Solid Tumors. Cancer
In Press.

13. McCredie, K.B., Freireich, E.J, Hester, J.P., and Vallejos, C.:
Leukocyte Transfusion Therapy for Patients with Host-Defense Failure.
Transplan. Proc. 5:1285-1290, 1973.

14. Rodriguez, V., Bodey, G.P., Horikoshi, N., Inagaki, J., and
McCredie, K.B.: Ticarcillin Therapy of Infections. Antimicrob.
Ags. Chemother. 4:427-431, 1973.

15. Simpson, J.F., Leddy, J.P., and Hare, J.D.: Listeriosis
Complicating Lymphoma.   Am. J. Med. 43:39-49, 1967.

16. Valdivieso, M., Horikoshi, N., Rodriguez, V., and Bodey, G.P.:
Therapeutic Trials with Tobramycin. Am. J. Med. Sci. 268:149-156,
1974.

17. Vallejos, C., McCredie, K.B., Bodey, G.P., Hester, J.P., and
Freireich, E.J: White Blood Cell Transfusions for Control of
Infections in Neutropenic Patients. Transfusion 15:28-33, 1975.

INFECTION IN ADULTS WITH ACUTE LEUKEMIA

Stephen C. Schimpff, M.D.

Baltimore Cancer Research Center, National Cancer
Institute at the University of Maryland Hospital,
22 South Greene Street, Baltimore, Maryland, USA

Until very recently, one new serious infection developed
about every two weeks in adults with acute leukemia undergoing
remission induction therapy. Nearly 25% had an associated bacteremia; death usually occurred within two to three days of the onset
of Gram-negative bacteremia. However, in the past few years
certain advances in diagnosis, therapy, and prevention have significantly reduced the number and severity of these serious
infections.

The predominant etiologic organisms are the Gram-negative
bacilli, especially Pseudomonas aeruginosa, Klebsiella pneumoniae,
and Escherichia coli, plus Staphylococcus aureus. Despite their
frequency in the general population, pneumococcal and Beta streptococcal infections are rarely encountered. Less common, but of
great importance because of their almost uniform lethality, are
disseminated Candida albicans infection and pneumonia caused by
Torulopsis glabrata, Aspergillus spp and Phycomycete spp.
Although known to occur, Cytomegalovirus, Pneumocytis, and Toxo-
plasma infection have been rather infrequent in adults with acute
leukemia.

Just as these relatively few organisms predominate, most
infections originate from relatively few sites. Pneumonias, perianal and perirectal lesions, pharyngitis and other oral lesions,
skin lesions, and urinary tract infections along with esophagitis
and viral hepatitis are the principal infections.

Pneumonias are most frequently caused by Gram-negative bacilli,
Staphylococcus aureus, and (in patients who have been granulocytopenic for prolonged periods of time and have received consi-

derable broad spectrum antibiotic therapy) fungi and yeasts.
Pneumonia has continued to be the most serious type of infection
in that it is difficult to diagnose, difficult to treat, and
remains the most frequent cause of infectious death. Perianal
and perirectal lesions usually begin at a small tear in the mucosa
at the anal opening and rapidly become infected with P. aeruginosa
and other Gram-negative bacilli. Septicemia secondary to these
lesions is exceedingly common. Pharyngitis is frequently caused
by normal oral flora, but also by P. aeruginosa, S. aureus, or
C. albicans.

     Skin lesions often begin in the axilla or groin, perhaps
because of moisture and the tendency to develop a minor folliculitis which progresses to a major cellulitis caused by S. aureus
or, occasionally, Gram-negative bacilli. Urinary tract infections
rarely occur in the absence of an indwelling urinary catheter or
an anatomic defect such as prostatic hypertrophy. Normal intestinal organisms, principally E. coli, cause most urinary infections. Esophagitis is common following prolonged periods of granulocytopenia. Although frequently assumed to be caused by Candida
spp recent data suggests that viruses such as Cytomegalovirus or
Herpes hominis (simplex) may initiate infection followed by Gram-
negative bacilli (e.g., P. aeruginosa) or yeasts (e.g.,Candida
spp).

     Finally, viral hepatitis continues to occur in patients with
acute leukemia despite the use of blood products screened for
hepatitis-antigen.   At the Baltimore Cancer Research Center
(BCRC) where the incidence has been approximately 80%, most cases
of hepatitis have features suggesting an agent other than types
A or B.

                          Predisposing Factors

     Granulocytopenia ($<1,000/mm^3$) is undoubtedly the major factor
predisposing to infection in adults with acute leukemia. It has
been well demonstrated that the incidence and severity of
infections rises in these patients as the absolute granulocyte
count declines. Granulocytopenia not only predisposes to
infection, but complicates diagnosis of infection. Overall, the
inflammatory response is markedly diminished such that the typical
signs and symptoms of infection are frequently absent, especially
in the early hours and days in the development of a lesion.

     Other major predisposing factors are those anatomic obstruc-
tions to natural passages such as lymph node enlargement or prostatic infiltration with leukemic cells. Damage to any natural
barrier will likewise encourage infection such as mucosal tears
or ulcerations in the oro-intestinal tract, hemorrhagic defects,
or the invasive procedures often necessary for adequate therapy

of the leukemia. Hospital acquisition of pathogens also represents a major predisposing factor; over one-half of the infections
are caused by hospital acquired organisms. Microbes reach the
patient through food and water (Gram-negative bacilli), personnel
(Staphylococcus aureus and Gram-negative bacilli), catheters, air
(Aspergillus spp) and by contact with other patients. In addition, alterations in microbial flora through the use of antibiotics, corticosteroids, and inadequate patient hygiene may lead
to an ascendency of organisms, which normally are in low numbers,in
the areas where infections most commonly occur. Finally, and
perhaps most important, are the iatrogenic procedures such as the
use of indwelling intravenous catheters or urinary catheters or
the use of any type of intravenous needle left in place for more
than 48 hours. Other problems are the use of contaminated intravenous solutions or blood products (Gram-negative bacilli and
hepatitis virus).

Prevention

The techniques used to prevent infection in adults with acute
leukemia are derived from a consideration of the types of infection which occur and their predisposing factors. First is to
bolster the damaged host defense mechanisms with agents such as
killed vaccines (influenza), passive immunization (hepatitis),
and relief of obstruction.

Avoidance of urinary catheters and venous catheters will
almost totally prevent urinary tract infections and markedly
reduce bacteremias. At the BCRC we use only butterfly type needles
and change the site every 48 hours.

To prevent skin infections, all patients are encouraged to use
hexachloraphene as both a bath soap and shampoo. A soft tooth-
brush, dental floss, and a povadine-iodine mouthwash solution is
used four times per day. Axillary shaving is discouraged as are
occlusive antiperspirants which might predispose to folliculitis.
Pathogen acquisition can be reduced by maintaining patients out
of hospital whenever possible and ensuring that they are not
placed in overcrowded wards. Reverse isolation (in laminar air
flow rooms) will reduce acquisition of new pathogens to a minimum.
Equally important is the use of pathogen-free infusions and blood
product transfusions.

Microbial suppression has also proven useful. As noted, hexachloraphene is used for bathing and povadine-iodine is used as a
mouthwash. In addition, oral non-absorbable antibiotics
(gentamicin, vancomycin, and nystatin given every four hours) are
very useful in suppressing the microbial flora of the oral-
intestinal tract with a consequent marked reduction in Gram-
negative infections including a 10X reduction in bacteremias.

A vigorous combined approach utilizing all of the methods referred to has clearly been proven to reduce, to a major degree, the frequency and the severity of infections. Ultimately however, the best infection prevention technique is induction of a complete remission with return of normal-host defense mechanisms.

Diagnostic Approach

It is essential to be exacting and thorough during the history to detect the subtle clues of a minimal inflammatory reaction associated with granulocytopenia, e.g. perianal discomfort, non-productive cough, dysphagia, or minimal dyuria. The examination must likewise be detailed, exacting and thorough. Subtle findings on examination such as a minimal inflammatory reaction at a perianal mucosal tear (erythema and tenderness) or pharynx (erythema with submandibular tenderness) usually represents serious infection. A urine sample should be examined personally by the physician for the presence of bacteria. Pyuria should not be expected because of granulocytopenia and probably for the same reason these patients have minimal other symptoms or signs of urinary tract infection.

Even if the patient has no pulmonary findings, a chest radiograph is essential and should be repeated daily if no other site of infection is found. The initial chest radiograph may be entirely negative but infiltrates may develop rapidly over the next few days.

The basic initial microbiologic samples should include, at least, two separate sets of blood cultures, a quantitative urine culture and surveillance cultures of nose, throat, axilla and rectum. In patients with pneumonia, examination of expectorated sputum has proven to be of minimal value because of scanty material and contamination with the posterior pharyngeal flora. Therefore a transtracheal aspiration or transtracheal brush biopsy is often extremely useful in obtaining adequate non-contaminated material for culture and histology.

Esophagitis can be initially diagnosed by symptomatology but a barium swallow followed by esophagoscopy with biopsy for histology and culture is essential to define the etiologic agent and guide proper management.

Techniques such as the limulus endotoxin assay, the nitroblue tetrazolium dye reduction test, and gallium scanning, while still under evaluation, have not yet proven of major value.

Therapy of Suspected Bacterial Sepsis in the Patient with Fever
and Granulocytopenia.

An adult with acute leukemia who suddenly develops a rising
temperature in the presence of granulocytopenia frequently has an
infection which may prove to be severe and even fatal if not
treated promptly and aggressively. Empiric antibiotic therapy has
therefore become a standard approach to management. It is
essential that the antibiotics chosen be given in their full
dosage intravenously to ensure adequate blood levels. The agent(s)
should be broad spectrum in nature and preferably bactericidal.
The specific agents used will depend upon the organisms known to
cause the majority of infections at any given cancer center. We
have been using various combinations of carbenicillin (or
ticarcillin), gentamicin (or tobramycin), and cephalothin
(or cephazolin) because P. aeruginosa, K. pneumoniae and S. aureus
are most common at the Baltimore Cancer Research Center.

Once the nature of the infecting organism is known adjust-
ments to these antibiotics can be made. For example, if P.
aeruginosa is the infecting organism then we would be inclined to
continue a combination of carbenicillin and gentamicin or cephalothin plus gentamicin when Klebsiella sp is found.

Generally, these antibiotics will be efficacious in most
patients who are granulocytopenic and infected. However, if host
defense mechanisms are so severely damaged that the patient does
not respond promptly to antibiotic therapy we attempt to obtain
HLA-matched granulocytes for transfusion. Available data indicates
that granulocyte transfusions will indeed salvage patients
who otherwise would not have survived. Some infections may not
clear fully until the granulocyte count spontaneously rises with
impending remission, however, most patients will now survive for
at least a few weeks (c.f. previously only a few days) which gives
the antileukemia drugs time to affect a complete remission.

Patients who develop fungal infections (Aspergillus, Phycomycete, Candida, Torulopsis, or Cryptococcus) should be treated
with amphotericin B. There is no data to support the use of
5-fluorocytosine in granulocytopenic patients. We institute amphotericin B in a dose of 0.3 ml/kg and increase to 0.6 ml/kg daily
thereafter. It is essential that the diagnosis of fungal infection
be made promptly so that amphotericin B can be instituted immediately in this situation increasing numbers of patients will
indeed survive fungal infection provided that they ultimately
achieve a complete remission of their leukemia.

Summary

A firm understanding of the etiologic agents and sites of
infection which occur most frequently in adult patients with acute
leukemia coupled with an application of the predisposing factors,
preventive measures, diagnostic techniques, and prompt efficient
management will ensure a reduced incidence of severe infection
coupled with a marked increase in the number of patients who will
survive those infections which continue to occur.

Therapy of infections in acute leukemia

Jean KLASTERSKY

Institut Jules Bordet, Rue

Héger-Bordet 1, 1000 Brussels, Belgium

Neutropenia is a major factor predisposing the patient
with leukemia to severe bacterial infections. In neutropenics,
bacterial infections are most often due to gram negative
bacilli (Ps. aeruginosa, E. coli, Klebsiella sp.) and originate
from sites such as lungs, pharynx, gastro-intestinal tract,
perineal region and skin. Very often bacteremia is associated with these infections.

Early therapy of severe infections in neutropenic patients
is probably of considerable importance. It is known that
over 50% of such patients will die from sepsis within 48
hours of its onset. Therefore, if one waits for the results
of the bacteriologic cultures and for the reports of the sensitivity of the isolated bacteria, there is a risk that a substantial proportion of the patients will be dead without having
had a chance for an adequate antimicrobial therapy.

This is the reason why Schimpff and his co-workers have
proposed to administer antibiotics to patients with fever and
neutropenia as soon as infection is suspected. (1)

However, the initial reports on empiric therapy with
carbenicillin plus gentamicin in cancer patients with fever
and neutropenia were not adequately controlled. It was not
clear whether the patients-many of whom had Pseudomonas
sepsis-responded favorably because of the early initiation of
antimicrobial therapy or because the new drug carbenicillin,
which is highly active when used alone in Ps. aeruginosa
infected patients, was a part of the empiric regimen.

Nevertheless, there are experimental data suggesting that

antimicrobial therapy of severe infections should be instituted early in order to secure optimal results.   Therefore,
many clinicians have adopted the principale of empirical
therapy of suspected sepsis in patients with severly impaired
natural mechanisms of defence against infection in spite of
the general consensus that it is usually not desirable to
treat an infection before having some knowledge about the
offending pathogen.

   Antimicrobial regimens to be used empirically in leukemia patients with fever and granulocytopenia should not only
represent an adequate coverage against the most frequently
encountered pathogens; in addition, their clinical effectiveness
should be reliable under the circumstances in which they
have been employed.
This is the reason why gentamicin and other similar aminoglycosides, in spite of their excellent anti-staphyloccal spectrum in vitro, should not be used as a single therapy in
severe infections in neutropenic patients.   The use of gentamicin in gram negative septicemia in granulocytopenics
results in a favorable outcome in only 20-30 % of the patients.
This is probably due to a narrow margin between the effective and the toxic concentrations of that drug (2).
No other single antibiotic can represent an adequate empiric
regimen on the basis of its antimicrobial spectrum. Therefore, one has to resort to the use of combinations of antibiotics for empiric therapy for patients with neutropenia and
suspected sepsis.
Many different associations of antibiotics have been proposed
for empiric therapy in patients with increased susceptibility
to infection.   Among them the combination of carbenicillin,
cephalothin and gentamicin probably represents the best
theoretical choice. However, it has been shown that the
triple combination carbenicillin-cephalothin-gentamicin is not
more effective clinically than that of carbenicillin and cephalothin without gentamicin.   In addition, nephrotoxicity has
been found in about 20% of the patients who receive the carbenicillin-cephalothin-gentamicin combination. While the combination carbenicillin-cephalothin is not nephrotoxic (3).   A
similar incidence of nephrotoxic reactions can be found with
the combination cephalothin-gentamicin. This latter association, in addition, does not represent an adequate coverage
against enterococci, Hemophilus sp. and Bacteroides sp. We
are thus left for empirical therapy in neutropenic leukemia
patients with suspected severe infection with the two combinations carbenicillin plus gentamicin and carbenicillin plus

cephalothin which appear to be equally effective from the
clinical point of view. Recent controlled clinical trials,
under the auspices of the EORTC (European Organization
for the Research on Treatment of Cancer) and which are
still in progress, indicate that these two regimens result in
about 88 % of favorable clinical responses in bacteriologically proven infection without bacteremia and in 63 % of the
bacteremic episodes (4).

The effectiveness of various combinations of antibiotics
may not only be related to their broad spectrum but also to
the occasional potentiation of one drug of the combination by
the other.

The significance of the in vitro synergism of the penicillin-
aminoglycoside combination is well known in streptcoccal
endocarditis. As far as gram negative infections are concerned, we have shown that, in patients with cancer and
bacteriologically demonstrated gram negative infections, the
use of synergistic combinations was associated with a better
clinical response than that of combinations that were not
synergistic against the pathogens responsible for the infections
considered (5). Combinations of antibiotics which are synergistic against the offending pathogen result in a higher antimicrobial activity in the serum and presumably in the tissues,
than the non-synergistic combinations. The antimicrobial
activity, which should be measured against the offending pathogen in the serum taken 1 hour after the administration of
the antibiotics to the patient, should be sufficient to inhibit
the microorganisms (10^5 microorganisms per ml) when diluted at 1:8. The titration of the antimicrobial activity of the
serum in antibiotic-treated patients represents a convenient
guide for adjustment of therapy (6).

As a result of the preceeding considerations, we recommend
at the present time to administer antibiotics to the neutropenic ($<$ 1000 granulocytes per mm3) patient as soon as infection is suspected (fever 38.5°C, with or without clinical
signs of infection, unless there is some reason for artificial
suppression of fever). Blood cultures and other cultures when
indicated should be obtained prior to the injection of the antibiotics.

The empiric regimen should consist of carbenicillin plus cephalothin. Both should be given intravenously at 6-8 hours
intervals. The daily dosage should be 500 mg/kg for carbenicillin and 1500 mg/kg for cephalothin. Hypokalemia may
be a complication of this type therapy but it responds to
the administration of supplements of potassium.

If a favorable response is obtained, therapy should be continued for 7-8 days. If a pathogen is available retrospectively, therapy may be restricted to carbenicillin or cephalothin alone, provided an adequate (1:8) antimicrobial activity of the serum of the treated patient can be demonstrated against that microorganism with the use of a single drug.

If no favorable response is obtained after 48 or 72 hours, the therapeutic attitude will depend on whether or not a pathogen is available.

If no pathogen can be isolated, the patient should receive gentamicin in addition to carbenicillin and cephalothin in order to cover the possibility of an infection caused by a microorganism resistant to both carbenicillin and cephalothin and to take advantage of a possible synergism between carbenicillin and gentamicin or cephalothin and gentamicin against the unknown pathogen. A favorable response may be observed under these circumstances (7). If no favorable response can be obtained then, the possibility of a fungal disease should seriously be considered, especially if the neutropenia has been prolonged, if multiple courses of antibiotics have already been given and chie fly if a pulmonary lesion has appeared. Microbiological documentation of disseminated fungal disease is notoriously difficult and serological diagnosis is still unreliable. Since fungal disease (especially candidiasis and aspergillosis) causes about 20 % of the deaths due to infection in leukemics, the empiric administration of antifungal therapy should be considered in the neutropenic patient who is not responding to the triple combination carbenicillin-cephalothin-gentamicin and in whom no pathogen has been isolated.

It has been postulated that the use of a combination of amphotericin B and 5- fluoro cytosine may be advantageous while decreasing toxicity through reduction of dosage of amphotericin B and by prevention of emergence of organisms resistant to 5-fluoro cytosine.

In addition, knowledge of the mechanisms of action of each drug suggests that amphotericin B might accelerate the entry of 5-fluoro-cytosine into to microorganism, thus potentiating their individual biological activities. Garriques et al reported on their experience in human disease with combined therapy and after treatment of 15 patients, they concluded that their results justified a "larger cooperative study" (8).

Transfusion of granulocytes may also be considered when no adequate clinical response can be obtained in a neutropenic patient with a broad spectrum antimicrobial therapy.

If a pathogen has been isolated (especially from blood cultures)

and the response to the initial combination carbenicillin-
cephalothin has not been satisfactory, antimicrobial therapy
should then be adjusted in such a manner that the antimicrobial activity of the serum would be at least 1:8 against the
pathogen. This can be done by selecting the most appropriate
antibiotics and synergistic combinations of antibiotics as
based on in vitro studies. If, after such an adjustment,
septicemia or signs of severe infection persist, a cryptic
focus of infection should be looked for, especially in the
gastro-intestinal, urinary and endovascular systems. New
scanning techniques using isotope-labeled granulocytes may
be useful here. In addition, a transfusion of granulocytes
may be necessary.

In summary, the approach of infections in patients with leukemia is not basically different from that used in the management of severe infections in other types of patients. It
should be stressed, however, that the neutropenic patients
mainly rely on antibiotics to eradicate infection. In addition,
in such patients, owing to the absence of the basic mechanism of defence, infection becomes rapidly extensive and
generalizes itself by invading the bloodstream.

These are the reasons why therapy should be undertaken early
with appropriate antibiotic combinations which are presumably active on most gram-negative pathogens. The adequacy
of the treatment must be substantiated, when feasible, by
in vitro sensitivity studies and back titration of the antimicrobial activity of the serum of the treated patient against
the isolated pathogen.

Finally, consideration should be given to early administration of antifungal agents when disseminated fungal disease
is a possibility and to transfusions of granulocytes in patients in whom sepsis cannot be controlled with antibiotics.

References.
1) Schimpff, S; Satterlee, W. S.; Young, V. M.; Serpick, A. A.
   (1971). Empiric therapy with carbenicillin and gentamicin
   for febrile patients with cancer and granulocytopenia.
   New. Engl. J. Med. 284: 1061-1065.

2) Bodey, G. P.; Middleman, E.; Umsawadi, T.; Rodriguez, V.
   (1972). Infections in cancer patients. Results with gentamicin sulfate therapy. Cancer 29: 1967-1701.

3) Klastersky, J.; Henri, A.; Hensgens, C.; Daneau, D. (1974)
   Gram negative infections in cancer. A study of empiric
   therapy comparing carbenicillin-cephalothin with and
   without gentamicin. J. A. M. A. 227: 45-48.

4) Gaya, H.; Klastersky, J.; Schimpff, S.; Fière, D.; Wid-
maier, S.; Nagel, G. (1975). Prospective randomly controlled trial of three antibiotic combinations for empirical therapy of suspected spesis in neutropenic cancer
patients. Europ. J. Cancer (in press).

5) Klastersky, J.; Cappel, R.; Daneau, D. (1972) Clinical
significance of in vitro synergism between antibiotics in
gram negative infections. Antimicrob. Ag. Chemother.
2 : 470-475.

6) Klastersky, J.; Daneau, D.; Swings, S.; Weerts, D.
(1974) Antibacterial activity in serum and urine as therapeutic guides in bacterial infections. J. Infect. Dis.
129: 187-193.

7) Rodriguez, V.; Burgess, M.; Bodey, G. P. (1973) Management of fever of unknown origin in patients with neoplasms and neutropenia. Cancer 32: 1007-1012.

8) Garrique, I. L.; Sande, M. A.; Utz, J. P.; Mandell, G. L.;
Warner, J. F.; Mc Gehee, R. F.; Shadomy, S. (1973)
Combined amphotericin B-flucytosine chemotherapy in
human cryptococcosis (abstract). Proceedings of the 13th
Interscience Conference on Antimicrobial Agents and
Chemotherapy.

INFECTION PREVENTION IN ACUTE MYELOID LEUKAEMIA: ORAL

NON-ABSORBED ANTIBIOTIC PROPHYLAXIS

HAROLD GAYA, BERYL JAMESON AND
RODERICK A. STORRING
ST. MARY'S HOSPITAL MEDICAL SCHOOL, THE ROYAL
MARSDEN HOSPITALS AND THE ROYAL POSTGRADUATE MEDICAL
SCHOOL, LONDON

Despite advances in cancer chemotherapy and supportive care,
infection remains the major cause of death in patients with malignant blood disease, more than a quarter of these patients dying
of infection before antineoplastic therapy has had an opportunity
to induce remission (1-3). The effective prevention of infection
in these patients should therefore improve the prognosis of the
primary disease by permitting more prolonged and more intensive
anti-leukaemic therapy and consequently result in better remission
rates and survival.

Several factors leading to neutropenia predispose patients with
malignant disease to infection, and in addition, some cytotoxic
agents cause intestinal mucosal ulceration and promote the spread
of intestinal organisms. There is a quantitative relationship
between the degree of neutropenia and the risk of bacteraemic
infection ("septicaemia") in patients with acute leukaemia, and it
is clear that as the neutrophil count falls below 1000 per µl. the
chances of infection occurring rise steeply (4,5). Thus the
patient, with severe neutropenia, as a result of primary bone
marrow disease or following therapy for malignancy, is particularly
at risk from infection since circulating neutrophils constitute an
important defence against bacterial invasion.

The prolonged neutropenia associated with the acute leukaemias
demands that attention be paid to possible sources and routes of
infection, and that measures be taken to prevent it (3,4,6-9).
Many infections are due to organisms acquired in the hospital
environment which colonize the patient, and his gastro-intestinal
tract may be the final pathway leading to infection (3,7,10). It is
thus rational to consider the use of oral non-absorbed antibiotics

for intestinal decontamination to prevent infection by organisms
from both endogenous and exogenous sources.

We are currently evaluating oral prophylaxis in a prospective,
randomized, controlled trial at the Royal Marsden Hospitals and
Hammersmith Hospital, supported by the Leukaemia Research Fund, and
our preliminary results are summarised here. A few other studies
of the value of such measures have been published (7-12) and, on
balance, it would appear that oral prophylaxis may contribute to
a reduction in the incidence of infection, even though there is
no consensus in this respect.

Schimpff and his colleagues (9) comparing oral prophylaxis in the
open ward and in reverse isolation with "unprotected" control
patients, showed that a combination of gentamicin, vancomycin, and
nystatin (GVN) reduced the incidence of infection and improved
the remission rate both in the open ward and in reverse isolation.
Klastersky and his co-workers (12) similarly report a reduction
in serious infection in adults with acute leukaemia compared with
"unprotected" control patients. Both these groups found that
laminar air flow plus oral antibiotic prophylaxis reduced infection
to about the same level as did the oral antibiotics alone. Yates
and Holland (8), found a significant reduction in infection in
patients nursed in reverse isolation, with and without GVN, but no
increase in remission rates. Patients nursed in single rooms and
receiving oral non-absorbed antibiotics showed no such reduction.
Levine et al (7), comparing isolation plus oral prophylaxis, oral
prophylaxis alone and "unprotected" control patients were unable
to show any reduction in serious infection attributable to oral
non-absorbed antibiotics. However, the three prospective,
controlled trials (7-9) agree that reverse isolation plus gut
decontamination will reduce infection while differing on the
value of gut decontamination alone. There is no agreement on the
effects of these measures on remission rates.

In our own study we are comparing patients with adult acute
myeloid leukaemia (AML) or one of its variants, nursed in single
rooms with clean food, and randomized to a gut and orificial
decontamination regimen or to a control group. Our aim has been
to reduce the number of variables in this study so that the only
difference between the groups is the use or otherwise of the
decontamination regimen.

GUT DECONTAMINATION REGIMEN
(FRACON)

FRAMYCETIN	500 mg	(tabs)	q.d.s.
COLISTIN SULPHATE	1.5×10^6 units	(tabs)	q.d.s.
NYSTATIN	$(0.5 \times 10^6$ units	(tabs)	q.d.s.
	and $(0.5 \times 10^6$ units	(syrup)	q.d.s.

This regimen was chosen in preference to GVN for two main reasons. The first was economic in that FRACON costs about one-tenth of the price of GVN and second was the problem of gentamicin resistance. We regard gentamicin as a valuable therapeutic agent and are loath to use it prophylactically and topically. The Baltimore team (13), have already reported the development of gentamicin resistant P. aeruginosa in some patients receiving oral gentamicin, and Klastersky and his colleagues in Belgium have also reported increasing resistance to gentamicin (12).

ORIFICIAL REGIMEN
(Self-administered by patient)

1. Chlorhexidine Cream (1%) to anterior nares   b.d.
2. Chlorhexidine Dental Gel (2.5cm.) to gums   b.d.
3. Chlorhexidine Gluconate (0.02% aqueous) mouthwash   q.d.s.
4. Chlorhexidine Gluconate (0.02% aqueous) spray to
   ears and throat, and intranasally after each mouthwash
5. Chlorhexidine Obstetric Cream (1%) to vagina and vulva   b.d.
6. Chlorhexidine Gluconate (0.02% aqueous) vaginal douche   mane.
7. Amphotericin B Lozenges (10mg.) sucked between meals   ad lib.

DETAILS OF PATIENTS STUDIED

	CONTROL	FRACON
NUMBER OF PATIENTS ENTERED	42	41
- FRACON INTOLERANT		4
- DIED BEFORE STUDY	1	3
NUMBER OF PATIENTS STUDIED	41	34
REMISSION	24(59%)	21(62%)
PARTIAL REMISSION	5	3
DIED OF INFECTION	4	0
DIED OF OTHER CAUSE	1	1
DRUG RESISTANT	7	9
- discharged	3	5
- died of infection	3	2
- died of bleeding		1
- died of both	1	
- died of other cause		1
	41	34

Patients classified as intolerant of FRACON included those who were too ill to co-operate, and so 41 control patients and 34 in the FRACON group were studied. Looking crudely at the final outcome for the patients in both groups, remission rates are essentially the same but there were no deaths from infection in those FRACON patients who were responding haematologically.

Generally speaking FRACON reduces the number of episodes of infection
and the difference in the incidence of septicaemia between treated
and control groups is significant. Also striking is the absence of
perianal infections in the FRACON group. These are particularly
troublesome and often severe in patients with AML and so we find
the absence of this type of infection particularly encouraging.

EPISODES OF INFECTION

	CONTROL	FRACON
SEPTICAEMIA	13	4
PNEUMONIA	5	2
PERIANAL ABSCESS/FISTULA	4	0
OROPHARYNGEAL INFECTION	3	4
SKIN CELLULITIS	8	7
URINARY TRACT INFECTION	33	12
	66	29

If one considers the septicaemia rate in relation to the neutrophil
count for both groups it can be seen that no septicaemias occurred
in the FRACON group at a neutrophil count over 100 per µl., and
at levels below 100, the FRACON group suffered only about half
as many septicaemias as the control group.

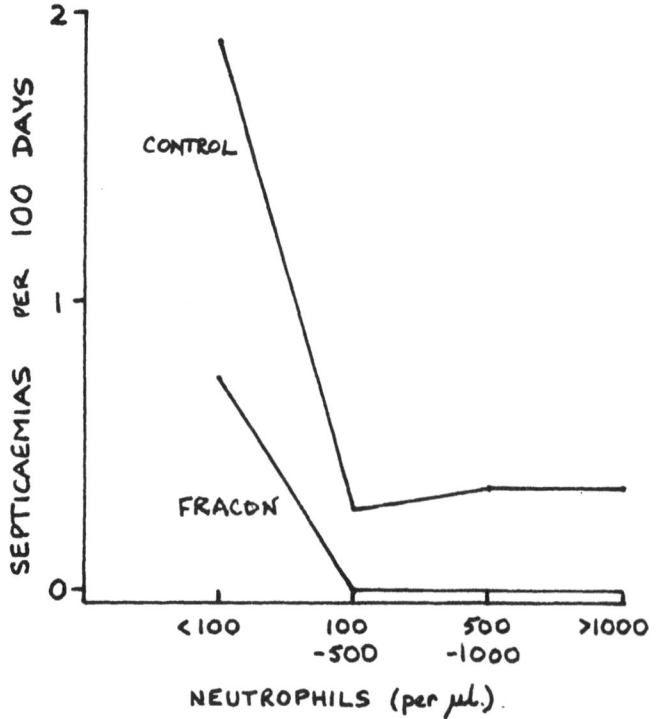

Fig. 1

PYREXIA AND ANTIBIOTICS

	CONTROL	FRACON
Days studied	1467	1272
Pyrexial Episodes $\geqslant$ 38°C	87	55
Pyrexial days $\geqslant$ 38°C	386 (26%)	249 (19%)
Days on antibiotics	906 (62%)	568 (45%)

Because the numbers with infection in both groups are relatively
small it is useful to consider the effect of FRACON on the occurrence
of pyrexial episodes and on systemic antibiotic usage. It is clear
that the FRACON group had fewer pyrexial episodes, fewer pyrexial
days and less antibiotic treatment. Thus hospitalisation was less
unpleasant for the FRACON patients and the cost of their prophylactic regimen was more than offset by the reduced usage of systemic
antibiotics.

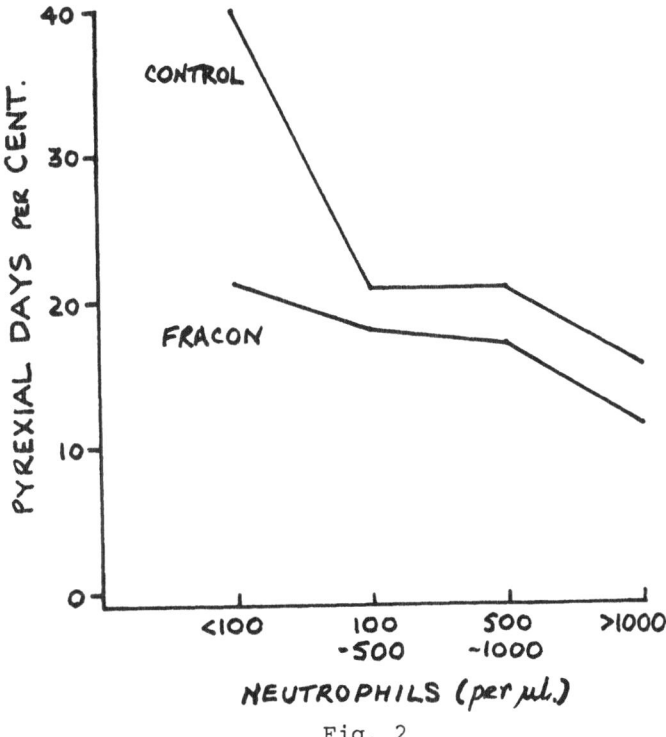

Fig. 2

When the numbers of pyrexial days spent by each patient are considered in relation to neutrophil count it is clear that as the
count falls below 100 per µl., the difference between the two
groups becomes highly significant statistically.

SUMMARY AND CONCLUSIONS

We feel our results with oral non-absorbed prophylactic antibiotics for gut decontamination are encouraging so far. The regimen is well tolerated. There are fewer deaths from infection in the FRACON group, there are fewer infections, especially septicaemia, and there are fewer pyrexial episodes in these patients than in the control group. Furthermore, there has been less usage of expensive systemic antibiotics in FRACON patients at a time when the efficacy of these agents is decreasing and new resistant strains of bacteria are emerging. Therefore gut and orificial decontamination is proving to be an important measure for the prevention of infection in patients with AML, not only allowing anti-leukaemic therapy to proceed in patients who would otherwise die of infection, but also improving the quality of life for those whose days are already numbered.

REFERENCES

1. Hersh, E.M., Bodey, G.P., Nies, B.A., Freireich, E.J., (1965). J. Amer, Med. Assoc., 193, 105
2. Levine, A.S., Graw, R.G., Young, R.C. (1972). Sem.in Haematol., 9, 141.
3. Schimpff, S.C., Young, V.M., Greene, W.H., Vermeulen, G.D., Moody, M.R., Wiernick, P.H. (1972). Ann.Int.Med., 77,707
4. Keating, M.J., Penington, D.G., (1973). Med. J. Aust., 2, 213
5. Bodey, G.P., Buckley, M., Sathe, Y.S., Freireich, E.J. (1966). Ann.Int.Med., 64, 328.
6. Jameson, B., Gamble, D.R., Lynch, J., Kay, H.E.M. (1971). Lancet, i,1034
7. Levine, A.S., et al. (1973). N.Eng.J.Med., 288, 477
8. Yates, J.W., Holland, J.F., (1973). Cancer, 32, 1490
9. Schimpff, S.C., Greene, W.H., Young, V.M., Fortner, C.L., Jepsen, L., Cusack, N., Block, J.B., Wiernick, P.H., (1975). Ann.Int.Med., 82, 351
10. Schimpff, S.C., Moody, M., Young, V.M. (1970). Antimicrob. Agents Chemother., 10, 240
11. Levine, A.S., Schimpff, S.C., Graw, R.G., et al. (1974) Sem.in Haematol., 2, 141.
12. Klastersky, J., et al. (1974). Path. Biol. (Paris), 22, 5.
13. Greene, W.H., Moody, M., Schimpff, S.C., et al. (1973). Ann.Int.Med., 79, 684

TREATMENT OF NEUTROPENIA WITH GRANULOCYTE TRANSFUSIONS

Donald J. Higby, M.D.

Roswell Park Memorial Institute

666 Elm Street, Buffalo, New York   14263

The treatment of the acute leukemias and other hematologic malignancies with currently available chemotherapeutic regimens frequently results in granulocytopenia. Infection accounts for 80% of deaths occurring in such patients (1). There is a quantitative relationship between the level of circulating granulocytes and the frequency of infection (2), and the duration of granulocytopenia is also implicated in the rate of acquisition of infection (3). Infections occurring in granulocytopenic patients are more difficult to treat than those occurring in patients with normal marrow reserves. It is likely that some potent antibiotics are less effective without the synergistic action of granulocytes (2).

Granulocyte replacement has become a useful therapeutic tool in the management of severe infections in neutropenic patients. Animal experiments had demonstrated the feasibility of this approach (4), but problems in acquisition of adequate quantities of human granulocytes delayed the exploration of this mode of therapy until the early 60's when buffy coats obtained from patients with chronic myelocytic leukemia were used to treat neutropenic patients (5). Such donors not being readily available, other sources of sufficient quantities of granulocytes for transfusion had to be developed.

METHODS OF GRANULOCYTE PROCUREMENT

Freireich and Judson designed the NCI-IBM Blood Cell Separator (6), a contemporary version of which is commercially available. Blood is pumped continuously from one arm of the donor into a spinning centrifuge bowl where it is separated into red cell, white cell and plasma layers. Separate pumps draw off the three layers. The red cell and plasma layers are recombined and re-infused into the patient and the white cell layer is collected in a storage bag. Thus, a large amount of blood can be processed continuously without volume depletion in the donor. Yields of granulocytes obtainable with this device are proportional to the skill of the operator, the amount of blood processed and the granulocyte counts of the donor. Median yields for a typical three hour run vary between 0.5 and 1.3 x 10^{10} granulocytes. The buffy coat fraction is variably contaminated by lymphocytes (7). If hydroxyethyl starch, dextran or other sedimenting agents are added to the blood to be separated, higher yields can be obtained (8). Premedication with steroids followed with glucocorticoids (8,9) or etiocholanalone (10) can also augment the yield by increasing the percentage of granulocytes available to the separation process. Benbunan, utilizing multiple small doses of hydrocortisone given during the procedure together with fluid gelatin as a sedimenting agent, has obtained median granulocyte yields of 5 x 10^{10} (11). Several improvements on the continuous flow centrifugal separator system are being explored. Automatic adjustment of bowl and pump speed and variations in the shape of the centrifuge bowl may greatly improve the efficiency of the system (12,13,14).

Filtration leukapheresis permits the collection of large numbers of granulocytes relatively uncontaminated by other cell types. Many variations of Djerassi's original system (15) are in use. In all systems, heparinized blood from the donor is passed through nylon wool and returned to the donor. Granulocytes reversibly adhere to the nylon wool fibers. At the end of a procedure, the nylon wool-containing "filters" can be eluted with solutions containing agents capable of chelating calcium.

Table 1 compares yields of granulocytes available from normal donors using currently available techniques.

TABLE 1

Comparison of Yields Reported
For Different Leukapheresis Methods

Method	Granulocyte Yield Per Hour of Time
Single unit 'pheresis	0.01 x 10^{10}
Continuous-flow centrifugation (CFC)	0.2 x 10^{10}
CFC with augmentation (max.)	2.0 x 10^{10}
Reversible leukoadhesion	2.5 x 10^{10}

EFFICACY OF GRANULOCYTES

Granulocytes obtained by plasmapheresis or continuous-flow centrifugation techniques are in all particulars comparable to granulocytes obtained directly from peripheral blood. The use of steroids to augment yields has been shown to reduce the bactericidal capacity of the granulocytes (16). Hydroxyethyl starch and probably other sedimenting agents have no irreversible effect on the cells obtained (17).

Factors effecting the functional integrity of granulocytes obtained by filtration leukapheresis, on the other hand, are not yet fully understood. These granulocytes undergo a possibly irreversible metabolic change in the process of leukoadhesion. Release of lysosyme into the supernatant of eluted granulocytes has been demonstrated (18). Morphology of granulocytes obtained by filtration leukapheresis suggests that many of the cells are injured by the process, as is evidenced by vacuolization, extrusion of nuclear material, and clumping of granules (19). Measurement of various functions of such granulocytes, however, has shown that bactericidal capacity is normal or only slightly decreased (19,20, 21,22) and that chemotactic activity may, in fact, be slightly increased (21). Table 2 shows the results of studies comparing filtration-procured cells with normal controls. Structural and functional integrity of granulocytes obtained by filtration leukapheresis is dependent upon factors such as the presence or absence of plasma in the eluting fluid (20), the length of time in which the granulocytes remained attached to the nylon fibers (23) and perhaps the method of propulsion of the blood through the system (21). What relationship in vitro measurements have to the clinical usefulness of such cells is still uncertain.

TABLE II

In Vitro Studies on Filtration-Procured (FL) Granulocytes

	Control	FL	Difference
Glucose oxidation with phagocytosis (21)	173.6 nM	188.8 nM	+8.7%
Protein iodination with phagocytosis (21)	2.8 nMI	2.6 nMI	−7%
Chemotaxis (21)	18.2 %	26.1 %	+43.6%
Radiolabeled phagocytosis (22)	21,502 cpm	19,560 cpm	−9%
Bactericidal capacity (22)	91.8 %	81.1 %	−11.7%

Brecher showed that granulocytes transfused into aplastic dogs migrated into areas of infection (4). Sophisticated studies by Epstein and his co-workers have demonstrated efficacy against infections in neutropenic dogs for both centrifugation-procured

and filtration-procured granulocytes, and that a single granulocyte transfusion can only produce transient clearing of septicemia,
implicating the reticuloendothelial system as a sanctuary for multiplying organisms (24,25). Experimental Pseudomonas pneumonia
induced in dogs made neutropenic by radiation has also been used
as a test system for granulocyte transfusions, with good results
(26).

The usefulness of granulocyte transfusions in infected, neutropenic patients is difficult to ascertain due to variation in
types of infections, the reluctance of investigators to withhold
granulocytes from such patients, the potential of bone marrow recovery during the neutropenic period, and the concomitant use of
all indicated anti-infective measures. Therefore, most investigators have sought to infer clinical response to granulocyte transfusions from post-transfusion increments, granulocyte survival in
the circulation of the recipient, changes in temperature, and improvement in clinical condition. A drop in temperature and improvement in clinical condition in association with granulocyte
transfusions from patients with chronic myeloid leukemia was demonstrated by Morse. Fifty-four percent of febrile patients had a
return to normal of temperature within 36 hours following transfusion. Resolution of other signs of infection were also noted in
several of these patients (5). Vallejos has recently reported a
large series of neutropenic patients receiving leukocyte transfusions from CML patients, of 179 infectious episodes 49% showed
clinical response. Episodes of cellulitis responded in 76% of
cases, while only 41% of patients with septicemia responded (28).
Graw's study, using chiefly granulocytes obtained by centrifugation,
showed resolution of septicemia in 12 patients receiving four or
more transfusions, whereas in 19 similar neutropenic, septicemic
patients who lived long enough to have received four or more transfusions, only five survived (29). Most recently, Lowenthal demonstrated a correlation between clinical response and total cell
dose given (30). It has been demonstrated that granulocytes obtained from donors having chronic myelocytic leukemia, when transfused into leukopenic patients without leukocyte antibodies, exhibit intravascular survival, extravascular migration, and phagocytic capacity similar to what has been observed in normal individuals. In patients with leukoagglutinins, poor post-transfusion
increments and severe transfusion reactions were noted (31).

Repeated leukapheresis in normal donors can be performed
safely. Donors complain most frequently of the discomfort of
having to lie in one place for a three-hour period of time (7).
Occasionally, fainting is observed but this is highly variable and
seems to depend on psychological factors as well as actual blood
volume changes. On rare occasions, rigors are noted during the
procedure. Some of these are undoubtedly due to the lowering of
body heat by exposure of blood to air conditioned rooms. Post

leukapheresis granulocyte counts are usually unchanged or only slightly decreased. The change in platelet count is from 0 to a drop of 50,000. Changes in hemoglobin are usually less than one gram percent (7). Repeat leukapheresis can result in gradual decreases of hemoglobin. Theoretical dangers of repeated continuous flow centrifugation include selected depletion of stem cells (32), and lymphocytes, and effects of long term administration of hydroxyethyl starch or other sedimenting agents.

Recipients of granulocytes obtained by continuous flow centrifugation have minimal complications if leukocyte antibodies and other transfusion incompatibility factors are not present (33). Marrow engraftment has been reported with granulocytes obtained from CML patients (28) and graft versus host reaction has been a rare complication of such transfusions (34).

Problems associated with continuous flow centrifugation include the high cost of the equipment, the relatively low efficiency in obtaining granulocytes both in terms of time expended and amount of blood processed, and the need for skilled operators.

Detailed studies on the usefulness of filtration procured cells in humans are limited. Schiffer noted definite clinical improvement in three recipients, stabilization of infection in nine and progression of infection in eight patients given cells obtained by reversible leukoadhesion. In addition, migration of granulocytes to skin windows was noted in four of six attempts (35). We have randomly assigned neutropenic infected patients to receive conventional therapy alone or conventional therapy together with a daily granulocyte transfusion for four days. These transfusions were obtained by filtration leukapheresis. In this study only five of 19 patients in the control group survived to 20 days, whereas 15 of 17 patients receiving filtration-procured cells and conventional therapy survived to 20 days (Table 3). At the time of analysis, some differences existed between the two groups, but were not of sufficient magnitude singly or in aggregate to account for the difference in survival (36). Post-transfusion increments with filtration-procured cells are about one-fourth that of centrifuge-obtained cells (22,37).

Donors undergoing filtration leukapheresis are subject to the same complications as those undergoing continuous flow centrifugation leukapheresis. Immediately after blood has passed through the filters and back to the donor's circulation, a brief but prolonged leukopenia followed by a gradual granulocytosis occurs. This reaction, similar to that noted in hemodialized patients, is thought to be due to effects of disrupted granulocyte contents (37). Buchholz has observed an elevation in SGOT following a multiply leukapheresed donor (7). Ruder described microscopic hematuria in 24% of her filtration leukapheresis donors and has noted slight

increases in bilirubin after the procedure (38). Our own studies
in which detailed analysis of pre- and post-procedure serum hemoglobin, serum haptoglobin, bilirubin and microscopic urinalysis
were performed indicating no suggestion of hemolysis or hematuria.
However, a slight decrease in fibrinogen in the post-filtered
blood prior to its return to the recipient is seen in some patients
towards the end of the procedure. This has not resulted in clinical
sequelae. In our own experience of over 600 filtration leukapheresis donations, there has not been even moderately serious
morbidity. The most commonly encountered problem is persistence
of bleeding from the intravenous puncture site after the procedure
is terminated and this is readily controlled by prolonged application of pressure.

In recipients, Schiffer (35) has described serious reactions
complicating 27% of leukoadhesion-procured granulocyte transfusions.
Our own experience has been more favorable, although we have seen
moderate fevers and rigors accompanying granulocyte transfusions
about 60% of the time. Since adopting a very slow rate of transfusion, our patients have never had life threatening complications
attributable to the procedure. The explanation for the wide variation in results both clinically and in vitro may have to do with
factors associated with leukocyte procurement and transfusion.
We have noted fewer obviously injured cells in the eluant when the
length of time the cells adhere to the fibers is minimized. The
composition of the eluting solution and the handling of the cells
following elution is also important in maximizing the functional
integrity of these cells (20). Finally, Djerassi has long advocated very slow infusions of granulocytes into recipients (39),
and we have observed patients who developed a febrile reaction
during the infusion but were able to receive the remaining cells
without further reaction if the rate of infusion was slowed following a brief rest period.

TABLE III

Results of a Prospective Randomized Study of The
Effectiveness of Filtration-Procured Granulocyte Transfusions

	Experimental	Control
Males/total	12/17	16/19
Days of fever, pre-entry	4.2 (2-10)	3.7 (0-8)
Granulocyte ct.: Day 1	30 (0-200)	36 (0-185)
Type of infection:		
Pneumonia	3	4
Septicemia	5	6
Abscess	8	4
Other	1	5
Alive, Day 20	15	5

FACTORS INFLUENCING THE RESPONSE TO GRANULOCYTE TRANSFUSIONS

That leukocyte antibodies impair post-transfused increments has already been mentioned (22). Graw has shown that the percent granulocyte recovery is related to the HL-A antigen match between donor and recipient and is impaired when there is an ABO mismatch (27). We have been unable to show a relationship between leuko-adhesion-procured cell increments and HL-A matching. However, this may be due to the wide variation in the severity and types of infection in the recipient population. It does appear both from our own data and from that of Hester (40), that granulocyte transfusions can be given when HL-A incompatibility is present with good clinical results over a short term. We have seen patients with markedly positive titers of leukocyte antibodies become clinically free of infection with an intensive course of randomly obtained granulocyte transfusions without serious side effects other than fever and chills.

CONCLUSIONS

Granulocyte transfusions are a welcome addition to the thera-peutic armamentarium. In recent years, the great strides made in the treatment of acute myelocytic leukemia can be partially attributed to the widespread adoption of granulocyte transfusion support by centers treating such patients. Granulocyte transfusion therapy also holds promise for dealing with aplastic crisis and bone marrow transplantation. As cancer chemotherapy becomes more vigorous, such ancillary therapy will undoubtedly play a role in the management of patients receiving treatment for other malignancies.

Prophylactic granulocyte transfusion therapy is just beginning to be explored (41). The possibility of using granulocyte transfusions to maintain a patient with neutropenia in an infection-free state is very attractive and obviously has relevance in the management of remission induction of acute leukemia.

Filtration leukapheresis is inexpensive, requires little technician training and little donor time. Large numbers of cells are obtainable. Complications to the recipient are manageable and clinical efficacy has been shown. Centrifugation leukapheresis while expensive and requiring trained operators, does produce un-impaired granulocytes. Advances in the technique and reduction in the cost of the equipment will further improve its usefulness. In addition, the apparatus, unlike leukoadhesion techniques, can be used for other inline continuous flow separation procedures. Most likely, both techniques will continue to be used for support of leukopenic patients in the future. We feel that for short term support, filtration leukapheresis is advantageous and can be

used almost anywhere. For those patients requiring support for
long periods of time, centrifugation leukapheresis probably is
advantageous in that transfusion increments are higher, transfused granulocytes remain in the circulation longer, and the
frequency of unavoidable, uncomfortable reactions is lower. These
issues, of course, need to be studied further.

     We have not yet seen a patient in whom there was a contra-
indication to granulocyte transfusion. Immunological, circulatory
and renal dysfunction can be managed and even rare allergic phenomena can be controlled. The long term results of granulocyte
transfusions are not yet fully understood. Whether or not patients
receiving such transfusions will develop immunologic disease at a
later time, or whether there is an effect of the transfusions on
remission duration is not known. The benefit of granulocyte transfusion, however, is so great that they should be made available
to all patients who are neutropenic and infected.

REFERENCES

1. Levine, A., Schimpff, S., et.al., Sem. Hemat. 1974, 11, 141.
2. Bodey, G., Buckley, M., et.al., Ann. Int. Med. 1966, 64, 328.
3. Yates, J., and Holland, J., Cancer 1973, 32, 1490.
4. Brecher, G., Wilbur, K., and Cronkite, E., Proc. Soc. Exp. Biol. Med. 1953, 84, 54.
5. Morse, E., Bronson, W., et. al., Clin. Res. 1961, 9, 332.
6. Freireich, E., Judson, G., and Levin, R., 1965, 25, 1516.
7. Buchholz, D., Schiffer, C., et.al., Transfusion, 1973, 2, 96.
8. Mishler, J., Higby, D.J., et.al., Transfusion, 1974, 14, 352.
9. Pfister, H., and Ruppert, W., Am. Assoc. Banks Annual Meeting, Washington, 1972.
10. McCredie, K., and Freireich, E., Proc. Amer. Assoc. Cancer Res., 1971, 58.
11. Benbunan, M., Bussel, A., et.al., Int. Symp. on Leukocyte Separation and Trans., 1974.
12. West, C., and Willis, D., Int. Symp. on Leukocyte Separation and Trans., 1974.
13. Krager, V., McCredie, K., and Freireich, E., Symp. on Leukocyte Separation and Trans., 1974.
14. Latham, A., and Kingsley, G., Int. Symp. on Leukocyte Separation and Trans., 1974.
15. Djerassi, I., Kim, J., Mitrakul, C., et.al., J. Med. (Basel), 1970, 1, 358.
16. Rubins, J., MacPherson, J., et.al., (Submitted for publication, May 1975).
17. Mishler, J., Higby, D.J., et.al., Int. Symp. on Leukocyte Separation and Trans., 1974.
18. Higby, D.J., Burnett, D., et.al., Int. Symp. on Leukocyte Separation and Trans., 1974.
19. Higby, D.J., Mazzone, T., et.al., Int. Symp. on Leukocyte Separation and Trans., 1974.
20. Sanel, F., Aisner, M., et.al., Int. Symp. on Leukocyte Separation and Trans., 1974.
21. Harris, M., Djerassi, I., et.al., Blood, 1974, 5, 707.
22. Herzig, G., Root, R., and Graw, R., Blood 1972, 39, 554.
23. Higby, D.J., Unpublished observations.
24. Epstein, R., Clift, R., Thomas, E., Blood, 1969, 34, 780.
25. Debelak, K., Epstein, R., Anderson, B., Blood, 1974, 43, 757.
26. Dale, D., et.al., J. Clin. Invest., 1974, 54, 664.
27. Cartwright, G., Athens, J., Wintrobe, M., Blood, 1964, 24, 780.
28. Vallejos, C., McCredie, K., et.al., Transfusion, 1975, 15, 28.
29. Graw, R., et.al., N.E.J.M., 1972, 287, 367.
30. Lowenthal, R., et.al., Lancet, 1975, 353.
31. Eyre, H., Goldstein, I., et.al., Blood, 1970, 36, 432.
32. Hill, N., Kahn, A., and Hill, J., et.al., Int. Symp. on Leukocyte Separation and Trans., 1974.
33. Ward, H., Ann. Int. Med., 1970, 73, 689.
34. Schwartzenberg, G., Mathe, J., et.al., Amer. J. Med. 1967, 43, 206.

35. Schiffer, C., Buchholz, D., et.al., Amer. J. Med., 1975, 58, 373.
36. Higby, D.J., Yates, J.W., et.al., N.E.J.M., 1975, 292, 761.
37. Schiffer, C., Aisner, J., and Wiernik, P., Int. Symp. on Leuko-
        cyte Separation and Trans., 1974.
38. Ruder, E., Hartz, W., Int. Symp. on Leukocyte Separation and
        Trans., 1974.
39. Djerassi, I., Kim, H., Suvansri, U., et.al., Int. Symp. on
        Leukocyte and Trans., 1974.
40. Hester, J., McCredie, K., Freireich, E., et.al., Int. Symp. on
        Leukocyte Separation and Trans., 1974.
41. Cooper, M., Pahak, T., Richards, F., et.al., Int. Symp. on
        Leukocyte Separation and Trans., 1974.

BACTERIAL FLORA ISOLATED DURING INFECTIOUS COMPLICATIONS IN PATIENTS WITH NEOPLASIA

G. Pacilio, D. Caruso, R. De Domenico, L. Campanella

Autonomous Department of General Antineoplastic
Chemotherapy, Cardarelli Hospital
Naples, Italy

Our study was carried out on 41 patients, 27 males and 14 females, the age ranging from 26 to 78. In 37 cases the patients had solid neoplasia (pulmonary neoplasia mainly) and lymphoma in 4 cases. All patients were hyperpyretic. The treatment was performed according to different schemes of antiblastic polychemotherapy.

At the beginning and at the end of treatments we made bacteriological examinations of bronchial secretions, expectorate, blood, pleural fluid and urines. In vitro sensitivity to various chemoantibiotic agents was studied on the isolated micro-organisms. The sensitivity was evaluated with the agar disc-plate method.

RESULTS

Table 1 shows number, quality and origin of the micro-organisms isolated from the patients examined. The bacterial flora is mainly formed by Gram-positive bacteria. Streptococci show the highest percentage (24%) followed by Staphylococcus aureus (17%). In two patients Diplococcus pneumoniae (5%) was isolated.

As reported in Table 2, testing in vitro sensitivity to various chemo-antibiotic agents the most effective drugs were found to be rifampicin, chloramphenicol, novobiocin, neomycin, bacitracin and erythromicin.

It is indeed necessary to underline the differences between the results obtained in our center as well as in other Italian hospitals and the results reported in other European countries.

In fact, as Anglo-Saxon and North-European countries denounce the net predominance of a Gram-negative bacterial flora, our results indicate an almost entirely Gram-positive flora. It is therefore of the utmost importance for the choice of the specific antibiotic therapy to consider the upstated geographical distribution of the bacterial flora responsible for infectious complications occurring to patients with neoplasia.

TABLE 1.   Sensitivity to various antimicrobial agents of microorganisms isolated from 41 patients with neoplasia.
VS = very sensitive; LS = lightly sensitive; R = resistant.

D R U G	S E N S I T I V I T Y %		
	VS	LS	R
Tetracycline	52.05	33.36	14.59
Gentamicin	33.35	16.64	50.01
Rifampicin	81.25	6.25	12.50
Chloramphenicol	77.09	8.32	14.59
Penicillin	37.50	12.50	50.00
Erythromycin	62.50	12.50	25.00
Novobiocin	83.36	8.32	8.32
Streptomycin	41.68	14.57	43.75
Neomycin	83.36	14.59	2.05
Colimycin	25.00	31.25	43.75
Bacitracin	70.83	10.42	18.75
Sulfamethoxy-pyridazine	39.58	16.66	43.76

TABLE 2.   Distribution of bacterial strains isolated from different organic fluids.

Micro-organisms	Nr. of positive strains	Blood	Bronchial secretion	Pleural fluid	Urines
Staphylococcus	7 (17%)	1 (14%)	4 (57%)	2 (29%)	- -
Streptococcus	10 (24%)	1 (10%)	7 (70%)	1 (10%)	1 (10%)
Pneumococcus	2 (5%)	--	2 (100%)	--	--
Non identified Gram-positive mixed flora	14 (34%)	--	11 (78%)	1 (7%)	2 (15%)
Gram-positive and Gram-negative mixed flora	8 (20%)	--	5 (62%)	1 (13%)	2 (25%)

ANTIBIOTIC MANAGEMENT OF SEPTIC COMPLICATIONS IN PATIENTS WITH MYELOID INSUFFICIENCY

E.LANG,* N. HONETZ, K. MITTERMAYER

I. MEDICAL UNIVERSITY CLINIC, VIENNA

A-1090 WIEN, LAZARETTGASSE 14

In a previous study we were able to demonstrate that the chance of survival for patients with myeloid insufficiency clearly improved on applying an intensive empirical antibiotic therapy, immediately after the first signs of infection, without waiting for the bacteriological findings.

Thus it was to a certain extent possible to avoid a foudroyant development of the infection with a mostly lethal end on the one hand and to constitute a basis for a cytostatic therapy on the other.

In the course of a prospective study of patients with myeloid insufficiency - the numbers of granulocytes were all under 1500/ μl - we have tried to ascertain the effectiveness of some antibiotic combinations and to improve the possibility of an appropriate antibacterial treatment, by means of regular bacteriological examinations. We did not administer systemic antibiotics prophylactically, due to the fact, that this usually leads to superinfections with highly resistant bacteria and fungi.

Over 90 % of the patients treated had acute leukaemia, the rest panmyelopathy and malignant growths.

The patients with granulocytopenia were carefully checked. Blood cultures, specimens of urine and stool, as well as throat swabs and vaginal smears were regulary taken.

These bacteriological checks were also carried out during the whole antibiotic therapy in order to recognize a change of infection in time.

Special attention was paid to oral hygiene. The interdental spaces were cleaned with a disinfecting spray to reduce unpleasant anaerobic infections onginating in the cavity of the mouth.

When there is reason to presume a septic complication, we start an empirical antibiotic combination therapy immediately after taking specimens for bacteriological examination. As a criteria of an infection we consider: temperature over 38° C, bacteraemia and other clinical signs.

The antibiotic combinations administered are shown in Table No. 1. The combination carbenicillin + gentamicin was used in our last study and will only be quoted here for reasons of comparison.

The antibiotic combination administered in the first approach, was cephalothin and gentamicin, lately also Cefazolin and Tobramycin. We expect the latter combination to increase the success rate considerably.
If there was no response to this therapy and the clinical symptoms deteriorated, or the causative agent has been isolated, we administered the combination No. 2 with carbenicillin + gentamicin (resp. Tobramycin) + Flucloxacillin.

Table No. 2 shows the isolated pathogens as well as the positive blood cultures. Enterobacteria dominate with nearly 80 %.

In 33,3 % of clinically manifest infections no pathogens could be isolated.

There were remarkably few side-effects. Apart from the well-known and frequent hypokalemias we had only two cases with impaired renal function. These were most likely due to hemorrhages which finally lead to the death of the patients.

We could not find the nephropathies in our patients, which were observed by other authors and which were attributed to administering a combination of gentamicin and cephalosporin. This is probably due to the

TABLE 1

ANTIBIOTICS	DOSAGE
CEPHALOTHIN + GENTAMICIN	2 (-3) x 4 g + 2 x 40 (-80) mg
CARBENICILLIN + GENTAMICIN	3 x 10 g + 2 x 40 (-80) mg
CARBENICILLIN + GENTAMICIN + FLUCLOXACILLIN	3 x 10 g + 2 x 40 (-80) mg + 2 (-3) x 1 g
CEFAZOLIN + TOBRAMYCIN	2 (-3) x 2 g + 2 x 80 mg

TABLE 2

ISOLATED PATHOGENS				
	TOTAL	%	FROM BLOOD	%
F. COLI	10	20,8	3	6,2
KLEBSIELLA	10	20,8	2	4,2
PSEUDOMONAS	7	14,6	5	10,4
PROTEUS	6	12,5	1	2,0
STAPH. AUREUS	4	8,3	1	2,0
STREPTOCOCCI (HAEMOLYTIC)	3	6,2	1	2,0
STREPTOCOCCI (VIRID.)	2	4,2	-	
ENTEROCOCCI	2	4,2	-	
CITROBACTER	2	4,2	-	
SALMONELLA TYPHI MUR.	1	2,0	1	2,0
PASTEURELLA MULTOCIDA	1	2,0	1	2,0
TOTAL	48		15	31
NO PATHOGENS ISOLATED	16	33,3	33	69

TABLE 3

ANTIBIOTICS	No OF TREATMENTS	SUCCESS RATE
CEPHALOTIN + GENTAMICIN	49	60 %
CARBENICILLIN + GENTAMICIN	57	59 %
CARBENICILLIN + GENTAMICIN + FLUCLOXACILLIN	17	82 %

fact that we administer gentamicin in far smaller
doses than is usual.

Additionally, we never give gentamicin as monotherapy,
because of the development of resistance, but always
in combination with β - lactam- antibiotics. Thus we
were able to delay an increase of resistance and also
a diminution of the efficacy of gentamicin such as has
been observed in Germany.

Table No. 3 again shows the combination of antibiotics
administered, also the number of cases and the success
rate of treatment.

The success of the treatment was judged by the following criteria: normal temperature over a ten day
period, improvement of the clinical picture and repeated negative bacteriological results.

We find that the reason for the surprising increase of
success when administering carbenicillin, gentamicin
and flucloxacillin - i.e. by merely adding flucloxacillin - is the fact that flucloxacillin protects the
non penicillinase-stable carbenicillin against being
neutralised by penicillinase. Thus its antibacterial
activity is maintained.

And now a few words regarding infections with fungi.
Two patients had a sepsis caused by fungi with coloni-
sations in the brain, liver, kidneys and lungs. This
diagnosis was made at the autopsy. All fungi cultures
intra vitam were sterile. Both patients had undergone
long periods of treatment with antibiotics, cytostatic
drugs and cortisone and had granulocytopenia for 12/
16 weeks respectively.

Systemic antimycotics, amphotericin B and 5-fluorocy-
tosin, were administered to one patient and achieved
a temporary success. At the autopsy scars of healed
hepatic abscesses were found. In the other case there
was a foudroyant sepsis caused by Aspergillus.

In summing up, we would like to draw a few conclusions, on the basis of the experience gained by this
study, for our future planning of treatment and which
could achieve more success without subjecting additional stress on the patient:

1. No prophylactic systemic therapy, but careful clinical and bacteriological control of the patients with granulocytopenia.

2. At the first signs of infection, immediate administration of an empirical antibiotic combination-therapy without waiting for bacteriological findings.

3. The combinations cephalothin + gentamicin and carbenicillin + gentamicin proved to be more or less equivalent, with a success rate of about 60 %.

4. According to our hitherto existing results the success rate could be increased to 82 % by adding flucloxacillin to carbenicillin and gentamicin.

Literature

1. G.P. Bodey, c.s. Infections in cancer patients. Results with gentamicin sulfate therapy. CANCER 29, 1967 (1972).

2. H. Gaya, The treatment of Infection in acute Leukaemia, British J. of Hospital Medicine, February 1975, 124.

3. E. Lang, Antibiotika-Therapie, Banaschewski-Verlag München, 1975

4. K. Metzger, Synergistische Wirkung der Kombination Ampicillin mit Isoxazolylpenicillin. ARZNEIM.-FORSCH! (Drug Res.) 24, 471 (1974)

5. S. Schimpff, W. Satterlee, V.M.Young and A.Serpick, Empiric therapy with carbenicillin and gentamicin for febrile patients with cancer and granulocytopenia. NEW ENGLAND J.MED. 248, 1064 (1971)

PARENTERAL TOBRAMYCIN AND CEPHALOTHIN IN THE TREATMENT OF

SUSPECTED SEPSIS IN NEUTROPENIC CHILDREN

Jesse D. Cohen, M.D. and Thomas D. Miale, M.D.

Dept. of Pediatrics, University of Florida College of

Medicine, Gainesville, Florida, U.S.A.

SUMMARY

A study of the safety and efficacy of parenteral tobramycin and cephalothin in the treatment of suspected sepsis in neutropenic children ($<$ 1000 polymorphonuclear leukocytes/mm^3 of blood) with various underlying malignancies was undertaken. Twenty episodes of suspected sepsis in 19 febrile children with cancer were treated with parenteral tobramycin and cephalothin for a total of one to 80 days. Each was followed closely for renal, hepatic, bone marrow, and auditory toxicity. In 14 of the 20 episodes of suspected sepsis, a favourable clinical response was achieved within five days of initiation of antibiotics. These included a Proteus mirabilis urinary tract infection and E.coli sepsis. No clinical improvement was noted in the remaining six episodes. In four of the six episodes, clinical deterioration was felt to be secondary to the underlying malignancies. The remaining two episodes included one with E.coli sepsis which ended fatally within six hours of admission, while the other included a nosocomial infection with Eikenella corrodens. No evidence of renal, auditory, hepatic, bone ma-row, or vestibular toxicity was noted either during or following antibiotic therapy. Results of this study suggest the safety and efficacy of combination tobramycin and cephalothin in the treatment of suspected sepsis in neutropenic febrile children with malignancies.

With the recent advances in the treatment of childhood cancer, children with previously uniformly fatal neoplasms now represent potential cures. Because the aggressive antineoplastic therapy required to achieve long-term survival is often associated with immunologic suppression, these children are susceptible to

117

overwhelming infection.   Such infections are usually caused by
gram-negative bacteria such as <u>Escherichia coli</u>, <u>Klebsiella
Enterobacter</u> species, and <u>Pseudomonas aeruginosa</u> (Klastersky
et al, 1973a).   Despite continued improvements in antimicrobial
therapy, the mortality rate from infection in children with cancer
remains high.   The major predisposing factor to infection in these
children is neutropenia, defined here as < 1000 polymorphonuclear
neutrophils (PMN's) per mm^3 of blood.   Neutropenia may result from
the underlying malignancy or may be secondary to radiotherapy or
chemotherapy.   Since neutropenic children frequently do not manifest the usual inflammatory response to infection, fever is often
the only presenting sign of serious infection (Yates, 1973).
Because fever in a neutropenic cancer patient may indicate possible sepsis and herald rapid clinical deterioration and death,
many institutions treat such patients with parenteral broad-
spectrum antibiotics after appropriate culturing but prior to
identification of a pathogen.   Although various combinations of
broad-spectrum antibiotics have been used to treat possible sepsis
in neutropenic cancer patients, none has been proved to be uniformly efficacious (Klastersky et al, 1973a).

        Tobramycin, an aminoglycoside antibiotic produced by <u>Strepto-
myces tenebrarius</u>, has been shown to be effective both <u>in vitro</u>
and <u>in vivo</u> against many strains of gram-negative organisms,
including some strains of <u>Pseudomonas aeruginosa</u> resistant to
gentamycin (Klastersky et al, 1973b- Valdivieso et al, 1974;
Naber et al, 1973).   Cephalothin is effective in its antimicrobial
activity against many pathogenic gram-positive organisms resistant
to tobramycin (Herrell, 1973).   In addition, tobramycin has been
shown to act synergistically with certain cephalosporins against
selected bacterial species (Hyams et al, 1974).   For these reasons,
it was decided to evaluate the safety and efficacy of the combination of tobramycin and cephalothin in febrile neutropenic
children with cancer and suspected sepsis.

                            MATERIALS AND METHODS

        Twenty episodes of suspected sepsis in 19 children with can-
cer, admitted to the Shands Teaching Hospital at the University
of Florida during a seven month period in 1974-75 were studied.
All patients had neutropenia, temperature of 101°F or greater,
and malignancies treated with chemotherapy and/or radiotherapy
prior to or during their febrile episode.   Subjects included
13 boys and six girls who ranged in age from five months to
13 8/12 years.   Thirteen were diagnosed with acute lymphoblastic
leukemia, three with acute myeloblastic leukemia, while one each
had chronic myeloblastic leukemia in blastic transformation,
Wilms' tumor,and Ewing's sarcoma.   The degree of neutropenia
initially present in all patients is shown in Figure 1.   No

Initial Neutrophil Count	Episodes	(Percentage)
$<100/\text{mm}^3$	8	(40%)
$101-500/\text{mm}^3$	10	(50%)
$501-1000/\text{mm}^3$	2	(10%)
	20	(100%)

FIGURE 1

DEGREE OF NEUTROPENIA

A. Clinical improvement within 5 days - 14 children (70%)

    1. Proven infection - 2 (10%), E. coli and P. mirabilis

    2. No infection documented - 12 (60%)

B. No clinical improvement within 5 days - 6 children (30%)

    1. No infection documented - 4 (20%)

    2. Treatment failure - 1 (5%), E.coli

    3. Nosocomial infection - 1 (5%), Eikenella corrodens

FIGURE 2

RESULTS OF 20 EPISODES OF SUSPECTED SEPSIS

patient was admitted to the study who had known renal impairment, hearing loss, or vestibular dysfunction secondary to previous antibiotic therapy, or whose fever was related to previous blood product transfusion. Blood and urine cultures were obtained prior to institution of antibiotic therapy and were repeated during therapy for temperature elevations greater than $101^{\circ}F$ as well as post-therapy. Other appropriate cultures, as well as chest x-rays, were obtained when clinically indicated. All bacterial isolates were tested _in vitro_ for susceptibility to tobramycin and cephalothin by the Kirby-Bauer disk sensitivity method.

Antibiotic therapy consisted of a combination of parenteral tobramycin and cephalothin. Tobramycin was administered in a dose of 5 mg/kg/day intramuscularly or intravenously, for cases of severe thrombo-cytopenia, in 200 ml of 5% glucose in water over two hours every eight hours. Cephalothin was administered intravenously every six hours in a dosage of 160 mg/kg/day. Both antibiotics were continued for a minimum of five days or until the absolute number of PMN's rose to greater than 1000/mm^3.

Patients were followed closely for signs of bone marrow, renal, hepatic, and auditory toxicity. Hemograms including differential and platelet count, BUN, creatinine, and urinalysis were obtained prior to, at weekly intervals during, and upon completion of antibiotic treatment. In addition, serum bilirubin, serum transamidinases, and alkaline phosphatase were monitored before and after each course of therapy. When possible, audiograms were obtained before, during and after antibiotics to detect auditory toxicity.

RESULTS

Patients who had documented clinical improvement within five days after initiation of antibiotics or who did without clinical or laboratory signs of infection were considered to have responded favourably to therapy. As can be seen in Figure 2, a satisfactory clinical response was achieved in 14 of the 20 episodes of suspected sepsis. This group included two patients with proven infection, one with Proteus mirabilis urinary tract infection and one with E.coli sepsis. No clinical improvement was noted in the remaining six episodes. In four of these six episodes, patients remained febrile, despite negative cultures and had progressive, deteriorating clinical courses secondary to their malignancies. These four episodes were not considered treatment failures since cultures remained negative. The remaining two episodes included one treatment failure in a chold with acute lymphoblastic leukemia with E.coli sepsis who did four hours after antibiotic institution as well as a patient with initially negative cultures who developed a superinfection with Eikenella corrodens 29 days after institution of antibiotics. In the

majority of children, no organisms were isolated from extensive
pretreatment cultures. The three initial bacterial isolates were
all sensitive to both tobramycin and cephalothin. However, antibiotic sensitivities of the Eikenella corrodens isolate were
not obtained due to the fastidious nature of the organism. All
three episodes of documented initial infection occurred in children with severe neutripenia ($<$100 PMN's/mm^3). No evidence of
renal, hepatic, bone marrow, vestibular, or auditory toxicity
was found either during or following tobramycin and cephalothin
administration.

DISCUSSION

In this study, only three of 20 episodes of suspected sepsis
(15%) were documented to be secondary to bacterial infection.
This is lower than the percentages reported in many studies that
deal primarily with adult cancer patients and may relate to the
high incidence of benign febrile viral infections in children as
well as the incidence of fever from neoplasia. Of note is the
fact that all three of the initial positive cultures were in
severely neutropenic children ($<$ 100 PMN's/mm^3) and that two of
the three infections responded to the tested antibiotic combination. This finding is in contrast to the report of the limited
efficacy of tobramycin alone in severely neutropenic cancer
patients (Valdivieso et al, 1974). Although systemic fungal infections were investigated in children with persistent fevers, none
was found. Despite reports of both nephrotoxicity and ototoxicity
following the use of parenteral tobramycin, no such toxicity was
noted in the 19 children involved in this study (Valdivieso et
al, 1974; Brumfitt et al, 1972). In addition, no bone marrow,
or hepatic toxicity was found.

In summary, this study was designed to test the safety and
efficacy of the combination of parenteral tobramycin and cephalothin in febrile neutropenic children with malignancies. Of the
20 episodes of suspected sepsis studied in such children, only
three were documented to be secondary to infection. All three
infections occurred in children with severe neutropenic, and in
two of the three infections, marked clinical improvement occurred
following tobramycin and cephalothin therapy, while one patient
died within four hours after institution of antibiotics. No bone
marrow, renal, hepatic, auditory, or vestibular toxicity was noted
during or following antibiotic therapy. These date suggest the
safety and efficacy of this antibiotic combination in such compromised children. However, additional experience is needed before
definite conclusions regarding the efficacy of tobramycin and
cephalothin can be reached.

REFERENCES

Brummett, R.E., Himes, D., Saine, B. and Vernon, J. (1972),
    Archives of Otolaryngology, 96, 505.

Herrell, W.E. (1973) Clinical Medicine, 80, 12.

Hyams, P.J., Simberkoff, M.S. and Rahal, J.J. (1974) Anti-
    microbial Agents and Chemotherapy, 5, 571.

Klastersky, J., Daneau, D., Henri, A., Cippel, R. and Hensgens, C.
    (1973a), European Journal of Cancer, 9, 407.

Klastersky, J., Daneau, D. and De Maertelaer, V. (1973b),Clinical
    Pharmacology and Therapeutics, 14, 104.

Naber, K.G., Westenfelder, S.R. and Madsen, P.O. (1973) Anti-
    microbial Agents and Chemotherapy, 3, 469.

Rodriguez, V., Burgess, M. and Bodey, G.P. (1973) Cancer, 32,1007.

Valdivieso, M., Horikoshi, N., Rodriguez, V. and Bodey, G.P. (1974),
    Americal Journal of the Medical Sciences, 268, 149.

Yates, J. (1973), Seminars in Drug Treatment, 3, 27.

EXPERIENCE WITH TOBRAMYCIN AND CEPHALOTHIN SODIUM IN INFECTED

PATIENTS WITH ACUTE LEUKAEMIA (AL)

P. C. Vincent, F. Jennis, R. Hilmer and Sharne Fabre

Medical Research Department, Sydney Hospital

Sydney, N.S.W. 2000, Australia

Bacterial infection - especially with Gram-negative organisms - remains a major cause of morbidity and mortality in patients with acute leukaemia and other pancytopenic blood disorders. In these patients fever has to be assumed to be due to bacterial infection and treatment with effective antibiotics must be instituted as soon as cultures are obtained. Intravenous therapy is necessary, not only because of the potential seriousness of infection but also because of the thrombocytopenia which is almost invariably present.

The recently introduced aminoglycoside tobramycin has been shown in vitro and in experimental animals to be effective against a wide range of Gram-negative organisms, particularly Pseudomonas (Black & Griffith, 1970; Del Bene & Farrar, 1972; Shadomy & Kirchoff, 1972; Saslaw et al 1972). For this reason we have studied its safety and efficacy in a group of patients with acute leukaemia or other diseases associated with pancytopenia.

PATIENTS AND METHODS
Thirty episodes of clinically diagnosed infection occuring in 15 patients were studied. Ten patients were suffering from acute leukaemia, 2 from malignant lymphoma, one from the acute phase of chronic granulocytic leukaemia, one from aplastic anaemia, and one from acute myeloid dysplasia. One patient (with acute leukaemia) was aged 11 and the remainder were adults. One patient who had been neutropenic had a normal neutrophil count at the time of study; the remainder were neutropenic, many of them profoundly so. The median pre-infection neutrophil count for all episodes was 230 per ul.

Fever greater than $38^{\circ}C$ of longer than 6 hours duration was taken as indicative of infection, and samples of blood and urine as well as swabs from nose, throat, skin, groin and axilla were collected for aerobic and anaerobic culture. Infected sites and sputum, if present, were also cultured. Antibiotic sensitivities were determined by a disc diffusion technique (Association of Clinical Pathologists, U.K.).

The antibiotics used in conjunction with tobramycin are summarized in Table 1. Cephalothin sodium was used with tobramycin in 27 of the 30 episodes; in 17 it was continued and in 10 carbenicillin was substituted after 2 to 4 days because of apparent failure to respond. Cultures of these apparent non-responders however subsequently revealed organisms in only 3, and of these the Pseudomonas and Klebsiella proved to be resistant to carbenicillin in vitro.

Table 1
Antibiotic Combinations and Dosage

Initial Antibiotic	No. of Courses	Dose mg/Kg/day	Route	Interval
Tobramycin	30	3 - 5	IV inf.	8h
Cephalothin	27	150 - 200	IV push	2h
Carbenicillin	2	500	IV push	4h
Methicillin	1	200	IV push	4h

Renal, auditory and vestibular functions were assessed before and after treatment, and no adverse effects were detected. No patients were in renal failure; the mean serum creatinine before treatment was 0.9 ± 0.2 mg/dl (mean $\pm$ sd) (range $0.4 - 1.4$) and after treatment was 0.8 ± 0.2 mg/dl (range $0.4 - 1.4$).

RESULTS

The concentration of tobramycin in β-lactamase inactivated serum samples (Waterworth, 1973) was estimated using a solid medium disc diffusion technique, by comparison with reference standards, in 13 course of treatment. The results are shown in Figure 2; at 30 minutes the mean concentration was 3.0 µg per ml, at 1 hour 2.5 µg per ml, and at 4 hours 1.0 µg per ml.

Positive cultures were obtained in only 17 of the 30 clinically diagnosed infective episodes. The clinical diagnoses, with the number in which cultures were positive, were as follows; septicaemia 9(5); upper respiratory tract 9(6); soft tissue 7(3); lower respiratory tract 3(3); peritonitis 1(0); and pyrogenic reaction (subsequently shown to have been due to daunorubicin) 1. In 12 episodes, patients were found to be infected with 2 pathogens. The organisms isolated were as follows; Klebsiella spp

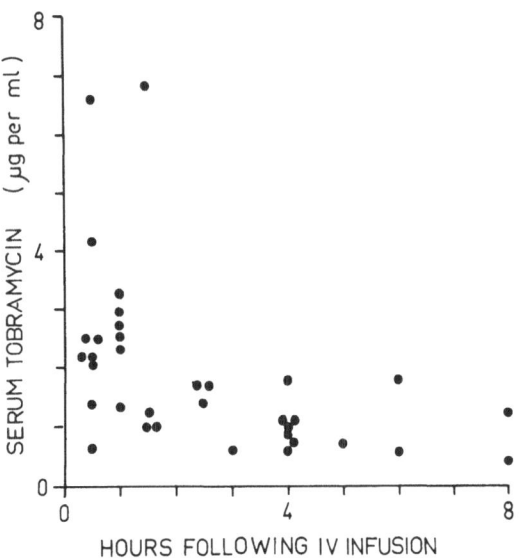

Figure 1: Serum tobramycin levels in 13 episodes of infection,
measured from the end of a 2 hour infusion of 80 mg tobramycin
intravenously.

(8 episodes); Pseudomonas aeruginosa (5); Haemophilus spp (4);
Escherichia coli (4); Staph. aureus (1); B-haemolytic Streptococcus, not group A (1). All of the pathogens except the Streptococcus were sensitive in vitro to tobramycin and gentamicin, and
all except the Pseudomonas isolates were sensitive to cephalothin.
The Klebsiella and Pseudomonas isolates, and 2 of the 4 Escherichia coli isolates, were resistant to carbenicillin and ampicillin
in vitro. Repeat cultures showed the elimination of the pathogen
in 9 episodes, while in another mixed infection Haemophilus was
eliminated but Klebsiella persisted. Organisms were shown to
persist in 4 episodes, while in 3 follow-up cultures were not
obtained.

In 21 of the 30 episodes the clinical response was satisfac-

tory, as judged by complete resolution of fever and disappearance
of signs of infection, while in 6 it was unsatisfactory and in 3
it was non-evaluable. These were 3 episodes in which, on review,
the fever could have been due to non-bacterial infection; one was
the pyrogenic reaction to daunorubicin, one was probably an
erythema multiforme and one was probably a viral infection. The
incidence of satisfactory clinical responses in patients with
positive cultures (14 out of 17) was similar to that in patients
in whom cultures were negative (7 out of 13). In patients with
positive cultures, the clinical response was satisfactory in those
in whom the organism was eliminated, and in three in whom persistence of the organism was demonstrated despite clinical improvement.
Although all patients except one were neutropenic before the onset
of fever, there was no apparent correlation between the degree of
neutropenia and the likelihood of clinical or bacteriological
response.

In this series, the toxic effects of tobramycin, usually in
combination with cepalothin, were minimal. Mild thrombophlebitis
was seen occasionally, but in no case was there any impairment of
auditory, vestibular, renal or hepatic function. Four deaths
occurred during or within 6 weeks of completing antibiotic therapy;
2 of these were due to infection, one to cerebral haemorrhage and
one to abdominal lymphoma with intestinal obstruction.

DISCUSSION

Antibiotic therapy for presumed infection in patients with
neutropenia should be effective against a wide range of Gram-
negative organisms, particularly Pseudomonas aeruginosa which is
a frequent cause of infection in this setting (Schimpff et al
1973; Tattersall et al 1973), and combinations of up to 5 antibiotics have been recommended (Tattersall et al 1973). In this
study we chose tobramycin because of its effectiveness against
Pseudomonas in combination with cephalothin, with the reservation
that carbenicillin would be substituted for cephalothin if there
was an apparent failure to respond. As it transpired Pseudomonas
aeruginosa was the pathogen in only 1 of the 10 courses in which
antibiotics were changed, and then it proved to be carbenicillin
resistant. Indeed, in this series all of the Klebsiella and all
of the Pseudomonas isolates were resistant to carbenicillin, as
were 2 of the 4 isolates of Escherichia coli. On the other hand,
all of the Gram-negative organisms were sensitive to tobramycin
and gentamicin, and all except the Pseudomonas isolates were
sensitive to cephalothin.

The problem of negative cultures in these patients has been
referred to by others (Schimpff et al 1971; 1972) In the present
series, retrospective analysis suggests that 3 of the episodes of
fever might have been non-infective; nonetheless there were still
10 episodes with clinical infection in which extensive cultures

(including anaerobic and fungal cultures) failed to define an organism.

Like all aminoglycosides, there is a risk of renal toxicity and ototoxicity with tobramycin, and care must be exercised in its use. The absence of any such toxicity in the present small series in which the drug was given intravenously justifies its further use by this route in patients, such as those with acute leukaemia or other causes of pancytopenia, in which its intramuscular use is contraindicated by thrombocytopenia. The mild thrombophlebitis which was seen occasionally was probably due to cephalothin rather than tobramycin, but because both antibiotics were used together initially in most cases this cannot be established from the present data.

SUMMARY
Intravenous tobramycin has been shown to be a safe and effective agent to use in combination antibiotic therapy in clinically infected patients with acute leukaemia or other profound pancytopenic states. In combination, usually with cephalothin, clinically satisfactory results were obtained in 21 out of 30 episodes of fever. Toxic effects were minimal and were limited to occasional mild thrombophlebitis.

ACKNOWLEDGEMENTS

This study was supported by Eli Lilly & Co., through the Medical Department of Lilly Industries Pty.Ltd. (Australia).

REFERENCES

1. Black, H. R. and Griffith, R. S. "Preliminary Studies with Nebramycin Factor 6". Antimicrobial Agents and Chemotherapy, p. 314, 1970

2. Del Bene, V. E. and Farrar, W. E. Jr. "Tobramycin: In Vitro Activity and Comparison with Kanamycin and Gentamicin". Antimicrobial Agents and Chemotherapy, 1(4):340, 1972.

3. Shadomy, S. and Kirchoff, C. "In Vitro Susceptibility Testing with Tobramycin". Antimicrobial Agents and Chemotherapy, 1(5):412, 1972.

4. Saslaw, S., Carlisle, H. N. and Moheimani, M. "Comparison of Tobramycin, Gentamicin, Colistin, and Carbenicillin in Pseudomonas Sepsis in Monkeys". Antimicrobial Agents and Chemotherapy, 2 (3):164, 1972.

5. Waterworth, P. M. "An enzyme preparation inactivating all penicillins and cepalosporins". J. Clin. Path., 26:596, 1973.

6. Schimpff, S. C., Greene, W. H., Young, V. M. and Wiernik, P. H. "Pseudomonas Septicaemia: Incidence, Epidemiology, Prevention and Therapy in Patients with Advanced Cancer".

Europ. J. Cancer, 9:449, 1973.

7.   Tattersall, M. H. N., Hutchinson, R. M., Gaya, H. and Spiers,
     A.S.D. "Empirical Antibiotic Therapy in Febrile Patients
     with Neutropenia and Malignant Disease". Europ. J. Cancer,
     9:417, 1973.

8.   Schimpff, S., Satterlee, W., Young, V. M. and Serpick, A.
     "Empiric therapy with carbenicillin and gentamicin for
     febrile patients with cancer and granulocytopenia".
     New Engl. J. Med., 284:1061, 1971.

9.   Schimpff, S. C., Young, V. M., Greene, W. H., Vermeulen,
     G. D., Moody, M. R. and Wiernik, P. H. "Origin of
     Infection in Acute Nonlymphocytic Leukemia". Ann. Int. Med.,
     77:707, 1972.

EXPERIENCE WITH GENTAMICIN AND CLINDAMYCIN IN THE

MANAGEMENT OF FEBRILE PATIENTS WITH BLOOD DYSCRASIAS

P.M. Wilkinson, I.W. Delamore, D. Gorst, T.A. Tooth

Department of Haematology, Manchester Royal Infirmary

SUMMARY

Thirty-two febrile neutropenic patients were treated with a nomogram or fixed dose of gentamicin; in addition all patients received Clindamycin by mouth. In 26 patieints the treatment response could be evaluated. Complete resolution of the febrile episode was observed in 6 of 13 (42%) of patients receiving fixed dose, and in 10 of 13 (77%) of patients receiving the nomogram dose of gentamicin. All patients who received the fixed dose were, with one exception under-dosed. There was no evidence of nephrotoxicity due solely to gentamicin. The efficacy of gentamicin may be increased when prescribed on a nomogram basis.

INTRODUCTION

Patients with blood dyscrasias, especially those with an associated neutropenia, frequently develop pyrexial illnesses. Neutropenic patients cannot respond to infection with a normal inflammatory response and classical signs of infection are often absent. A pyrexial illness in such patients, therefore, is generally regarded as infective in origin.

Gentamicin used singly or in combination has proved effective in the management of such episodes (Rodriguex et al. 1973, Atkinson, Kay, and McElwaine, 1974). The dose prescribed is usually on an empirical basis or related to body weight.   Recently prescribing aids for Gentamicin have been devised (Mawer et al. 1974) which provided therapeutic concentrations but minimised toxicity.

The purpose of this study was to assess whether the administration of Gentamicin on a nomogram basis was more effective than a fixed daily dose in the management of febrile patients with blood dyscrasias.

PATIENTS AND METHODS

Patients with either acute myeloid leukaemia (A.M.L.), acute lymphatic leukaemia (A.L.L.), aplastic anaemia (A.A.), lymphoma or iatrogenic neutropenia, were eligible for entry when a pyrexia developed.   The pyrexia was defined as an oral temperature of more than 38°C persisting for more than 4 hours, not related to blood transfusion or blood products.

Patients were carefully examined for the source of infection.   Blood cultures were taken on 2 or 3 occasions during the first 24 hours and bacterio-logical culture of sputum, nose, throat, urine, faeces and relevant skin lesions were obtained.   Chest radiograph, haematological and biochemical tests were performed routinely.   Viral screening tests were also performed in some instances.   The majority of patients received therapy within 24 hours, after completion of the relevant bacteriological tests.

Drugs

Patients were randomly allocated to 2 groups: Group F: received Gentamicin at a fixed dose of 80 mg 8 hourly; and Group N: received a predicted dose obtained from the prescribing aid.

Each dose was administered intravenously by injection into the last 100 mls of infusion fluid, given over 30 minutes.   To cover anaerobic organisms, each patient received in addition, Clindamycin 300 mg 6 hourly by mouth.

Assessment

The patients were examined daily; pulse and temperature were recorded 4-6 hourly.   Patients who failed to respond were treated with modified anti-biotic therapy in the light of clinical and bacteriological findings.

RESULTS

Thirty-two patients were admitted to the study. Three patients were withdrawn from the analysis due to administration of additional antibiotics not specified in the proforma. The details of the remaining patients are given in Tables 1(a) and 1(b). Fifteen patients received the fixed dose and 14 patients a nomagram dose of Gentamicin. Two patients in the former group were not evaluable; patient no. 14 developed a drug allergy 12 hours after therapy and was treated with alternative antibiotics; patient no. 15 developed a fatal gastro-intestinal haemorrhage 36 hours after entry to the trial. One patient on the nomagram regime was considered inelligible for the evaluation due to modification of therapy in the light of blood culture findings. There was no significant difference in the remaining 2 groups regarding age, sex, nature and type of disease, pre-treatment total and peripheral neutrophil counts.

Response

Complete resolution of the febrile episode was observed in 6 of 13 (42%) patients in Group F and 10 of 13 (77%) patients in Group N ($x2 = 1.0$ not significant). Excluding those patients in whom no cause of infection was identified, complete resolution was observed in 3 of 9 (33%) patients in Group F and 7 of 10 (70%) in Group N ($p = 0.17$).

Source of Infection

In 20 of 29 (70%) of patients a source of infection was identified. Six (21%) had respiratory infection, 5 (18%) septicaemia, 3 (12%) peri-anal infections, 3 (12%) peri-oral infections and 3 (12%) urinary tract infections. In the remaining 8 patients no cause was identified. In 6 of these resolution was complete; in 1 patient (no. 9) Gentamicin was prescribed on a nomogram basis with resolution, and 1 patient (no. 11) failed to respond to additional antibiotics.

Three patients died, 2 the direct result of sepsis.
Patient No. 10 (Group F). A 55 year old male with iatrogenic marrow hypoplasia and reticulum cell sarcoma. Klebsiella was isolated from 2 culture media. The patient died 4 days after commencing therapy.
Patient No. 24 (Group N). A 38 year old male with acute A.M.L. E. coli was isolated from the urine and the pyrexia settled with therapy. Two days after resolution the patient became oliguric and later collapsed and died. Post mortem revealed a large gastro-intestinal haemorrhage;

Table 1a.   DETAILS OF 15 PATIENTS TREATED WITH A FIXED DOSE OF GENTAMICIN AND CLINDAMYCIN

Case No.	Age (7)	Sex	Diagnosis	Source of infection	Daily dose Gent. mg.	Neutrophil count/mm^3	Response
1	28	F	A.M.L.	Not found	240	820	Complete recovery
2	16	M	A.L.L.	Urinary infection – E. coli	240	100	Complete recovery
3	9	F	A.A.	Not found	240	300	Complete recovery
4	55	M	A.M.L.	Pneumonia	240	22	Complete recovery
5	15	F	A.M.L.	Respiratory infection	240	300	Complete recovery
6	49	M	A.M.L.	Not found	240	680	Complete recovery
7	16	F	A.L.L.	Staphylococcus septicaemia	240	7,400	No response – eventually resolved with Chloramphenicol
8	58	F	A.M.L.	Pneumonia	240	0	No response – eventually resolved with Septrin
9	24	M	A.M.L.	Not found	240	380	No response – settled with increased dose of Gentamycin
10	59	M	Lymphoma	Klebsiella septicaemia	240	1,090	Died
11	22	F	A.A.	Not found	240	50	No response
12	54	M	A.M.L.	Perianal abscess	240	240	No response
13	38	M	A.M.L.	Respiratory infection	240	1,160	No response – eventually resolved
14	17	F	A.M.L.	Respiratory infection	240	1,380	Not evaluable – drug allergy
15	28	F	A.M.L.				Not evaluable – died 36 hours after entry with massive G.I.T. haemorrhage

Table 1b.   DETAILS OF 14 PATIENTS TREATED WITH GENTAMICIN (ON A NOMOGRAM BASIS) AND CLINDAMYCIN

Case No.	Age (7)	Sex	Diagnosis	Source of infection	Daily dose Gent. mg.	Neutrophil count/mm^3	Response
16	16	M	A.M.L.	Perianal abscess	360	4,000	Complete recovery
17	23	M	A.L.L.	Not found	480	300	Complete recovery
18	20	M	A.L.L.	Broncho pneumonia	480	40	Complete recovery
19	15	F	A.M.L.	Perioral infection	360	10	Complete recovery
20	33	F	A.M.L.	Perioral infection	360	24	Complete recovery
21	67	F	A.M.L.	Perioral infection	240	70	Complete recovery
22	16	M	A.L.L.	Anal fissure, Perioral infection	360	60	Complete recovery
23	16	F	A.L.L.	Not found	240	16	Complete recovery
24	38	F	A.M.L.	Pyelonephritis	240	100	Complete recovery
25	18	M	A.M.L.	Not found	480	3,000	Complete recovery
26	22	F	lymphoma	Urinary infection	360	–	No response
27	34	F	lymphoma	Septicaemia (Bacteroides frasilis)	360	300	Not evaluable – therapy changed in view of culture findings
28	21	F	A.A.	Septicaemia	480	120	Initial response, antibiotics modified in view of culture findings
29	64	M	A.M.L.	Septicaemia	240	600	No response – died

infection was still present in the right kidney.

Patient No. 29 (Group N). A 64 year old male with A.M.L. Two organisms were isolated from blood culture (E. coli and moraxellae). After 2 days therapy Cephaloridine and 1 day later Pyopen and Cloxacillin were added. The patient died 6 days after commencing therapy. Terminally he developed oliguria and renal failure.

Side Effects

One patient (no. 14) developed a marked urticaria due to Clindamycin. In 2 patients impaired renal function was observed. Patient no. 24 developed terminal oliguria associated with the documented abnormalities of renal function found in A.M.L. Patient no. 29 developed terminal renal failure and the antibiotic combination was partly responsible.

Dose of Gentamicin

The total daily dose of Gentamicin administered to Group N was significantly greater than that administered to Group F ($T = 4.8$, $DF = 26$). Patients in Group F with one exception received inadequate doses of Gentamicin according to the nomogram predictions ($T = 8.4$, $DF = 11$)

DISCUSSION

The neutropenic patient is continually at risk from infection and infection is now the major cause of death in acute leukaemia (Levine, Graw and Young 1972). The majority of patients (80%) in this study had neutropenia (neutrophil count $1,000/mm^3$ or less); 4 of the 6 remaining patients had A.M.L. with normal peripheral neutrophil counts but neutrophil function is abnormal due to extrinsic and intrinsic factors.

The aetiology of the fever may not always be apparent and therefore current management is to treat all febrile episodes as presumed bacterial infection. In patients with leukaemia and lymphoma, infection is ultimately proven in 70-80% of febrile episodes. The majority are bacterial in origin, usually infections of the oropharynx, septicaemias, pneumonitis, anal-rectal lesions and urinary tract infections. Such were the findings in this series. The most dangerous of these is septicaemia and therefore antibiotic combinations have evolved to cover the patient against organisms commonly giving rise to septicaemia as well as covering other common sources of infection.

Gentamicin was chosen in this study because of its antibacterial spectrum. Clindamycin was added to cover the patient against infection with anerobic organisms whose recognition is assuming increasing importance. The latter drug, however, has no activity against gram negative organisms and only moderate activity against gram positive cocci.

Whilst Gentamicin is commonly used in combination with other antibiotics, it is usually administered as a fixed dose without taking into account the various parameters known to influence the body's handling of this drug. The patients who received Gentamicin on a fixed basis were, with one exception, under-dosed. This is reflected in the results obtained, which although not significant, suggest that those patients who received a nomogram dosage fared better.

It is debateable whether antibiotics should be given to patients with no evidence of bacterial infection. Present evidence suggests however that such episodes should be treated as a cause will eventually be identified in 50% and may eventually prove fatal (Rodriguex, Burgess and Bodene, 1973).

Five patients (18%) had bacteriological evidence of septicaemia, 2 of whom died. Septicaemia is frequently fatal, survival ranging from 7/100% according to the series study (Levine, Graw and Young 1972). One patient (Group N) had infection with 2 organisms and such infections are invariably fatal (Tattersall, Spears and Daniel 1974). The other patient (Group F) had a Klebsiella septicaemia sensitive to Gentamicin in vitro.

Antibiotics should be mandatory for the neutropenic patient who develops a febrile illness. The combination of Gentamicin and Clindamycin proved effective in 77% of such episodes when the former drug was administered on a nomogram basis. It would seem reasonable, therefore, to assess this combination further.

REFERENCES

Atkinson, K., Kay, H.E.M. and McElwain, T.J. (1974). Brit. Med. J:
    3, 244-247.
Levine, A.S., Graw, R.G. and Young, R.C. (1972). Seminars in
    Haematology: 9, 141-179.
Mawer, G.E., Ahmad, R., Dobbs, S.M., McGough, J.G., Lucas, S.B.
    and Tooth, J.A. (1974). Br. J. Pharmac: 1, 45-50.
Rodriguez, V., Burgess, M. and Bodey, G.P. (1973). Cancer: 32,
    1007-1012.
Tattershall, M.N., Spiers, A.S.D. and Darrell, J.H. (1972). The Lancet:
    1, 162-165.

CLINICAL EXPERIENCE IN THE TREATMENT OF STAPHYLOCOCCAL SEPTICEMIAS IN ORPTHOPEDIC PATIENTS

Gr. N. Tsekos, M. Constantinidou and A.S. Dontas

Dept. of Medicine, Accident Hospital, Kifissia, GREECE

The treatment of staphylococcal septicemias has been a therapeutic challenge, ever since Barber described in 1947 the increase in resistance of staphylococcal strains isolated from patients in British Hospitals. Presently, the number of staphylococcal infections within and out of Hospitals increases year by year, and the strains resistant to Penicillin - G vary between 50 % and 80 % in cases cultured from Hospitals. Finland and Jones stated in 1956 that since the advent of antibiotic therapy the frequency of septicemias from staphylococci had quadrupled, that from Gram-negative bacteria had increased six - fold, and mortality had also somewhat increased. The use of chemoprophylaxis, according to Barnes et al . (1959), while not affecting the frequency of post - surgical infections, has been one of the main factors involved in the emergence of resistant microbial strains.

Factors related with the recent increase in septicemias reported from various orthopedic centers are : the use of broad-spectrum antibiotics, frequently given as a prophylactic or pre-operative measure for short periods, common skin lesions, frequent surgical manipulations, and usually advanced age of the patients. We have studied and report herein all cases of staphylococcal septicemias referred to us over a two-year period (1972 - 74) in the Accident Hospital of Kifissia, the largest Orthopedic-Traumatology Center in Greece.

SUBJECTS - METHODS

Thirty-one patients were studied, 18 males and 13 females, of whom 24 were post-surgical or post-traumatic, and the remaining had common

TABLE 1

STAPHYLOCOCCAL STRAINS RESISTANT IN VITRO

TO VARIOUS PENICILLINS

	BENZYL-PENICIL.	METHICIL.	OXACIL.	CLOXA-CIL.	DICLOXA-CIL.
TOTAL STRAINS	26	26	26	26	26
RESISTANT STRAINS	17	3	-	2	2
	65%	11.6%	-	7.7%	7.7%

TABLE 2

CHARACTERISTICS OF 31 CASES OF STAPH. SEPTICEMIAS

POST-OPERATIVE	20
POST-TRAUMATIC	4
COMMON CUASES (ABSCESSES etc.)	7
TOTAL	31

BLOOD CULTURES POSITIVE (CASES)	26
" " NEGATIVE "	5
	31
MICROORGANISMS ISOLATED	
STAPH. ALBUS "	24
STAPH. AUREUS "	2
	26

RESULTS OF THERAPY		
CURED	23	(74.2 %)
NOT IMPROVED	3	(9.7 %)
DEATH	5	(16.1 %)

causes of their infection. They were aged 14 – 80 years with a mean of 38 years.

Twenty of the above patients had been subjected earlier to empiric broad-spectrum or penicillin chemotherapy, prophylactically or therapeutically because of fever of unknown etiology. In 26 of the 31 cases serial blood cultures in our clinic (three to five), obtained after two days or more without chemotherapy, yielded coagulase-positive staphylococci, of which 17 were resistant to benzyl-penicillin, but all sensitive in vitro to oxacillin (Table 1). All 31 cases had leucocyte counts ranging from 9,000 to 16,000/mm^3, predominantly polymorphonuclear, and evidence of hypochromic anemia.

Cloxacillin (9 cases) and dicloxacillin (22 cases) were given i.m. or i.v. dosages of 3,0 to 4,0 gm./day for about 45 days, followed by one or two months of oral treatment by the same agent. The above synthetic penicillins were chosen because : a) both have bactericidal action, b) both are resistant significant untoward effects, and can be given parenterally every six or eight hours.

RESULTS

This treatment resulted in clinical and laboratory healing in 23 cases (74.2 %), and clinical temporary improvement followed by relapse in three (9.7 %). Of the five (16.1 %) deaths during the study, two were due to a neoplasm, and in three several open fractures and severe cardiopulmonary complications were present (Table 2).

The decrease in temperature occurred gradually, by steps of 0.2 - 0.3 C per day, and it was uncommon to observe minor spikes after apyrexia had been already achieved for some days. In two cases where therapy was discontinued after a relatively short period, a relapse appeared some two or three months later with the same strain of staphylococcus. This necessitated a second much longer period of dicloxacillin administration, to attain clinical and laboratory healing. Cloxacillin, used alternately with dicloxacillin in the first 18 cases, proved somewhat less effective that the latter, so that the remaining patients were treated with dicloxacillin.

DISCUSSION

Empiric administration of antibiotics, especially bacteriostatic for chemoprophylaxis or chemothrapy, pre- or post-operatively, and for short periods of time, leads to : 1. Falsely negative blood cultures. 2. Resistant infections or strains. 3. False clinical healing followed by relapses of septicemias or superinfections. 4. In orthopedic patients, it may conceal acute bone infections, which can lead to chronic osteomyelitis.

In the present series the administration of dicloxacillin proved more efficient than cloxacillin in eradicating the staphylococci from the blood stream. The reasons for the better effectiveness of dicloxacillin are probably related to its higher (at least 2-fold) and much longer lasting blood concentrations when given in equal amounts (Gravenkemper et al 1965). This phenomenon must be associated with the smaller renal clearance rate of dicloxacillin, and probably overrides its higher protein-binding, compared to that of methicillin, oxacillin and cloxacillin (Rosenblatt et al., 1968).

On six of our patients a local wound infection accompanying the septicemia was present. Cultures of the wound exudate yielded a variable flora, mostly of Gram-negative organisms, for whom a variety of antibiotics had been employed prior to the referral of the patients to our service. After discontinuation of such treatment, blood cultures revealed the underlying staphylococcal infection. It appears that the staphylococci residing in the skin can invade traumatic surfaces by enzymic activity, and thus induce a blood-borne infection, whereas the local infections and only rarely do they result in Gram-negative septicemias. In conclusion, synthetic penicillin therapy in staphylococcal septicemias must be given early, in adequate doses i.v. or i.m., and for a minimum of two months.

SUMMARY

Out of thirty-one cases of Staphylococcal septicemias (24 post-operative or post-traumatic) nine were treated with cloxacillin and 22 with dicloxacillin, administered i.m. or i.v. for 45 days, and then orally for one to two further months. Twenty of the above had been sudjected earlier to empiric broad-spectrum chemotherapy for prophylaxis or post-surgical fevers of unknown etiology. Twenty-tree patients were healed with this treatment, whereas three showed no change. Two patients with underlying neoplasms and three with several open fractures died within 4 - 5 weeks of onset of treatment.

REFERENCES

1.   Barber, M. : Staphylococcal infection due to penicillin resistant strains. Brit. Med. J. 2, 863, 1947.

2.   Barnes, J., Page, W.C., Trump, D.S., and Ellison, E.H. : Prophylactic prostoperative antibiotics. A.M.A. Archives of Surgery 79, 190, 1959.

3.   Finland, M. and Jones, W.F. : Staphylococcal infections currently encountered in a large municipal hospital : Some problems in evaluating antimicrobial therapy in such infections. Annals of the New

York Academy of Sciences 65, 191 , 1956.

4. Gravenkemper, C.F., Bennett, J.V., Brodie, J.L., and Kirby, W. M.M. : Diclocacillin in vitro and pharmacologic comparisons with oxacillin and cloxacillin. A.M.A. Archives of Internal Medicine 116, 340 , 1965.

5. Rosenblatt, J.E., King, A.C., Brodie, J.L., and Kirby, W.M.M.: Mechanisms responsible for the blood level difference of isoxazolyl-penicillin. A.M.A. Archives of Internal Medicine 121 , 345 ,1968.

THE RECENT TREND OF CLINICAL GRAM-NEGATIVE BACILLARY ISOLATION

IN JAPAN*

Masaaki Ohkoshi[†] and Ueda Yasushi[††]
[†]Dept. of Urology, Tokai University
Isehara, Kanagawa Prefecture
[††]Dept. of Internal Medicine, Jikei University
Nishishinbashi, Tokyo

That the incidence of gram-negative bacilli as causative organisms of infection in man recently has been on the increase is a worldwide tendency, and Japan is not an exception to this trend. I already described this on the occasion of the 6th International Congress held at Tokyo in 1969.

The present communication deals with a statistical survey on the trend of clinical isolation of gram-negative bacilli in this country over the ensuing years, based on the statistics of data obtained through questionnaires from medical institutions throughout the country, data from the Urological Department of Keio University and those of sepsis and pyelonephritis from the Department of Internal Medicine of Jikei University.

I. Summarization of Nationwide Data Obtained Through Questionnaires

Figure 1 illustrates the yearly percentages of gram-negative bacillary strains to total numbers of clinical bacterial isolates. The figures are based on the data obtained through questionnaires sent to a number of medical institutions throughout the country

---

*This paper appears here in abridged form. In several places graphic or tabular presentations of data have been deleted to keep the report within the allocated length. These places have been marked in the text by three asterisks(***).

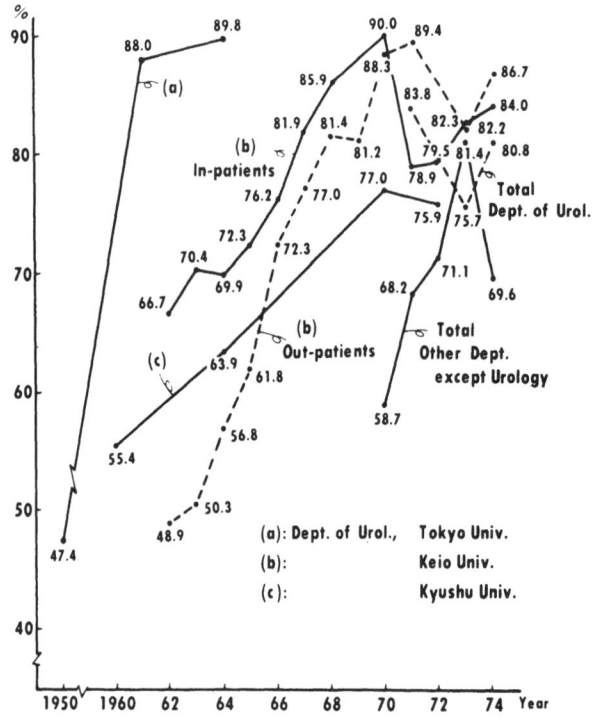

Figure 1.   Isolation ratio of gram-negative bacteria in Japan

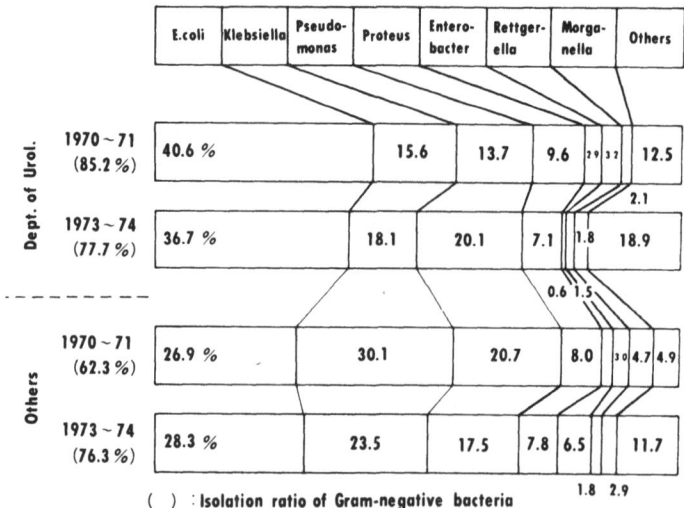

Figure 2.   Distribution of gram-negative bacteria isolated in Japan

and those reported from the urological departments of a few university hospitals. The isolation of gram-negative bacilli from urinary tract infections are particularly high in incidence.

Notably frequent are E. coli strains among the variety of bacterial genera isolated from cases of urinary tract infection throughout the country. Moreover, when compared between the two period from 1970-1971 and from 1973-1974, the incidence of E. coli involvement in urinary tract infection has been on the decrease with a trend of pseudomonas to increase (Fig. 2).

II. Statistics on Organisms Obtained at the Department of Urology, Keio University Hospital

As shown in Figure 3, gram-negative bacilli accounted for 81.7% and 84.1% of all bacterial isolates from hospitalized cases respectively during the 1970-1971 period and the 1973-1974 period. The corresponding rates of gram-negative bacillary isolated from outpatients were 88.05% and 82.6%; thus no conspicuous difference. Among the various genera of gram-negative bacilli isolated from outpatients, E. coli was most frequent accounting for approximately three-quarters of all gram-negative bacillary isolates, in contrast only one-fifth to a quarter for E. coli among the gram-negative bacillary isolates from inpatients. Such genera as Pseudomonas and Klebsiella were obtained with notably high frequency instead from inpatients, at rates virtually to that of E. coli. Proteus showed the highest incidence of isolation next to the foregoing three.

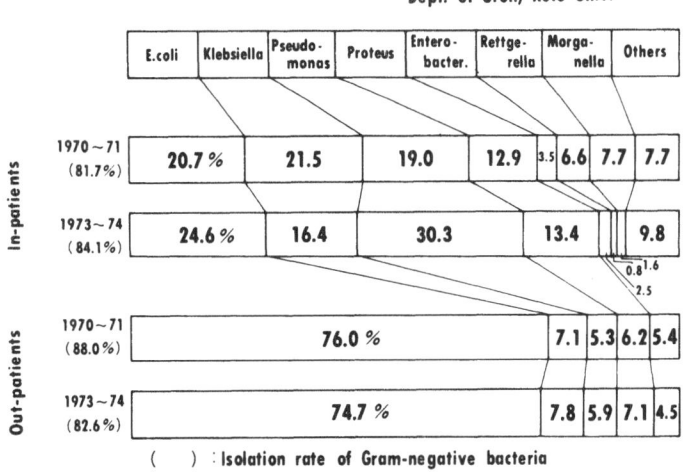

Figure 3. Distribution of gram-negative bacteria isolated from in- and out-patients

Rates of isolation of gram-negative bacilli from outpatients, classified by sex and bacterial species, have been determined.*** Noteworthy is that E. coli isolation was by far the most frequent (86.2) from female patients. This would be ascribed to the fact that cystitis is common in female ambulatory cases for the considerable proportion of which the causative organisms are identified as E. coli.

Disc tests for antimicrobial susceptibiltiy carried out with eleven different chemotherapeutic agents have demonstrated that, generally, the gram-negative bacilli isolates from outpatients were more sensitive to various antibiotics than from inpatients. The data concerning sensitivity of E. coli, Proteus, Klebsiella and Pseudomonas isolates*** indicate this trend, being prominent with E. coli and with Proteus. When viewed with respect to individual antimicrobial agents, the tendency is most pronounced with the B-lactam antibiotics, followed by kanamycin. Naridixic acid displays this trend only for the E. coli isolates.

A further data analysis by comparison of yearly variation in antimicrobial susceptibility between the 1970-1971 group and the 1973-1974 group has revealed a general trend for the latter group, rather than the former, to exhibit an increase in susceptibility.*** This tendency was prominent particularly with Proteus isolates the susceptibility of which generally increased for 7 out of the 11 drugs. The trend of increased susceptibility was observed frequently for such agents as streptomycin, tetracyclines and chloramphenicol, the first in particular.

		ABPC	CBPC	CER	GM	KM	SM	CL	CP	TC	NA	Sulfa
Decrease of susceptibility (In-patients to Out-patients)	E.coli	↓↓↓	↓↓↓	↓↓↓		↓↓↓			↓↓		↓↓↓	
	Klebsiella	↓	↓	↓↓		↓			↓			
	Pseudo-monas					↓	↓					
	Proteus	↓	↓	↓					↓	↓		
Increase of susceptibility (1973 74 to 1970 71)	E.coli						↑↑		↑	↑	↑	
	Klebsiella					↑	↑↑					
	Pseudo-monas						↑↑		↑	↑		
	Proteus	↑↑	↑	↑		↑	↑		↑	↑		

Figure 4.   Change of the susceptibility to antibiotics classified by out- and in-patients, and years

The findings heretofore described are summarized in Figure 4.
It would follow that the phenomenon may be interpreted as implying
the antimicrobial susceptibility of an organism is lowered with increasing chance of its contact with the antimicrobial agent or enhanced if the chances are slender.

III.   Statistics on Bacteremia and Pyelonephritis   (Dept. of
       Internal Medicine, Jikei University)

In Figure 5, the clinical data on 25 cases of bacteremia experienced during the period from 1965 to 1974 at the Third Department of Internal Medicine of the Jikei University School of Medicine
are summarized.

Gram-negative bacteremia was higher in incidence from 1970 on,
as compared with the period from 1965 to 1969. The most frequent
gram-negative organisms causative of bacteremia among the 25 cases
were Pseudomonas and Klebsiella and the former characteristically
has shown a progressive increase since the year of 1970.

The portals of entry of organisms in 20 cases of gram-negative
bacteremia included: the respiratory tract, biliary tract, urinary
tract, operation, burn, arterio-venous shunt and so forth.*** The
most frequent was the external arteriovenous shunt encountered in
8 cases, in 7 out of which the causative organism was Pseudomonas
or Acinetobacter.

In the development of bacteremia with gram-negative bacilli,
underlying diseases, antibiotic therapy and/or steroid therapy are
universally recognized to be largely involved. As assessed according to the classification proposed by McCabe and Jackson, there
were rapidly fatal diseases such as aplastic anemia or acute leukemia in 5 cases and ultimately fatal diseases such as chronic renal

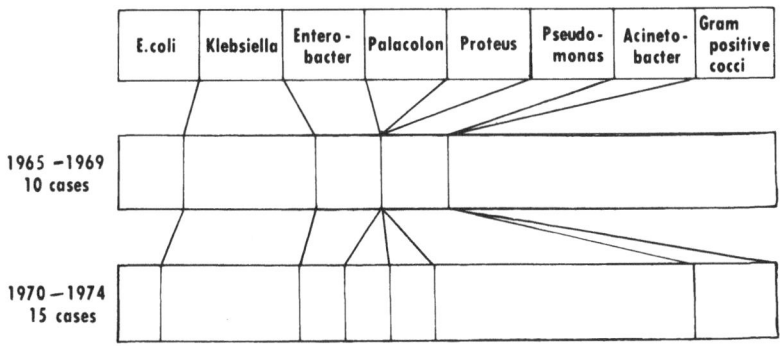

Figure 5. Isolation rate of bacteria isolated from Bacteremia

Table 1

Gram-negative Bacteremia and Hospital Infection

	No. of Cases	Non-Hospital Acquired	Hospital Acquired
E. coli	2	2	
Klebsiella	5	3	2
Enterobacter	2		2
Paracolon	1	1	
Proteus	1		1
Pseudomonas	7		7
Acinetobacter	2		2
	20	6	14

failure or lupus erythematosus as the underlying disease in 10 out
of the 20 cases studied; hence fatal underlying diseases in two-
thirds of the cases and non-fatal diseases in 5 cases. Eleven
patients were receiving or had been given within 2 weeks prior to
onset of bacteremia, antibiotic therapy and/or steroid therapy.

With a view to clarifying the interrelationship between gram-
negative bacteremia and hospital infection, the data were analyzed
by classifying the cases into two groups: cases of "non-hospital
acquired infection" in which bacteremia developed within 2 weeks
after admission and those with "hospital acquired infection" in
which onset of bacteremia was later than 2 weeks of hospitalization.
The results obtained are presented in Table 1. As can be seen,
14 out of the 20 cases were of hospital acquired infection, and

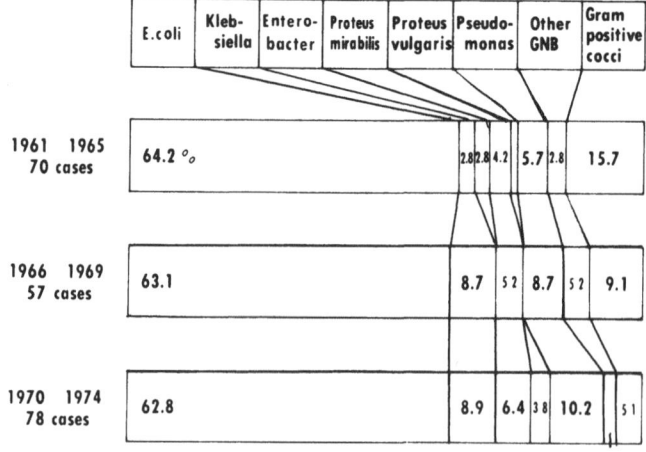

Figure 6. Distribution of bacteria isolated from pyelonephritis

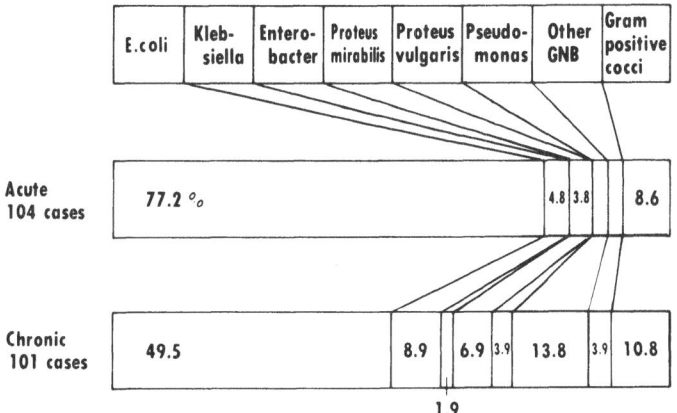

Figure 7. Distribution of bacteria isolated from acute- and
           chronic-pyelonephritis

Enterobacter, Pseudomonas and Acinetobacter were the organisms
isolated from the case of hospital acquired infection alone.

     In the meantime, bacteremic shock was encountered in 7 cases
or 35% of the cases studied. Shock due to bacteremia occurred in
patients over 30 years of age and was particularly high in incidence among those over 50 years, 4 out of 5 cases. No significant
interrelationship, nevertheless, was noted to exist between any
specific genus of causative organism or underlying disease and
shock.

     In Figure 6 are summarized the data on causative organisms
isolated from a total of 200 cases of pyelonephritis experienced
between 1961 and 1974. Of these 200 cases, 180 cases, or 90 per
cent were due to infection by gram-negative bacilli, among which
E. coli was the most frequent pathogen, followed, in order by
Pseudomonas, Klebsiella and Proteus mirabilis. Although no significant change in the yearly rate of isolation could be observed
with any of the species or genera of causative organisms during
the 13 year period, Klebsiella and Pseudomonas showed an increase
from 1966, onwards. The frequency of isolation of bacterial pathogens differed between acute and chronic pyelonephritis; E. coli
infection was demonstrated in 80 per cent of acute cases in contrast to as low as 50 per cent for chronic cases (Figure 7). The
findings are consistent with the reports by other investigators.

CLINICAL STUDY OF GRAM NEGATIVE RODS (GNR)

SEPTICEMIA AT KEIO UNIVERSITY HOSPITAL

Mitsuto Hasegawa, Susumu Tomioka, Yoshio Kobayashi

School of Medicine, Keio University

35 Shinanomachi, Shinjuku-ku, Tokyo, Japan

Summary
1. A tendency of infectious organisms of GNR septicemia and the
sensitivity distribution of strains recently isolated were described.
2. Therapeutic results of GNR repticemia revealed the clinical
availability of the combined use of B-lactam antibiotics and Gentamicin or Tobramycin.
3. The synergetic effects was observed by the combined use of
Cefazoline and Gentamicin in bacteriostatic and bactericidal action
in in vitro antibacterial activity test.

One hundred and ninety-four cases of gram negative rods (GNR)
septicemia encountered at Keio University Hospital during 15 years
from 1960 to 1974 were reviewed. Changes of infectious organisms of
GNR septicemia and the sensitivity of the detected strains were
examined. The chemotherapeutic results of GNR septicemia in recent
years were also analyzed. Minimum inhibitory concentration (MIC)
of the drug was measured by agar dilution method.

Status of the incidence of GNR septicemia in the last 15 years
was investigated. The incidence of GNR septicemia had remarkably
increased in and after 1972. There were 58 cases with GNR septicemia
in 1974. E.coli, Klebsiella, Enterobacter and Pseudomonas were
representative as the infectious organisms in the last few years.
Besides, cases with mixed infection caused by Serratia and Bacteroides attracted our attention. According to the chronological
changes of infectious organisms, strains of E.coli had strikingly
increased in 1974. Enterobacter septicemia also increased.
Klebsiella or Pseudomonas septicemia have not increased after 1973.
In addition to these 3 cases of septicemia caused by Pseudomonas
cepacia were observed after 1973.

Table 1. Prognosis of GNR Septicemia* Complicated
with Hematologic Disorders

Organisms	No.of Cases	No.of Deaths	Mortality (%)
E.coli	11	7	63.6
Klebsiella	5	2	40.0
Enterobacter	4	3	75.0
P.aeruginosa	19	9	47.4
Total	39	21	53.8

*1959-1974, Department of Medicine of Keio Univ. Hosp.

Changes of pathogenic organisms were analized from the yearly amount of antibiotics used at Keio University Hospital. The results reveals that the rate of Klebsiella septicemia has reduced and that of Pseudomonas and Enterobacter septicemia has clearly increased in accordance with the increase of the amount of Cephalosporins used. Besides, the rate of Pseudomonas septicemia has decreased in accordance with the increase of the use of Carbenicillin, Sulbenicillin and Gentamicin. On the other hand, E.coli septicemia occupied 30% of GNR septicemia in 1974. One of the causes of these changes is considered to be due to the fact that about 60% of E.coli strains isolated from blood in and after 1972 were resistant to Ampicillin, Carbenicillin and Cephaloridine.

Mortality of this disease was examined by infectious organisms. Subjects were limited to the cases with hematologic disorders as underlying diseases. The examination revealed a high mortality in all cases with septicemia caused by E.coli, Klebsiella, Enterobacter and P.aeruginosa.

Almost all cases were fatal before 1972, but the mortality was

Table 2. Prognosis of Pseudomonas aeruginosa Septicemia Associated with Hematologic Disorders in Keio University Hospital

Year	No.of Cases	No.of Deaths	No.of Deaths complicated with Shock	Mortality (%)
1961-1971	5	5	3	100
1972	4	3	2	75
1973	7	2	0	28.6
1974	6	2	2	33.3

Table 3. Susceptibility of Pseudomonas aeruginosa
(1972-1974)

Antibiotics	Sourses	\ MIC(ug/ml)							
		12.5	25	50	100	200	400	800	1600<
Carbenicillin	Blood		3	8	9	2	2	1	1
	Others		1	28	10	12	3	1	4
Sulbenicillin	Blood	1	4	13	3	3			2
	Others		7	30	12	4	1	1	4

Inoculum: 1/100 x HIB culture fluid

extremely low even including 2 dead cases of shock in and after 1973 as shown in Table 2. Chemotherapeutic effect was observed here.

Then, we examined the therapeutic results in recent years of Pseudomonas aeruginosa septicemia associated with hematologic disorders. The results are as follows; single administration of 160mg/day or 240mg/day of Gentamicin or 240mg/day of Tobramycin could not inhibit the occurrence of P.aeruginosa septicemia either. However, all the cases received whichever 4 kinds of combined use; a large dose of Carbenicillin or Sulbenicillin and 160mg/day of Gentamicin or 240mg/day of Tobramycin, have been cured at present. On the other hand, no chemotherapeutic effect was observed in any kinds of combined use of Carbenicillin or Sulbenicillin and under a dose level of 120mg/day of Gentamicin or Tobramycin or under 200mg/day of Dibekacin. Here, we confirmed the availability of combined use of drugs clinically and at the same time, the effective doses of Gentamicin and Tobramycin for this combined use was suggested. The sensitivity of P.aeruginosa isolated from blood of these patients to Carbenicillin and Sulbenicillin were examined and the results are shown in Table 3. There was no difference in sensibity to Carbenicillin or Sulbenicillin between the strains of P.aeruginosa detected from blood and those from other than blood at present. MIC of Carbenicillin was between 50-200ug/ml and that of Sulbenicillin was between 25-100ug/ml and the antibacterial activity of the latter was a little stronger than that of the former.

The therapeutic result of P.aeruginosa septicemia was advanced. Whereas all the effective cases of septicemia caused by E.coli, Klebsiella and Enterobacter consisted of one case with E.coli septicemia who were affected by singly administration of Gentamicin and all the remaining cases received combined use of B-lactam antibiotics and Gentamicin or Tobramycin. Many cases who received a single

dose of Gentamicin because of having been resistant to B-lactam
antibiotic were not improved and died despite a dose of 160mg/day
of Gentamicin. Also here, we could recognize the availability of
combined use of B-lactam antibiotics and Gentamicin or Tobramycin.

In vitro antibacterial activity of the combined use of Cefazolin
and Gentamicin was studied on Klebsiella by agar dilution method.
There was the prominent synergetic effects in the combined use of
0.2-0.78ug/ml of Gentamicin and 0.78-3.13ug/ml of Cefazolin.
Besides, the synergetic effects were observed in bactericidal effect.
Bactericidal effect was obtained by dropping Cephalosporinase on the
plate on which MIC of the drug was measured and then by recultivating
organisms following breakdown of Cefazolin. Clinically, one of the
cases with Klebsiella septicemia associated with AML was relieved
by the combined use of 12g/day of Cefazolin and 160g/day of
Gemtamicin.

CLINICAL AND CHEMOTHERAPEUTIC STUDIES OF

PSEUDOMONAS INFECTIONS IN INFANTS AND CHILDREN

T. NISHIMURA, Y. KOTANI AND R. YOSHIDA

DEPARTMENT OF PEDIATRICS, OSAKA MEDICAL COLLEGE

2-7, DAIGAKUMACHI, TAKATSUKI, OSAKA, JAPAN

The clinical and chemotherapeutic studies were made in 37 infants and children with Pseudomonas infections in our hospital for 1955 to 1974. Of the 37 patients, 10 had septicemia; 13, respiratory infections; 8, skin and muscular infections; 1, urinary tract infection; and 5, postoperative infections. These patients ranged from 2 days to 11 years of age: 22 were under 3 months of age and 9 were especially under 15 days of age. Of the total patients, 29 had underlying diseases. Especially hypoplasia of thymus, asplenia, spina bifida, leukemia, aplastic anemia, etc. were encountered in 9 of the 10 patients with septicemia. In serotyping of Pseudomonas aeruginosa isolated from patients, Type 8 was 37.0%, followed by Type 5. Gentamicin, Colistin, Carbenicillin, Tobramycin and Dibekacin were given to 4 patients with septicemia and 12 with respiratory infections. Although 28 patients were given antibiotics sensitive to Pseudomonas, 2 with septicemia and 3 with respiratory infections died. Of the 37 patients, 16 died and especially of the 10 patients with septicemia 9 died.

With the recent great advances in chemotherapy, changes in bacterial infection patterns have been increasingly observed in children and infants. Infections due to gram-negative bacilli, particularly Pseudomonas are now one of the main targets of chemotherapy. For Pseudomonas infections, there are still many problems in therapy and prognosis.

Special attention has been paid to the role of Pseudomonas in superinfections and opportunistic infections associated with serious underlying diseases or complications.

In the pediatric field, Pseudomonas often causes systemic in-

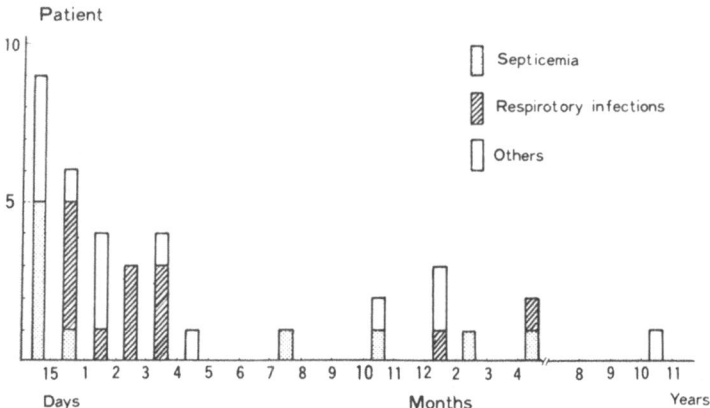

Fig. 1. Age distribution in patients with Pseudomonas aeruginosa
         infections.

fections. Pseudomonas produces terminal infections in patients
with leukemia or malignant tumor and easily leads to death-causing
diseases such as septicemia or meningitis. The outbreak rate of
Pseudomonas infections is high in newborn and infants and the death
rate of pediatric patients with septicemia or meningitis, not to
mention patients with terminal infections, is extremely high.

We would like to report here clinical and therapeutic problems
in 37 patients with Pseudomonas infections treated in our hospital
between 1966 and 1974, paying special attention to the underlying
diseases, complications, role of antibiotic therapy and prognosis.
Of these 37 patients with Pseudomonas infections, 10 had septicemia; 13, respiratory tract infection; and 14, other infections.

Fig. 1 shows the age distribution in patients with Pseudomonas
infections. Twenty six, that is, 70.3% of the 37 patients were 4
months or younger and 40.5% of them was one month old or less.
Septicemia was most commonly encountered within 15 days after
birth. In older patients, septicemia with complications of leukemia, aplastic anemia or malignant tumor was noted.

Table 1 shows the clinical findings in patients with septicemia due to Pseudomonas. The patients consisted of 6 males and 4
females ranging from 2 days to 4 years of age. As shown in this
table, underlying diseases or complications were present in 9 of
the 10 patients. The first clinical signs were mostly non-specific in the newborn. In 5 patients, Pseudomonas was isolated from
blood and in the others, it was identified in pathological materials by the fluorescent antibody technique.

TABLE 1
FINDINGS IN PATIENTS WITH PSEUDOMONAS SEPTICEMIA

Case No	Patient	Age	Sex	First clinical sign	Complication or underlying disease	Serotype of P aeruginosa	Prognosis
1	N H	2 Days	F	Cyanosis Dyspnea Abdominal distention	Thymic hypoplasia		Died
2	K I	4 Days	M	Vomiting Convulsion Abdominal distention	Thymic hypoplasia Hypoplasia of muscular layer of Intestine	8	Died
3	S M	6 Days	F	Poor feeding	Spina bifida	6·7	Died
4	M T	8 Days	M	Abdominal distention Poor feeding	Thymic hypoplasia	8	Died
5	S N	9 Days	F	Abdominal distention Poor feeding	Thymic hypoplasia Asplenia Cor biloculare		Died
6	Y S	27 Days	F	Abdominal distention Wheezing	Esophageal atresia	8	Survived
7	Z K	7 Months	M	Dyspnea		3	Survived
8	K.H	10 Months	M	Fever	Aplastic anemia	10	Died
9	K H.	2 Years	M	Fever, Diarrhea	Retinoblastoma	5	Died
10	A N	4 Years	M	Fever	A L L	5	Died

Table 2 gives the histopathological findings in patients who died of septicemia. The chief findings were vasculitis, hemorrhage and necrosis. Cellular reaction was poor in immunologically impaired hosts.

Table 3 shows the patients with Pseudomonas respiratory tract infections. Of the 13 patients, 9 had pneumonia; 2 empyema; 1, lung abscess; and 1, laryngitis. The age of the patients ranged from 17 days to 4 years. Underlying diseases and complications were encountered in 8 of the 13 patients. Four patients had Pseudomonas respiratory tract infections complicated by Staphylococcal infections. These diagnoses were confirmed by roentgen findings and positive sputum-throat-stool cultures. Wheezing was the most common of the clinical signs.

Table 4 shows other Pseudomonas infections. Of the 14 patients, 5 had postoperative infections; 3, abscess; 2, omphalitis; 1, urinary tract infection; 1, decubitis; 1, thermal burn. Underlying diseases and complications were present in 7 of the 14 patients.

Table 5 shows the serotypes of Pseudomonas aeruginosa isolated from patients. For serotyping, 14 different types of Pseudomonas aeruginosa antiserum supplied by Dr. Homma (Homma et al., 1970,

TABLE 2
CHIEF PATHOLOGICAL FINDINGS AT AUTOPSY OF PATIENTS
WITH PSEUDOMONAS SEPTICEMIA

Case No	Vasculitis	Hemorrhage	Necrosis	Cellular reaction
1	+	++	−	++
2	+++	+++	++	+
3	+++	+++	−	++
4	+++	++	−	−
5	+	+++	++	−
9	++	++	−	−
10	++	++	−	−

4 : Thymic hypoplasia
5 : Thymic hypoplasia, Asplenia
9 : Retinoblastoma
10 : ALL

TABLE 3
PSEUDOMONAS RESPIRATORY INFECTIONS

Case No	Patient	Age	Sex	Disease	Complication or underlying disease	Source	Serotype	Prognosis
1	R S	17 Days	F	Pneumonia		Throat Sputum Feces	NA	Survived
2	H Y	26 Days	M	Pneumonia		Throat Sputum Feces	10	Died
3	M S	26 Days	M	Pneumonia	Staphylococcal osteomyelitis	Throat Sputum Feces	3	Survived
4	K M	35 Days	F	Empyema	Staphylococcal empyema	Pleural fluid Throat Feces		Survived
5	M N	2 Months	M	Lung abscess	Staphylococcal empyema	Throat Sputum Feces	4	Survived
6	K N	2 Months	M	Pneumonia		Throat Sputum Feces	8	Survived
7	M H	2 Months	F	Pneumonia	Hydrocephalus Cleft palate	Throat Sputum Feces	8	Died
8	T U	3 Months	M	Pneumonia	Down's syndrome, Prematurity	Sputum Feces	6	Died
9	N S	3 Months	M	Pneumonia		Sputum	8	Survived
10	M F	3 Months	F	Pneumonia	Cerebral palsy Prematurity	Sputum Urine	9	Died
11	I I	1.4 Years	M	Pneumonia		Sputum	8	Survived
12	M A	4 Years	M	Empyema	Staphylococcal empyema	Pleural fluid		Servived
13	T H	29 Days	M	Laryngitis	Congenital deformity of larynx	Throat Feces	4	Survived

NA : not agglutinable

TABLE 4
OTHER PSEUDOMONAS INFECTIONS

Case No	Patient	Age	Sex	Disease	Complication or underlying disease	Source	Serotype	Prognosis
1	Y.F.	10 Days	F	Submaxillar abscess	Pyloric stenosis Otitis media Prematurity	Throat Pus Feces	7	Survived
2	T.Y.	1 Month	M	Lumbal abscess	Tetralogy of Fallot	Pus	NA	Died
3	Y.N.	1.8 Years	F	Occipital abscess	Letterer-Siwe syndrome	Pus		Survived
4	M.N.	7 Days	M	Omphoritis	Staphylococcal septicemia	Pus	5	Survived
5	M.S.	1 Month	F	Omphalitis		Pus	6	Survived
6	M.I.	10 Months	M	Sinusitis	Staphylococcal septicemia	Pus		Survived
7	T.O.	1.5 Years	F	Decubitus	Hydrocephalus	Pus	5	Survived
8	Y.I.	3 Months	F	Urinary tract infection	Cerebral palsy Vesial palsy	Urine	5	Survived
9	T.M.	10 Years	M	Thermal burn		Pus		Survived
10	M.K.	2 Days	F	Postoperative infection	Spina bifida	Pus	8	Died
11	G.H.	3 Days	M	Postoperative infection	Gastric perforation	Pus	6	Died
12	S.M.	29 Days	M	Postoperative infections	Cleft palate	Pus Throat Feces	NA	Survived
13	Y.M.	1 Month	M	Postoperative infection	Meningocele	Pus	8	Died
14	M.Y.	4 Months	F	Postoperative infection	Klippel-Feil syndrome Antresia ani	Pus		Survived

N.A : not agglutinable

TABLE 5
SEROTYPES OF PSEUDOMONAS AERUGINOSA ISOLATED FROM PATIENTS

Source	Strain	Serotype 4	5	6	7	8	9	10	4·8	6·7	NA
Throat Sputum	15	2	2	1	1	5	1	1	1		1
Pus	8		2	2		3					1
Blood	5					3	1		1		
Urine	1		1								
	29	2	5	3	1	11	1	2	1	1	2

NA : not agglutinable

TABLE 6
RELATIONSHIP BETWEEN UNDERLYING DISEASE
OR CLINICAL CONDITIONS AND FATALITY

	Conditions		survivors/total patients %
Septicemia 10 cases	Thymic hypoplasia		0/4
	Asplenia		0/1
	Aplastic anemia		0/1
	Acute lymphatic leukemia		0/1
	Others		1/2
		Total	1/9 (11.1)
Respiratory Infections 13 cases	Staphylococcal infections Empyema Osteomyelitis		4/4
	Others		1/4
		Total	5/8 (62.5)
Other infections 14 cases	Postoperative condition		2/5
	Others		6/7
		Total	8/12 (66.7)
		Total	14/29 (48.3)

Fatalities : 16/37 (43.2%)

Patients with underlying diseases and clinical conditions   15 29 51 7%
Patients without underlying diseases and clinical conditions   1   8   12 5%

TABLE 7
ANTIBIOTIC THERAPY AND PSEUDOMONAS INFECTION:
SURVIVAL RATE IN PSEUDOMONAS INFECTIONS

	survivors total patients %		survivors total patients %
Septicemia		Other infections	
Gentamicin Dibekacin and Carbenicillin	1/1	Gentamicin Fosfomycin and Sulbenicillin	1/1
Gentamicin and Fosfomycin	1/1	Gentamicin and Carbenicillin	1/1
Dibecasin and Carbenicillin	0/1	Gentamicin and Fosfomycin	1/1
Gentamicin	0/1	Gentamicin	3/4
No anti-Pseudomonas therapy	0/6*	Carbenicillin	1/1
Total patients	2/10 (20)	Sulbemicillin	2/2
Respiratory infections		Colistin	1/1
Gentamicin and Carbenicillin	4/5	Polymyxin B	0/1
Gentamicin and Colistin	1/1	No anti-Pseudomonas therapy	0/2
Gentamicin	0/1	Total patients	10/14 (71.4)
Carbenicillin	2/2		
Sulbenicillin	1/1		
Colistin	1/2		
No ant-Pseudomonas therapy	0/1		
Total patients	9/13 (69.2)		

* Includes three patients who died

shortly after admission

1971) were used. Serotype 8 was the most prevalent, followed by
Serotypes 5 and 6. Despite remarkable progress in antibiotic therapy, the outlook for surviving patients with Pseudomonas infections
is still bad. The prognoses of these patients were affected by age
and underlying diseases.

Table 6 shows the relationship between underlying diseases or
clinical conditions and fatality. Of the 10 patients with septicemia, 9 had underlying diseases, and only one survived. The survival rate of patients with respiratory tract infections and others
were 62.5% and 66.7% respectively. The efficacy of antibiotics
against Pseudomonas in general, and in the immunologically compromised hosts in particular, remains a major problems in the
management of Pseudomonas infections.

Table 7 shows the antibiotic therapy and survival rate of patients with Pseudomonas infections. The survival rate slightly
improved when antibiotics were given in combination.

From the above clinical and therapeutic results we concluded
that the therapeutic effect of the antibiotics depends largely on
the severity of the underlying diseases. We must still search for
the most effective means of conquering immunological derangements
due to underlying diseases and must study new antibiotic therapies
for septicemia.

REFERENCES

1) Homma,Y.J., Kim,K.S., Yamada,H. and Ito,M. (1970), Japanese
   of Experimental Medicine, 40, 347.
2) Homma,Y.J., Shionoya,H., Yamada,H. and Kawabe,Y. (1971),
   Japanese Journal of Experimental Medicine, 41, 89.
3) Nishimura,T., Takagi,M. and Kotani,Y. (1973), Japanese
   Journal of Experimental Medicine, 43, 43.

POLYMYXIN METHYLENE SULFONIC ACID (AREMYXIN)

IN THE TREATMENT OF INFECTIONS WITH GRAM-NEGATIVE ORGANISMS

J. MODAÏ ; F. VACHON and J. FROTTIER

CLAUDE BERNARD HOSPITAL

PARIS

SUMMARY

Polymyxin Sulfonic Acid (Aremyxin) was administered to 40 patients suffering from infections due to gram - organisms (24 cases of urinary infection and 16 of septicaemia). At a dose of 20,000 to 30,000 U/kg/day, cure was obtained in 31 patients, 15 of which were cases of septicaemia. In 12 cases it was used together with another antibiotic (carbenicillin or aminoside). Failures were due either to microbial resistance or to a change of organism. Renal impairment, present in 5 patients, resolved completely in all cases when treatment was discontinued. The substance may be given at lower doses to patients with renal insufficiency.

Polymyxin Sulfonic Acid (P.M.S.A.) is a semi-synthetic derivative of Polymyxin B. It is bactericidal against the majority of gram - organisms. Two injections daily are sufficient to provide a serum level in excess of the M.I.C. of sensitive organisms. P.M.S.A. is excreted in the active form via the kidney, and experimentally its renal tolerance is better than that of the other polymyxins.

These properties induced us to investigate the activity and tolerance of this antibiotic in a number of infections due to gram - organisms.

MATERIAL AND METHODS

1. SELECTION of PATIENTS

40 patients were treated in hospital with P.M.S.A. : 20 men and 20 women aged between 15 and 83 years.

In 24 cases, the diseases treated were urinary infections (bacteriuria $\geq$ 1 x 10^5 organisms/ml) and in 16 they were septicaemias (positive blood cultures). The organisms responsible are shown in the table below.

All the strains underwent bacteriological investigation, including identification, and their bacteriostatic antibiogram, and this was followed, in the septicaemia cases, by the determination of the bactericidal potency of combinations of antibiotics.

2. MODE of ADMINISTRATION

In 37 out of the 40 cases, P.M.S.A. was administered intramuscularly, twice daily. It was administered as a slow intravenous infusion in 3 cases.

The daily dose varied between 20,000 and 30,000 units per kilogram body weight. The dosage was reduced to 4000 U/Kg/day in 3 patients who were suffering from renal insufficiency before beginning treatment.

P.M.S.A. was administered alone in 28 cases. In 2 cases, however, P.M.S.A. was given together with Gentamycin (8 patients), Carbenicillin (2 patients) or Tobramycin (2 patients) because of the severity of the infection and on the basis of the antibiogram results.

The duration of treatment varied with the severity of the infection and tolerance of the product, and lay between 4 and 20 days, with a mean of 10 days.

3. CRITERIA of EFFECTIVENESS

The criteria adopted were clinical (temperature curve, general condition, the course of any local or functional signs present) and microbiological (blood cultures and bacterial examination of urine).

4. INVESTIGATION of TOLERANCE

This was carried out by examination of the skin (rash, or pain at the injection site), renal function (determination of serum creatinine and of blood and urinary levels of urea and potassium), and of the neurological state, with regard to the changes previously reported following the administration of polypeptide antibiotics (peribuccal dysaesthesia, vertigo and muscular hypotonus).

RESULTS

1. CURE

Thirty one patients were cured of their infection. This result was the more remarkable in that this group includes fifteen cases of septicaemia, in patients who were in many cases old or debilitated by a preceding general infection or a recent surgical operation, or who were submitted to assisted respiration.

2. FAILURE

These deserve further details :

a) They were due in 3 cases to resistance of the organisms to the antibiotic:

- one case of urinary infection due to enterobacter aerogenes.
- one case of urinary infection due to klebsiella, in a patient suffering from ureteric stone.
- one case of endocarditis on a Bjork aortic valve, due to p. aeruginosa.

b) There was a change in organism in three cases : these were cases of urinary infection, two due to E. coli and one to pseudomonas aeruginosa, in whom a resistant organism was found after treatment with P.M.S.A. : streptococcus, staphylococcus and providencia respectively.

c) The failure of treatment was due in two cases to a functional disturbance (cirrhosis of the liver) or to an organic lesion (urinary stone).

d) The injections were painful in one case, and treatment had to be discontinued on the 5th day.

3. TOLERANCE

a) In general, local tolerance was good. Pain at the injection site necessitated the discontinuance of treatment in one case only.

b) Renal impairment developed in five patients (a rise in the blood urea, and in one case a fall in the serum potassium). This disappeared in the three weeks following the discontinuance of treatment. It should be pointed out that the dose was high in two cases (40,000 to 60,000 U/Kg), that P.M.S.A. was given together with an aminoside in two cases, and that three of the patients were aged over 70. Renal biopsy showed tubular necrosis and interstitial oedema in one. Reduced doses (4,000 ; 7,000 and 12,000 U/Kg/day respectively) were used in three cases of overt renal insufficiency, without any worsening of the renal impairment.

c) Neuropsychic tolerance was excellent. Only one patient experienced malaise at the time of injection, but there were no objective neurological manifestations.

TABLE I - <u>SELECTION OF PATIENTS</u>

- 40 patients (20 female, 20 male)
- Age : between 15 and 83 years
      Mean age : 47 years.
- Urinary Infection : 24 cases (Bacteriuria $\geqslant 1 \times 10^5$/ml)
- Septicaemia : 16 cases.

TABLE II - <u>ORGANISMS RESPONSIBLE</u>

- Escherichia coli   16 cases (4 of septicaemia)
- Enterobacter cloacae   7 cases (4 of septicaemia)
- Enterobacter aerogenes   1 case
- Klebsiella   7 cases (4 of septicaemia)
- Pseudomonas aeruginosa   8 cases (3 of septicaemia)
- Septicaemia due to multiple gram - organisms   1 case

TABLE III - <u>ADMINISTRATION OF PRODUCT</u>

- Route of Administration
  I.M.   37 cases
  I.V.   3 cases

- Daily Dose
  Normal renal function 20,000 to 30,000 U/Kg/day
  Renal insufficiency (3 cases) 4,000 U/Kg/day

- P.M.S.A. given alone   28 cases

- P.M.S.A. given together with
  Gentamycin   8 cases
  Tobramycin   2 cases
  Carbenicillin   2 cases

- Duration of Treatment
  Between 4 and 20 days.
  Mean duration of treatment : 10 days.

TABLE IV - <u>CRITERIA OF EFFECTIVENESS</u>

- Clinical criteria :
  Pyrexia
  Functional signs
  Local signs

- Bacteriological criteria :
  Blood culture
  Cytobacteriology of urine.

TABLE V - <u>CRITERIA OF TOLERANCE</u>

- Cutaneous tolerance :
  Allergic manifestations
  Pain at injection site.

- Renal tolerance :
  Urea
  Serum Potassium
  Serum creatinine

- Neuropsychic tolerance :
  Peribuccal dysaesthesia
  Vertigo
  Muscular hypotonus
  Hyporeflexia

TABLE VI - <u>OVERALL RESULTS</u>

- Cure   31 cases (15 of septicaemia)
- Failure
  . Resistance of organism to antibiotic (Klebsiella)
                                                   3 cases
  . Change in organism   3 cases
  . Functional or organic lesion   2 cases
  . Local intolerance   1 case

TABLE VII - <u>GENERAL TOLERANCE</u>

- Pain at injection site leading to discontinuance of
  treatment   1 case
- Rise in blood urea   5 cases
- Sensation of general malaise   1 case

TABLE VIII - <u>RENAL TOLERANCE</u>

1. <u>Renal function previously normal (37 patients)</u>
   - Development of renal impairment   5 cases
     . high dosage   2 cases
     . P.M.S.A. given together with
       an aminoside   2 cases
     . patient aged over 70 years   3 cases

   - Recovery in all cases in three weeks.

2. <u>Pre-existing renal insufficiency (3 patients)</u>
   - Low dosage
   - No deterioration in renal function.

STUDIES ON ENDOTOXIN SHOCK

S. Ishiyama, I. Nakayama, H. Iwamoto, S. Iwai,
T. Kawabe, I. Murata
Department of Surgery, Nihon University School of
Medicine
8, 1-chome, Kandasurugadai, Chiyoda-ku, Tokyo, Japan

We observed 68 cases of septic shock, in the past 10 years. The diagnosis of these shock cases were determined by the criteria of Baue's triad.

Our experimental study on the endotoxin shock, which was performed with the purpose of investigating the pathogenesis of septic shock through endotoxin.

Materials and Methods

The healthy Sprague-Dawley male rats weighing about 200g were used in all our experiments. We used the DIFCO endotoxin prepared from Escherichia coli 0127 : B8. 5mg per kg of endotoxin was intravenously injected to each rat. Blood was drawn from inferior vena cava. Endotoxin in the rats plasma was assayed by Levin's chloroform method (Limulus Test). As to the coagulation factors; Prothrombin was measured by Owren's method. Fibrinogen was made by Sharp's method. V, VIII, IX and VII-X complex factors were measured, using free plasma. Serum histamine was analyzed by the Shore's method using clumn chromatography. Blood serotonin was assayed by Bogdanski's fluometric method.

Serum GOT and GPT, alkali phosphatase, glucose and cholesterol were measured with a Rapid Blood Analyzer. Serum transaminase was made by Reitman-Frankel method. Alkali and acid-phosphatase were measured by modified Kind-King method. Glucose was made by o-toluidine borate method. Cholesterol was measured by Zurkowski's method. Acid phosphatase in the lysosomes of the liver cells was studied with histochemical electronmicroscopy. It was performed by means of Barka's method.

The endotoxin clearance of normal rat after receiving endotoxin was measured with the Limulus Test. (Figure 1). It was dis-
closed in concentrations of 1.0 μg/ml during the first one hour
and rapidly decreased from 1.0 to 0.01 μg/ml for a period of 6
hours and it increased up to 0.1 μg/ml at the 7 and 8 hours levels
and decreased very slowly for a total 42 hour period after administration.

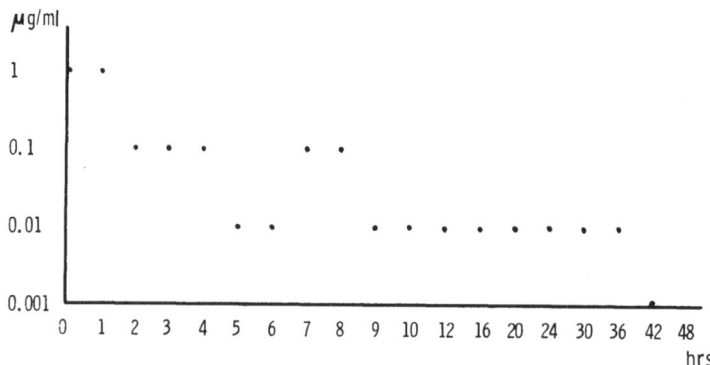

Figure 1.   Plasma Endotoxin Concentration

Effects on coagulation system was studied with a thrombelastgram. Each coagulation factor was measured after injection
of endotoxin. The reaction time was shortened and indicated the
hypercoagulability at the end of 2 hours after and in the contrast,
the reaction time was prolonged at 4 and 6 hours after endotoxin
administration. The coagulation velocity follows the reaction
time in its pattern. The maximum amplitude of the thrombelastgram continuously decreased in its width, from the onset, to the
end of reaction. The maximum elasticity accordingly decreased
continuously during the 6 hours after administration (Table 1).

Table 1.   Influences of Endotoxin to Rat's Thrombelastgram

			control	2 hrs	4 hrs	6 hrs
r:	reaction time	(min)	5.2	4.1	5.3	6.1
k:	coagulation velocity	(min)	2.1	2.4	4.1	2.9
ma:	maximal amplitude	(mm)	72.8	69.0	55.8	52.2
me:	maximal elasticity	(%)	272.3	223.0	133.8	115.8

   Fibrinogen slowly decreased during the 6 hour period, and it
showed 62%, 6 hours after administration. Prothrombin, IX, VII-X
complex factors also dropped until the end of 6 hours. Factor V
decreased during the first 4 hours and it recovered slightly.
Factor VIII rapidly decreased during the first 2 hours, it have a
value of 17%, and it continued for the 6 hours period. (Figure 2).

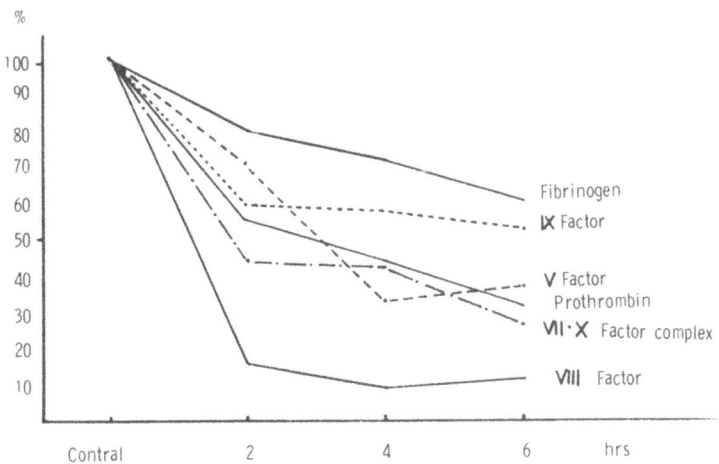

Figure 2.   Influences of Endotoxin to Rat's Coagulation Factor

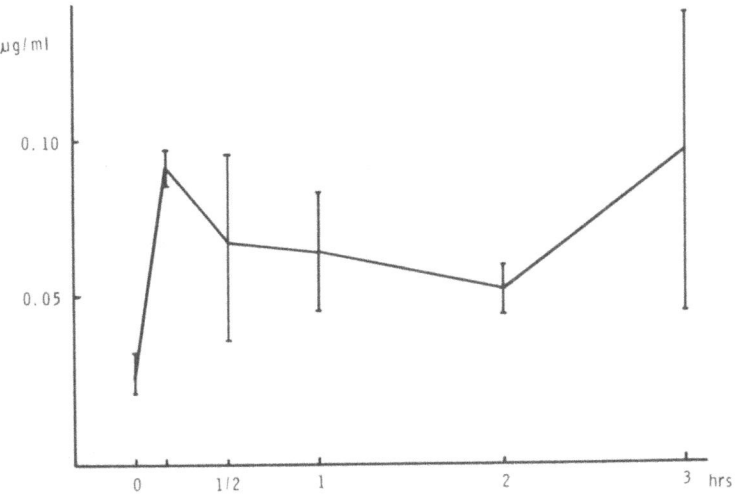

Figure 3.   Concentration of Histamine in Serum

Chemical mediators played important role on shock and they were assayed after initiation of endotoxin. Serum histamine concentration rapidly rose during the first 10 minutes and gradually dropped 2 hour period, but rose again later (Figure 3).

The rapid injection of endotoxin produced a sudden fall of the blood serotonin levels. They recovered rapidly during a one hour period and decreased again gradually (Figure 4).

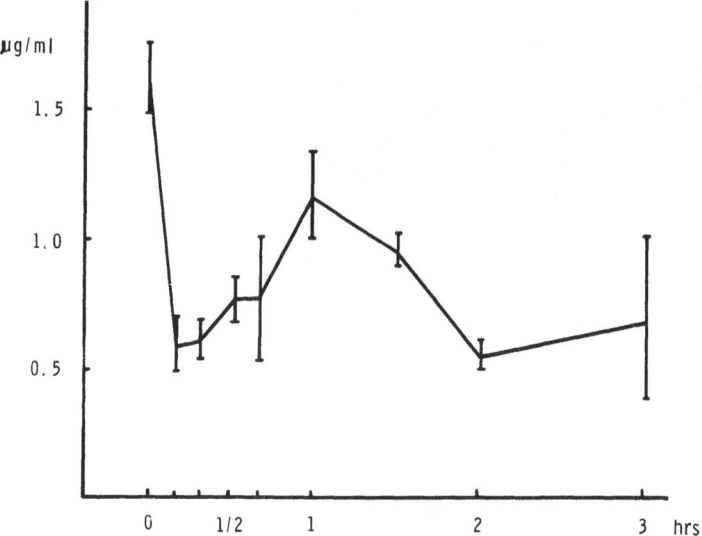

Figure 4.   Blood Concentration of Serotonin

Endotoxin influences the cells and metabolism. Changes of enzymes, glucose and cholesterol were studied after endotoxin injection. Serum GOT and GPT continuously increased after injection. Alkali phosphatase evidenced the peak value of 49 KAU at 2 hours, gradually decreased for a period of 6 hours, and increased again gradually. Acid phosphatase markedly rose within the first two hours and it quickly dropped afterward until it showed the normal value at 8 hours after injection. Serum glucose rapidly rose to the level of 293 mg/dl during the first one hour (hyperglycemia) and decreased quickly by the end of 2 hours follow by hypoglycemia at 4-8 hours after administration. Serum cholesterol showed the level of 71 mg/dl in normal rats. It gradually rose to the concentration of 94 mg/dl during a 6 hour period and dropped later. (Figure 5)

Electronmicrospic histochemically, in normal rats, the contour of the lysosomes was round and well maintained. Acid phosphatase activity was not activated. At one hour after administration, lysosomes were destroyed and the acid phosphatase activity elevated as it was released into the cells.

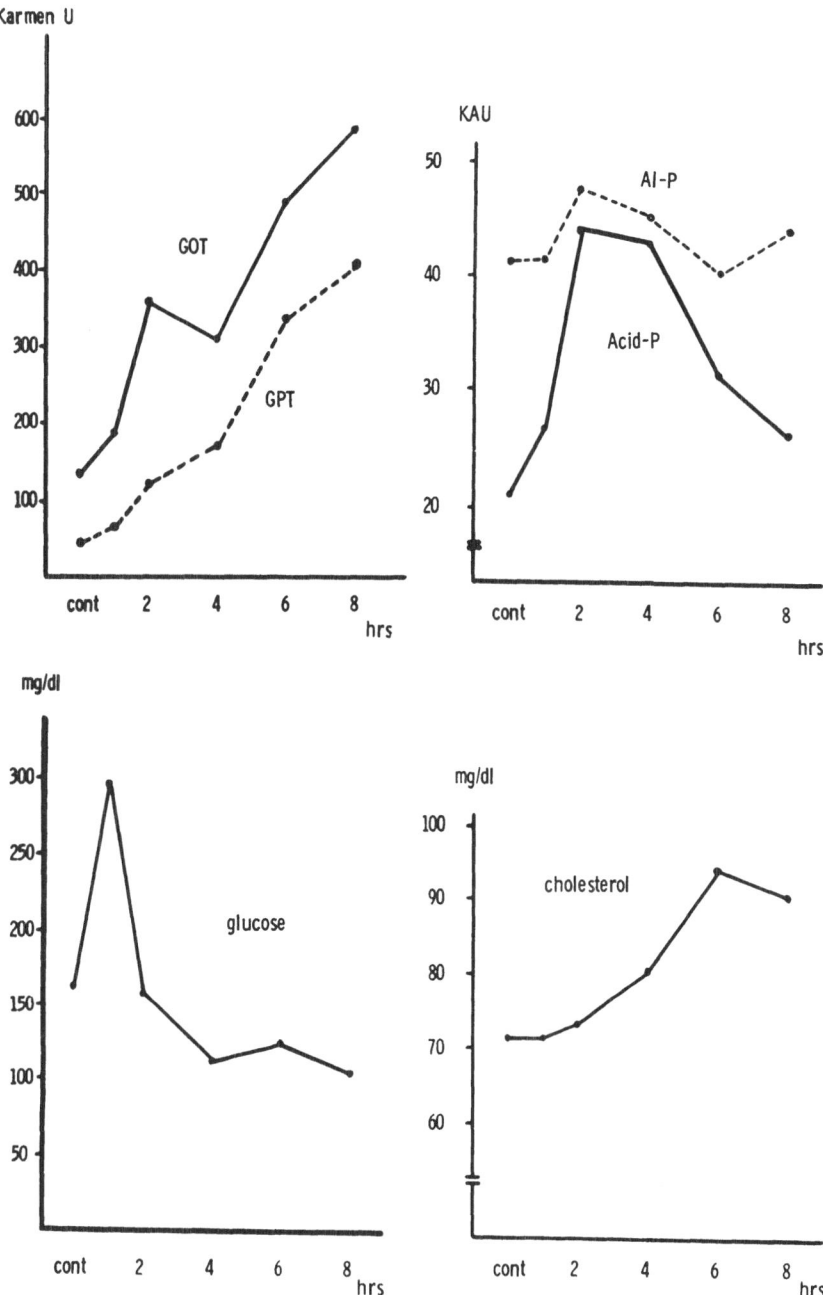

Figure 5.   Changes in Rat's Serum by Intra-Venous Administration

IN SUMMARY

1. Plasma endotoxin was detectable for a total of 42 hours after administration.
2. Hypercoagulability was seen in early stages and hypocoagulability occured in later stages.
3. Serum histamine increased and blood serotonin decreased immediately following endotoxin administration.
4. Serum transaminase, glucose, acid phosphatase and cholesterol evidenced remarkable changes.
5. Activity and release of acid phosphatase by lysosomes was studied with histochemical electron microscopy

LITERATURE

1) Baue A.E.: The treatment of septic shock : A problem intensifiedby advancing science, Surgery 65 : 850, 1969.
2) Levin J., et al : Detection of endotoxin in human blood and demonstration of an inhibitor, J. Lab. Clin. Med. 75 : 903, 1970.
3) Hinshaw L. B., et al : Prevention of death in endotoxin shock by glucose adminstration, S. G. O. 139 : 851, 1974.
4) Boler R. K., et al : An Electron Microscopic Study of the Liver of Endotoxin-Shocked Dogs Treated with a Combination of Propiomazine and Levarterenol, Lab. Invest. 20 : 319, 1969.

CEREBROSPINAL FLUID LACTATE DETERMINATION: A NEW PARAMETER FOR THE DIAGNOSIS OF ACUTE AND PARTIALLY TREATED MENINGITIS

G. Controni, W.J. Rodriguez, C.A. Deane, J.M. Hicks &
S. Ross

Children's Hospital National Medical Center, Washington
D.C. 20009 and George Washington School of Medicine
Washington, D.C.

SUMMARY

The lactic acid level in the cerebrospinal fluid of 250
patients with or without bacterial involvement was determined
using Gas Liquid Chromatography (GLC). This recently rediscovered
technique proved effective and reliable in distinguishing between
bacterial (21 cases) and non bacterial (179 cases) meningitis.
There were no false positives nor false negatives in either category. Partially treated meningitis had elevated CSF lactate on
admission. The duration of elevated CSF lactate correlated with
the clinical response to therapy. This simple and rapid technique
warrants further evaluation as a parameter to detect bacterial
central nervous system invasion.

INTRODUCTION

Purulent meningitis occurs quite frequently in children under
5 years of age; Lewin, 1974, reported that 18,000 cases are reported annually in the United States. From 45 to 50% of these patients
had received some form of antimicrobial therapy preceding the
initial lumbar puncture for the diagnosis of the disease. Such
prior antibiotic therapy often brings a drastic decrease in the
positivity of some diagnostic tests for bacterial meningitis.
This obviously makes the diagnosis of bacterial meningitis difficult.

Levinson, in 1917 demonstrated that bacterial meningitis
results in a depression of spinal fluid pH. Nishimura, in 1924
reported that the lactate content of cerebrospinal fluid (CSF) is

elevated in bacterial meningitis. This observation was confirmed
by Mollaret and Pocidallo in 1964. Since a report of Sudre and
Reiss in 1969, this finding of an increased lactate content of CSF
has been used to attempt a differentiation of viral from bacterial
or tuberculous meningitis. Previous measurements of lactate were
performed using an enzymatic spectrophotometric method. (Bland,
et al, 1974) (Sudre & Reiss, 1969)

The GLC is an extremely sensitive technique, capable of
separating and detecting many of the acids of the Kreb's Cycle,
even at the nanogram level. Acids, such as lactic acid, that are
not detected by GLC can be methylated to render them volatile and
therefore detectable by this method. The study that is described
here was undertaken to determine if gas chromatography can evaluate therapeutic efficiency of antibiotics in bacterial meningitis
by analysis of CSF lactate content during different stages of
therapy.

MATERIALS AND METHODS

One hundred and seventy nine spinal fluid specimens were
tested from patients whose spinal fluids showed a normal cell count,
a negative bacterial culture and normal protein and glucose values.
The majority of these samples were taken from patients suspected
of having bacterial meningitis or to rule out this condition. CSF
specimens from twenty one patients with proven bacterial meningitis
by culture were also tested for lactate levels at different stages
of antimicrobial therapy.

One ml portions of CSF were acidified with 0.2 ml of 50%
sulfuric acid as soon as they were received in the laboratory.
The specimen was well mixed and refrigerated to inhibit cellular
metabolism. Prior to analysis, 1 ml of methanol was added to the
mixture which was then placed in a 100°C temperature block for
5 minutes. After the incubation period and when the sample was
cold, 0.5 ml of chloroform was added and mixed by gentle inversion
20 times. The chloroform layer was drawn into a Hamilton syringe
and 14 uL were injected into the gas chromatograph column.

All the studies were performed on a Capco-Dohrman gas chromatograph equipped with a thermal conductivity detector and a strip
chart recorder of 1 millivolt sensitivity. A 1/4 inch by 6 feet
stainless steel column, packed with 15% CPE 2225 on chromosorb
A/AW, 45/60 mesh was used. The detector and column temperatures
were maintained at 120°C. The injection port temperature was
held at 145°C. The detector current was set at 85 milliamperes
with 1 X attenuation. The carrier gas was helium at a flow rate
of 120 ml/minute. A lactate standard was run at the same time as
the specimens. The peaks obtained from the CSF samples were

identified as lactic acid if they had a retention time equal to
that of the lactate standard. Quantitation was made by referring
to the standard curve.

RESULTS

Figure I illustrates a typical chromatogram obtained from
the CSF of a patient with H. influenzae meningitis and a chromatogram from the CSF of a patient having no bacterial involvement.
The figure also illustrates a chromatogram of the 30 mg/100 ml
lactate standard.

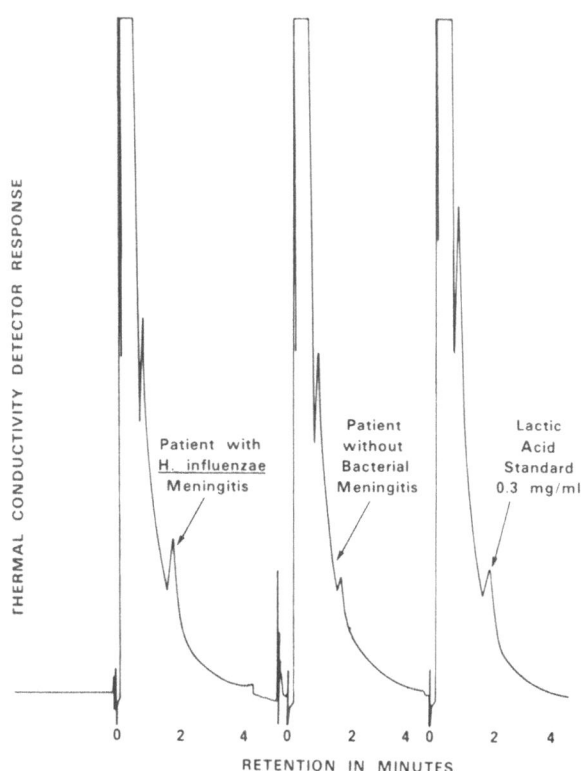

Figure I – Lactic Acid Determination in Spinal Fluid

Figure II illustrates a standard curve of peak heights from
chloroform extracts plotted against series of know concentrations
of methylated lactate in distilled water. Peak heights bear a
linear relationship to the concentration of lactate.

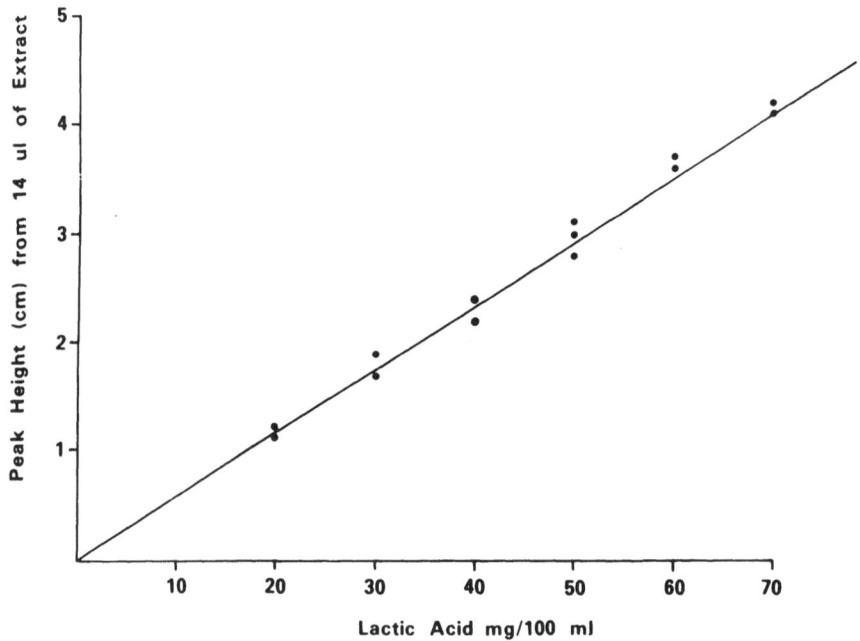

Figure II – Lactic Acid Standard Curve

All the patients with bacteriologically proven meningitis
yielded consistently high lactate levels. Past studies indicate
that the normal range of CSF lactate is less than 20 mg/100 ml.

Twelve of the children with bacterial meningitis were infected with H. influenzae, Type B, four with Beta Hemolytic Streptococcus Group B, one adult and two children had Streptococcus
pneumoniae meningitis and another adult had a Klebsiella meningitis. One child had a Listeria meningitis. The approximate
distribution of the spinal fluid lactate levels from these patients
are shown in Figure III.

All the patients with meningitis, including five which had
been pre-treated, had elevated lactate levels while the spinal
fluids from the 179 patients with no bacterial meningitis showed
lactate levels that were within normal limits.

The typical lactate changes seen during the course of effective therapy in bacterial meningitis are shown in Figure IV. The

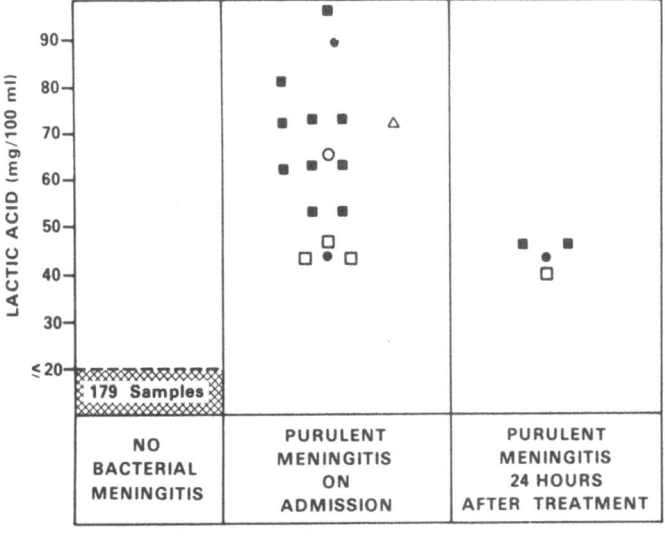

H. influenzae
Beta Streptococcus Gr. B
Klebsiella pneumoniae
Streptococcus pneumoniae
Listeria monocytogenes

Figure III - Concentration of Lactic Acid in Cerebrospinal Fluid

specimen was taken from a 13 month old white female that had been
pre-treated with 1 dose of penicillin and erythromycin three times
a day for 8 days, one week prior to admission. The patient was
admitted to the Infectious Disease Ward with a temperature of
105°F and a history of a few episodes of vomiting, diarrhea and
anorexia. Interestingly, her spinal fluid glucose value was
within normal limits. The gram stain did not reveal any organisms,
but the spinal fluid culture grew H. influenzae, Type B. The
spinal fluid protein was moderately elevated and the LDH value
was not consistent with bacterial meningitis. By the first day
of therapy, the lactate level was still elevated but had declined
dramatically and the glucose value remained normal while the
protein concentration was decreasing. On the third day of carbenicillin therapy, the spinal fluid lactate level of this patient
was responding clinically to therapy. She had become afebrile
and was tolerating liquids well.

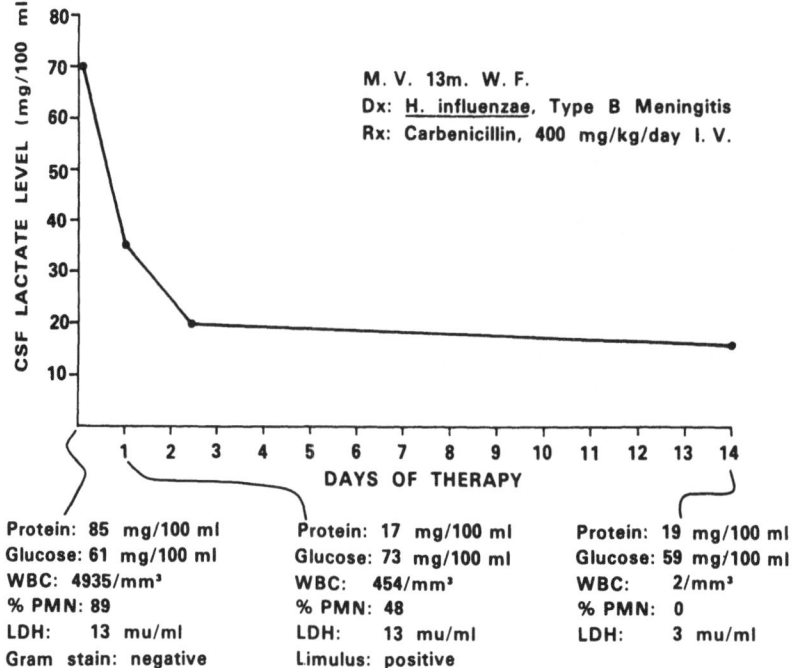

M. V. 13m. W. F.
Dx: <u>H. influenzae</u>, Type B Meningitis
Rx: Carbenicillin, 400 mg/kg/day I. V.

Protein: 85 mg/100 ml	Protein: 17 mg/100 ml	Protein: 19 mg/100 ml
Glucose: 61 mg/100 ml	Glucose: 73 mg/100 ml	Glucose: 59 mg/100 ml
WBC: 4935/mm³	WBC: 454/mm³	WBC: 2/mm³
% PMN: 89	% PMN: 48	% PMN: 0
LDH: 13 mu/ml	LDH: 13 mu/ml	LDH: 3 mu/ml
Gram stain: negative	Limulus: positive	

Figure IV – CSF Lactate Changes During Therapy

In another patient with <u>Streptococcus pneumoniae</u> meningitis, who was admitted in a semi-comatose condition and seizing with left hemiparesis, the CSF lactate remained elevated for several days. This patient had repeated taps for subdural effusions and maintained an intermittent fever until the 8th day. The CSF lactate remained elevated until the 8th day of treatment when it dropped to a normal level. After this time, the patient was well clinically and remained afebrile and was very active.

The results in Figure V show some examples that the value of spinal fluid lactate as determined by GLC is a useful parameter to detect meningitis. It detected all the meningitis cases caused by gram positive and gram negative bacteria. The Limulus test was, however, only able to detect thirteen out of twenty-one cases. Since gram positive bacterial do not possess endotoxins, the gram stain did not detect any bacteria in four pre-treated cases. One definite advantage of the lactate test over the Limulus test and gram stain has been that it has not failed to detect a partially treated or purulent meningitis; likewise, a negative result has had a total correlation with the absence of bacterial meningitis. Neither a negative Limulus nor gram stain, on the other hand, definitely precludes this possibility of non bacterial involvement.

No. of Patients	Organism	Number Positive by Indicated Test		
		GLC Lactate	Limulus Lysate	Gram Stain
3	S. pneumoniae	3	0	2
12	H. influenzae, type B	12	12	9
4	Streptococcus Gr. B	4	0	4
1	K. pneumoniae	1	1	1
1	L. monocytogenes	1	0	1
179	No bacterial growth	0	0	0

Figure 5 - Comparison of Methods for the Detection of Bacterial Meningitis

DISCUSSION

These studies have demonstrated that spinal fluid lactate levels rise significantly in bacterial meningitis and return slowly to normal levels during the course of effective therapy. Stone, as early as 1908, demonstrated that the brain and blood can maintain independent lactate concentrations. The slow clearance of lactate from the spinal fluid as demonstrated by Prockop, 1968, offers a reasonable explanation for the persistent lactate elevation in partially treated patients when the glucose has often returned to normal levels.

Our studies also demonstrate that in bacterial meningitis, lactate levels have a direct relationship to the response of antimicrobial treatment. In partially treated patients suspected of having bacterial meningitis, an elevated CSF lactate level strongly suggests an attenuated bacterial meningitis. The most likely mechanism of elevated CSF lactate concentrations in bacterial meningitis was postulated to be due to hypoxia of the brain induced by increased intracranial pressures with a resultant reduction of cerebral blood flow and incomplete oxygenation of glucose as shown by Kopetsky, et al, 1933, and Plum in 1907. Paulson, in 1972, demonstrated that in acute pyogenic meningitis, the cerebral blood flow is greatly reduced. In mammalian tissues, excess lactate is related to bothe glycolysis and tissue hypoxia.

CONCLUSION

This study demonstrates that lactate levels at different stages of antimicrobial therapy offer a useful parameter to evaluate drug therapy in meningitis. The rapid diagnosis and effective

therapeutic management of meningitis by the GLC lactate test
appears to be both a practical and useful procedure.

BIBLIOGRAPHY

1. Bland, R.D., Lister, R.C. and Ries, J.P. (1974), American
    Journal of Diseases of Children, 128, 151.

2. Kopetsky, S.J. and Fishberg, E.H. (1933), Journal of Labora-
    tory and Clinical Medicine, 18, 796.

3. Levinson, A. (1917), Journal of Infectious Diseases, 21, 556.

4. Lewin, E.B. (1974), American Journal of Diseases of Children,
    128, 145.

5. Mollaret, P., Pocidalo, J.J., Gaudebaut, C., Blayo, M.C.,
    Vachon, F. and Vic-Dupont(1966), Bulletins et Memoires da la
    Societe Medicale des Hopitaux de Paris, 11, 117.

6. Nishimura, K. (1924), Proceedings of the Society for Experi-
    mental Biology and Medicine, 21, 556.

7. Paulson, O.B., Hansen, E.L., Kristensen, H.S., Brodersen, P.
    (1972), Acta Neurologica Scandinavica, 48, 407.

8. Plum, F. and Posner, J.B. (1967), American Journal of
    Physiology, 212, 864.

9. Prockop, L.D. (1968), Neurology, 18, 189.

10. Stone, W.E. (1938), Biochemical Journal, 32, 1908.

11. Sudre, Y. and Reiss, D. (1969), Bordeaux Medical, 10, 2045.

MONITORING OF BLOOD CULTURE COMPARING INTENSIVE CARE PATIENTS WITH AND WITHOUT ANITBIOTIC PROPHYLAXIS

H.Pichler[1], F.Lackner[2], W.Haider[2], G.Krystof[2], M.Rotter[3], G.Wewalka[3], H.Bankl[4]
Chair of Chemotherapy[1], Intensive Care Unit of the Institute of Anaesthesiology[2], Hygiene-Institute[3] and the Institute of Pathology[4] of Vienna University, Austria Spitalgasse 23, A - 1090 Wien

Severe bacterial infection resulting into septicemia is one of the most life threatening complications we are facing in intensive care (2,). Previous studies have established that antibiotic prophylaxis in a compromised host has lead to an increase of infectious pulmonary complications and has neither been able to influence septicemia nor mortality rate (1,3,). However firstly the nature of groups studied then is not corresponding to the mainly traumatically injured respectively postoperative patients we have dealt with and secondly both dosage and choice of antibiotics given prophylactically are different from our concept calling for high dose administration of combinations of bactericidal compounds in immunologically impaired critical care patients (4). Therefore the aim of our study was to evaluate antibiotic prophylaxis prospectively with regard to the incidence of septicemia and bacterial complications.

132 patients of a non specialized intensive care unit, who upon admission had no symptoms of bacterial infection were at random divided into two groups. Group I received antibiotic prophylaxis immediately after admission with high dose penicillin combinations respectively in case of penicillin allergy, inflammatory, degenerative or traumatic cerebrospinal diseases cephalosporines if necessary supplemented by aminoglycosides. Group II had no antibiotic prophylaxis upon admission. Antibiotic therapy was administered only in case of proved or suspected bacterial infection in course of intensive care.

Routinely patients had a superior vena cava and an indwelling urinary catheter, if necessary an endotracheal tube was put in place.

In all patients the following bacteriological monitoring was performed: blood cultures were drawn whenever the basal temperature exceeded 38,5°C however if this did not occur, they were studied at least once a day for a period of seven consecutive days. Later on blood was only sampled for culture if the temperature exceeded 38,5°C. Every patient was thus observed for the length of his stay in the intensive care unit. Simmultaneously a quantitative and qualitative sampling of urine was carried out. Later on urine cultures were checked once a week or whenever there was evidence of urinary infection. Whenever bacterial counting in the urine revealed a significant number of urinary pathogens the bladder was irrigated with a solution containing gentamycin (80mg/l) and amphotericin B (50mg/l) twice daily. Pharyngeal respectively endotracheal swabs were investigated bacteriologically upon admission and during the stay at least three times weekly. In case of death it was attempted to obtain a detailed post mortem study including bacteriological and histological results.

Our criteria for septicemia apart from the typical clinical picture were either at least two isolations of the same bacteria with identical pattern of susceptibility or the proof of the same pathogen with identical susceptibility out of the blood plus another sample of the patients body.

The diagnoses of 132 patients studied are shown in table one. Age varied from 6 to 84 years (median 48 years). 74 (56%) patients were males and 58 (44%) were females. The median value of the duration of stay was seven days.

Table 1 Diagnoses of 132 Patients Studied

INTENSIVE CARE FOR	N = 132
POLYTRAUMA	46 (35 %)
DRUG INTOXICATION	33 (25 %)
COMPLICATED SURGERY	18 (14 %)
BLEEDING OESOPHAGEAL VARICES	15 (11 %)
CEREBROSPINAL DISEASES	11 (8 %)
VARIOUS DISORDERS	9 (7 %)

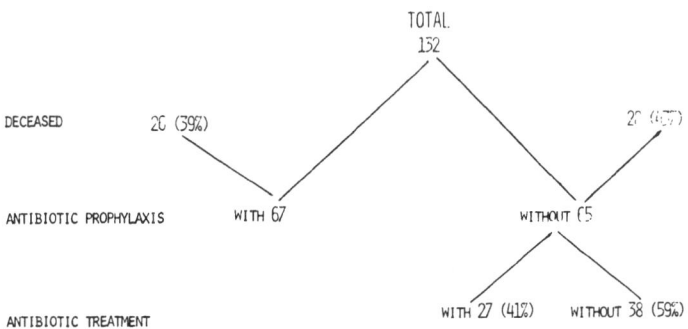

Fig. 1. Fate of 132 Patients Studied

Fig. 1 shows the fate of the patients studied at the intensive care unit itself. It is obvious that the mortality rate shows no significant difference in patients receiving antibiotic prophylaxis as compared to those without antibiotic prophylaxis. In 27 (41%) out of 65 patients without antibiotic prophylaxis antibiotic treatment had been supplied due to clinical, radiological or bacterial evidence of infection.

Table 2 Incidence, Day of Onset and Mortality of 30 Patients with Septicemia

PATIENTS	INCIDENCE OF SEPTICEMIA	DAY OF ONSET	MORTALITY
WITH ANTIBIOTIC PROPHY- LAXIS (N = 67)	9 (13%)	6	8 (89%)
WITHOUT ANTIBIOTIC PRO- PHYLAXIS (N = 65)	21 (32%)	4	17 (81%)

The overall rate of septicemia was 23 % (Table 2). 9 patients with antibiotic prophylaxis as opposed to 21 patients (p $<$ 0,05) without antibiotic prophylaxis acquired septicemia, with the onset on the 6th day in the group receiving antibiotic prophylaxis respectively on the 4th day in the group without. There was no difference in the mortality rate of septicemic patients in both groups.

Table 3   Organisms Causing Septicemia and their Susceptibility to Antibiotics in 9 out of 67 Patients with Antibiotic Prophylaxis

BACTERIA	NUMBER OF STRAINS	P	OXA	A	CARB	CEPH	G	CHLORO
KLEBSIELLA AERUG.	4	--	--	--	--	1	4	1
KLEBSIELLA PNEUMONIAE	1	--	--	--	--	1	1	1
E.COLI	1	--	--	--	--	--	1	--
CITROBACTER	1	--	--	--	1	1	1	1
PROTEUS MIRABILIS	1	--	--	--	--	--	1	--
PSEUDOMONAS AERUG.	1	--	--	--	1	--	1	--
SERRATIA LIQUEFACIENS	1	--	--	--	--	--	1	--

The organisms causing septicemia and their susceptibility to anti-biotics are enlisted in Table 3. It is obvious that all bacteria causing septicemia in patients with antibiotic prophylaxis do be-long to the family of enterobacteriaceae or pseudomonaceae. In one case a mixed infection with pseudomonas aerug. and klebsiella aerug. was found. All strains were resistant to the antibiotics administe-red routinely. Only to gentamycin all strains were susceptible.

Opposed to this the pattern of organisms causing septicemia in patients without antibiotic prophylaxis is quite different. Table 4 shows that in more than 50 % gram positive strains were respon-sible for septicemia namely 11 times staph.aureus and once entero-coccus. Nearly all those strains were sensitive to the antibiotics tested. The pattern of gram negative organisms and their suscepti-bility to antibiotics shows no difference in both groups. After appropriate therapy of staph.aureus respectively pseudomonas aerug. superinfection with pseudomonas aerug. respectively candida was observed in two patients.

Table 4   Organisms Causing Septicemia and their Susceptibility to Antiobiotics in 21 out of 65 Patients without Antibiotic Prophylaxis

BACTERIA	NUMBER OF STRAINS	P	OXA	A	CARB	CEPH	G	CHLORO
STAPH.AUREUS	11	9	11	9	9	11	11	11
ENTEROCOCCUS	1	1	--	1	1	--	--	1
E.COLI	2	2	--	2	2	2	2	2
KLEBS.AEROGENES	2	--	--	--	--	1	2	--
CITROBACTER	1	--	--	--	--	--	1	--
PROTEUS MIRABILIS	1	--	--	--	--	--	1	1
KLEBS.PNEUMONIAE	1	--	--	--	--	1	1	1
KLEBS.OXYTOCA	1	--	--	--	1	1	1	1
ENTEROBACTER CLOACAE	1	--	--	1	1	--	1	1
PSEUDOMONAS AERUG.	1	--	--	--	1	--	1	--
CANDIDA	1							

In Table 5 the attempt was made to investigate the apparent portal of entry in 30 patients with septicemia. In 12 (40%) patients the pulmonary system and in 3 (10%) patients the urinary tract were the source of infection. In another 3 (10%) cases osteomyelitis, septic thrombophlebitis, respectively wound abscess were the apparent source of septicemia. In 12 (40%) patients the origin of septicemia could not be identified.

Table 5   Apparent Source of Infection in 30 Patients with Septicemia

PULMONARY TRACT	12 (40%)
URINARY TRACT	3 (10%)
OSTEOMYELITIS	1 (3,3%)
SEPTIC THROMBOPHLEBITIS	1 (3,3%)
WOUND ABSCESS	1 (3,3%)
UNKNOWN	12 (40%)

Table 6 shows the results of post mortem study with respect to signs of bacterial infection. Here it can be seen that in 14 (54%) of 26 deceased patients with antibiotic prophylaxis the bacterial infection played an additional role for mortality as opposed to 22 (79%) of 28 deceased patients without antibiotic prophylaxis. The median periode of survival in deceased patients without bacterial infection irrespecitve wether they have prophylaxis or not was identical namely four days. Comparing the median survival time of patients classified as having died from the underlying condition (four days) respectively underlying disease plus bacterial infection (6-7 days) appears to be a distinct difference.

Table 6   Significance of Bacterial Infection in 54 Deceased Patients

DECEASED PATIENTS	UNDERLYING DISEASE	UNDERLYING DISEASE + BACTERIAL INFECTION
WITH ANTIBIOTIC PROPHYLAXIS (N=26)	12 (46%)	14 (54%)
WITHOUT ANTIBIOTIC PROPHYLAXIS (N=28)	6 (21%)	22 (79%)

Summarizing we may state that prophylaxis using high dose bactericidal antibiotics could reduce the rate of septicemia significantly in intensive care patients. It was clearly demonstrated that the predominant organisms causing septicemia in patients without prophylaxis was staph.aureus which has never been observed in the group which routinely had penicillin combinations. However it was evident that septicemia caused by gram negative organisms could not be favourably influenced by antibiotic prophylaxis.

References

1. Mc.Cabe, WR, Jackson CG: Gram-negative bacteremia. I.Etiology and ecology. Arch Intern Med 110:847-855, 1962
2. Manz, R., Feifel G, Drost R, Wendt S: Infektionsprobleme auf einer Intensivpflegestation, Der Anaesthesist, Bd. 19, Heft 3, 105-109, 1970
3. Petersdorf, RG, Curtin JA, Hoeprich PD, Peeler RN, Bennett IL: A Study of Antibiotic Prophylaxis in Unconscious Patients, The New Engl.J.of Med., Vol 257, No 21, 1001-1009, 1957
4. Spitzy KH: Antimikrobielle Chemotherapie mit besonderer Berücksichtigung der Sepsis, Intensivstation, -pflege, -therapie, 231-244, Georg Thieme Verlag, Stuttgart, 1972

GENTAMICIN IN ALLOARTHROPLASTIC OPERATIONS;

CLINICAL AND EXPERIMENTAL RESULTS

Wahlig, H., Dingeldein, E.

E. Merck, Medical Research, Dep. of Chemother.

61 Darmstadt, Frankfurter Str. 250, Germany

Operations of long duration, organ-transplants, and those where heterogenic material is implanted, all entail a particularly high risk of infection and consequent severe complications. The prophylactic use of ' antibiotics is therefore indicated in these situations.

Certain preconditions are important for antibiotic prophylaxis to be effective; these include that

1. Administration of the antibiotic should be started before or during operation so that high serum concentrations of the antibiotic are attained at the operation site;

2. The dose used should be sufficiently high;

3. The antibiotic used should be bactericidal and should possess a broad spectrum against common grampositive and gramnegative pathogenic bacteria.

The importance of sufficiently high levels of antibiotic at the site of operation has been demonstrated experimentally and the efficacy of antibiotic prophylaxis has been confirmed in various prospective double-blind clinical studies, and the aim of this study was therefore to obtain information on the antibiotic concentrations attainable in the area of the wound.

Table 1   Gentamicin concentration (ug/ml) in wound exudate after total hip replacement using Gentamicin Palacos R in 16 patients

Gentamicin in Palacos R		collection periods after operation		
		0 - 6 hours	6 - 24 hours	24 - 48 hours
1.25 %	mean	11.5	5.6	2.7
	range	1.9 - 16.4	0.65 - 11.4	0.1 - 6.2
2.5 %	mean	23.4	11.6	2.9
	range	10.8 - 49.8	2.4 - 22.8	1.2 - 5.5

An animal model was used first; the shaft of the canine femur was filled with gentamicin-Palacos$^{(R)}$R so that wound exudate could be collected from a cavity in the cement. Gentamicin concentrations in the exudate ranged between 1 and 54 µg/ml.
Koschmieder and Ritzerfeld described similar results using a modification of our technique in pigs.

Since the concentrations of antibiotic in the wound exudate provide information about the concentrations in the infection-endangered part of the operation area, the antibiotic concentrations in wound exudate and in serum of patients undergoing hip joint endoprosthesis surgery under parenteral prophylaxis with gentamicin[*] were determined, as well as the local application of gentamicin incorporated into the bone cement Palacos$^{(R)}$ R.

Ten patients were given 8o mg gentamicin i.m. concurrently with the induction of anaesthesia, and two further 8o mg injections at 12 hr intervals. Serum samples were obtained at the end of each exudate collection period, namely 4 and 6 hours after the first injection and 2 and 4 hours after the third injection.

The wound exudate was collected in fractions and specimens for the evaluation of gentamicin levels were drawn simultaneously with the blood specimens.

The results of this study are summarized in table 1 and show that gentamicin concentrations in the wound exudate were always less than the corresponding serum concentrations.
The higher concentration in wound exudate on the day of surgery, as compared with those observed the following day, are probably due to an additional amount of blood.
In a second group of 16 patients gentamicin was applied locally with the bone cement in total hip replacement. In 8 patients the gentamicin concentration in the cement was 1.25 %, and for the other 8 patients the gentamicin dose was 2.5 %.
Wound exudate was collected in fractions 6, 24, and 48 hours after implantation, together with blood samples drawn at the same time.

In table 2 mean gentamicin concentrations in wound

[*]Refobacin$^{(R)}$, E. Merck, Darmstadt

Table 2a   Gentamicin concentrations (ug/ml) in serum and wound exudate after injection of 80 mg in 10 patients

		time after injection of 80 mg Gentamicin i.m.					
		2 hours		4 hours		6 hours	
		serum	exudate	serum	exudate	serum	exudate
operation day	mean			1.26	0.85	0.67	0.51
	range			0.6-2.1	0.3-1.7	0.4-1.6	0.3-1.1
postoperative day	mean	1.81	0.34	0.96	0.51		
	range	1.1-3.1	0.2-0.5	0.6-1.9	0.2-1.0		

Table 2b   Amount of Gentamicin (mg) in wound exudate after total hip replacement

		collection periods after operation			
Gentamicin in Palacos R		0 - 6 hours	6 - 24 hours	24 - 48 hours	total
1.25%	mean	2.21	1.0	0.42	3.56
	range	0.37 - 4.1	0.01 - 2.28	0.01 - 1.40	1.08 - 4.69
2.5%	mean	6.45	1.9	0.23	8.49
	range	3.76 - 10.22	0.17 - 4.98	0.01 - 0.82	5.39 - 15.20

exudate are summarized. No gentamicin activity was
detectable in serum samples (the lowest level of gentamicin detectable with the technique used was o.o5
µg/ml), but the levels in wound exudate 6 hours after
application reached 11.5 µg/ml and ranged from 1.9 to
16.4 µg/ml when the concentration of gentamicin was
1.25 %. With the 2.5 % concentration the mean level
was 23.5 µg/ml, ranging from 1o.8 to 49.8 µg/ml.

Comparison between drug levels after either parenteral
or local gentamicin administration, show substantially
higher gentamicin concentrations in the wound exudate
of those patients who received gentamicin in the cement.
The high gentamicin levels in wound exudate following
this route of administration indicate high concentrations at the site of release of the antibiotic from
the cement, i.e. the interface between cement and
surrounding tissue.

Estimations of gentamicin concentration in human
tissues were made in 5 cases about 6 months after implantation of total hip prostheses using gentamicin-
Palacos$^{(R)}$R. Levels between 6 and 22 µg/g were found
close to the cement in callus, spongiosa and connec-
tive tissue samples and even in compacta gentamicin
concentrations ranged from o.3 to 1.4 µg/g.

High gentamicin concentrations in wound exudate and
tissues indicate that certainly at the time of operation and possibly for much longer all pathogenic bacteria sensitive to the drug should be inhibited.

LINCOMYCIN BONE CONCENTRATIONS DURING TOTAL HIP REPLACEMENT

R.L. PARSONS, J.P. BEAVIS, G.M. PADDOCK &
G.M. HOSSACK

Department of Clinical Pharmacology

Guy's Hospital Medical School. London. SE1.9RT

Introduction Empirical antibiotic regimes given during
total hip replacement (THR) are now widely used by most
orthopaedic units to reduce the incidence of postoperative
infections. In an elderly patient who has already under
gone one operation, an infection is a therapeutic disaster
since it requires a second operation to remove the prosthesis in a patient who is already debilitated, and
therefore at risk. Thus, it is of the utmost importance
that the antibiotics used are shown to provide adequate
concentrations in bone.

Subjects & methods 12 patients (7 males & 5 females)
mean age (58.83 ± 3.33 years) height (166.94 ± 3.23 cm)
and weight (69.15 ± 2.94 kg.) were studied. 10 patients
had osteoarthrosis of the hip joint and 2 had avascular
necrosis of the head of the femur.

The patients received an empirical regime of
parenteral lincomycin. 600 mg. was given by intramuscular
injection 6 hours before operation. This was followed by
an intravenous infusion (600 mg. given over 30 minutes)
at the time the head of the femur was being removed.
Postoperatively, lincomycin (600 mg. i.m. 12 hourly was
continued for up to 72 hours until removal of the drains.

Venous blood samples were collected prior to dosing,
immediately pre & postoperatively, after the lincomycin
infusion, and for up to 72 hours postoperatively.

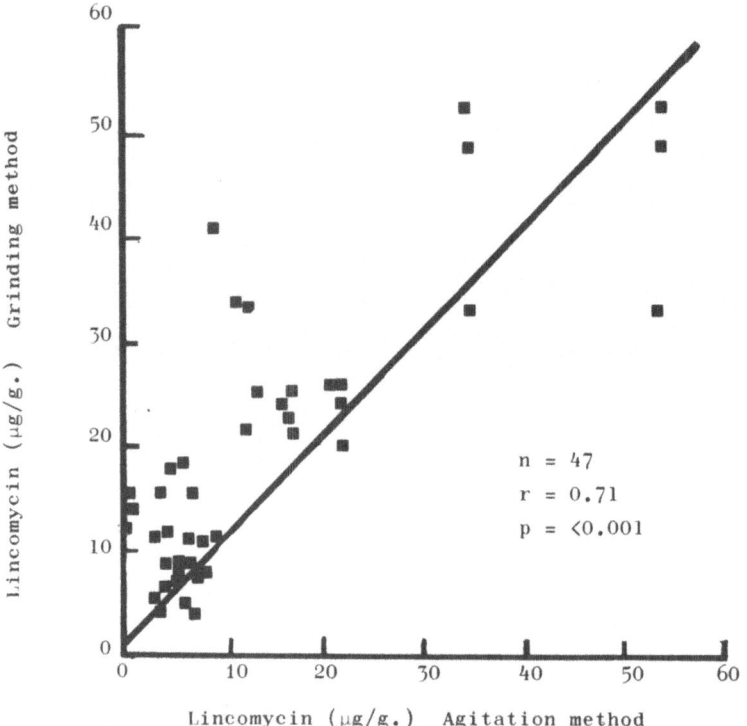

Figure 1:   Correlation between Assayed Concentration of
Lincomycin in Bone Estimated by Grinding and Agitation
Methods of Analysis.

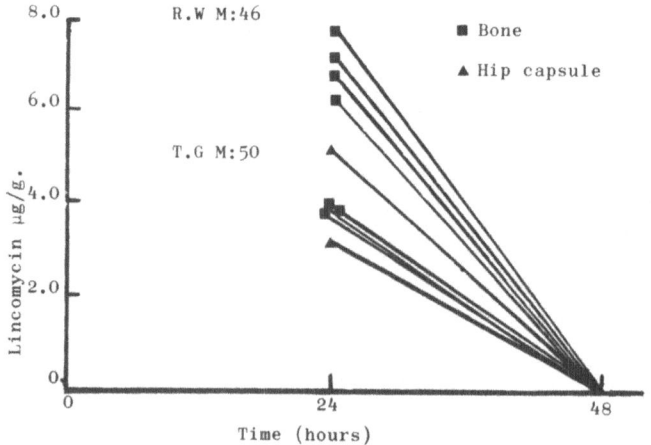

Figure 2:   Degree of Extraction of Lincomycin from Bone
and Hip Capsule.

Samples of cortical, cancellous & mixed cortical-cancellous bone, hip capsule and synovial fluid (when available) were collected during the operation prior to the lincomycin infusion.

The bone & capsule samples were agitated for up to 48 hours in a mixture of dipotassium hydrogen phosphate (16.7 g. L^{-1}) at pH 7.9. Adjacent samples of bone were ground into a paste with a pestle & mortar.

These samples were analysed for their lincomycin content by small plate microbiological assay(1). Standard concentrations of lincomycin hydrochloride solutions in the same phosphate buffer ranging from 8 > 0.25 µg/ml were used to plot a standard curve. This enabled the lower limit of the assay in the bone (using 4 ml of fluid for agitation and bone fragments weighing from 0.1<1.0 g.) to be as low as 0.5 µg/g.

Results The mean ($\pm$ SEM) plasma, bone, hip capsule, synovial fluid & drain fluid concentrations of lincomycin, together with the concentration range in the bone samples are given in the table.

The mean $\pm$ SEM plasma lincomycin ranged from 6.56 $\pm$ 0.86 µg/ml (preoperatively) to 58.7 $\pm$ 8.19 µg/ml (immediately postoperatively after the infusion). The concentrations of lincomycin in plasma, bone, hip capsule & drain fluid were almost all in excess of the M.I.C. of lincomycin against penicillinase producing Staph. aureus (2.8 µg/ml)(2), but there was individual variation in the concentration of lincomycin between samples of bone taken from adjacent sites.

We were concerned that the agitation method should accurately measure the concentrations of lincomycin in bone. Figure I shows that there was a good correlation (r = 0.71, P<0.001) between the estimated concentrations of lincomycin measured by the grinding method (ordinate) compared with those measured by the agitation of adjacent bone samples (abscissa).

We found by trial & error that the optimum period of agitation to obtain the maximum yield of lincomycin was 24 hours, no increase in the concentration in the agitation fluid occurring after this time. Agitation of the bone samples in fresh phosphate buffer for a further 24 hours also yielded no extra lincomycin. (Fig. 2).

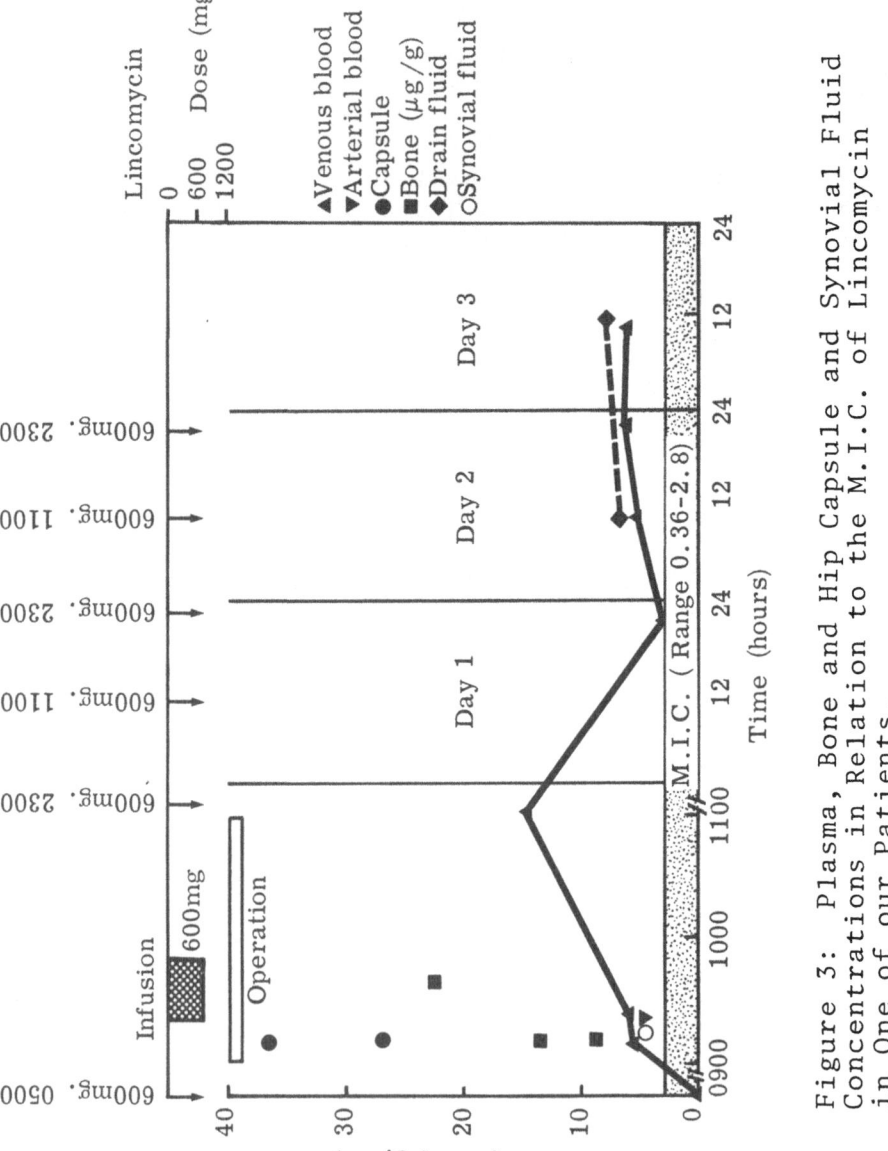

Figure 3: Plasma, Bone and Hip Capsule and Synovial Fluid Concentrations in Relation to the M.I.C. of Lincomycin in One of our Patients.

Table: Concentrations of Lincomycin in Plasma, Bone,
Joint capsule & postoperative drain fluid

Timing	Mean ± SEM plasma concentration
	μg/ml
Preoperative	6.56±0.86
Preinfusion	6.91±0.90
Postinfusion	58.67±8.19
Postoperative	13.36±1.50

Sampling site	n	Mean ±SEM	range (μg/g.)
Cancellous bone	30	8.90±1.91	(1.83-53.75)
Cancellous/cortical	8	8.58±2.44	(2.83-23.31)
Cortical	2	8.00±0.11	(7.89- 8.11)
Hip capsule	14	7.80±2.53	(0.2 -32.55)
Synovial fluid	3	5.43±3.51	(2.75- 8.11)

Timing	Mean ± SEM	PLASMA	DRAIN (μg/ml)
24 hour postop.		7.54±1.83	5.81±0.77
48 hour postop.		9.52±1.25	5.33±1.47

Discussion

An important analytical problem was to ensure that
the extraction of lincomycin from the bone samples had
been complete. Dissolving the bone into acid would have
enabled measurement of all the drug bound to bone. Since
this would inactivate lincomycin, it was not possible to
solve this problem by this method, we adopted an indirect
approach.

Fresh bone fragments were taken from patients who
had not previously been exposed to antibiotics. These
fragments were suspended in buffer solutions containing
the appropriate concentrations of lincomycin that had
previously been extracted from the patients' samples.
Since there was no change in the concentration of lincomycin in the buffer after agitation of these samples for
up to 48 hours, there was no indirect evidence of binding
sites for lincomycin remaining within the bone.

Thus, the good correlation between the two analytical
methods, with a regression line extending back through the
origin suggests that the extraction of lincomycin from

bone had been complete. This suggestion is confirmed by the findings in the last experiment.

We decided to use parenteral drug for this study, rather than orally administered capsules. This was done partly because of the poor oral absorption of lincomycin compared with its 7 chlorderivative clindamycin, and mainly because of the interpretation problems that would have arisen as a result of erratic oral absorption. Intestinal motility might have also been altered as a result of anxiety about impending surgery.

2 patients developed pseudomembranous colitis after this regime. Their clinical details have been reported elsewhere (3) in the proceedings of this congress.

We conclude that the prophylactic parenteral regime of lincomycin given during this study provided effective concentrations of this antibiotic in the majority of bone and hip capsule samples taken from patients undergoing THR.

References

1). Grove, D.C. & Randall, W.A. Assay methods of antibiotics: A laboratory manual. Medical Encyclopedia Inc. New York (1955).

2). Garrod, L.P., Lambert, H.P. & O'Grady, F.O. Antibiotic & Chemotherapy, 4th ed. p. 207. (1973). Churchill Livingstone, Edinburgh & London.

3). Parsons,R.L., Salfield, J. & Beavis, J.P. Antibiotic induced diarrhoea & colitis in orthopaedic in patients. Proceedings of the 9th International Congress of Chemotherapy. in press (1975).

CEPHRADINE BONE CONCENTRATIONS DURING TOTAL HIP REPLACEMENT

R.L. PARSONS, J.P. BEAVIS, GILLIAN M. PADDOCK,

& GILLIAN M. HOSSACK

Departments of Clinical Pharmacology &

Orthopaedics. Guy's Hospital Medical School

London. SE1. 9RT. U.K.

Introduction We have previously reported the concentrations of lincomycin achieved in aseptic bone (1.2)
after an empirical parenteral prophylactic regime of this
antibiotic given during total hip replacement (THR).

Cephradine is a broad spectrum cephalosporin (Fig.1)
which may be given orally or parenterally. It resembles
cephalexin in being a zwitterion, but possesses a cyclo-
hexadienyl ring in place of the terminal 6 aminobenzyl
portion of the 7 ACA nucleus. Since after oral administration, cephradine is well absorbed, it was considered
that this antibiotic might be a useful alternative when
lincomycin was contraindicated (e.g. pseudomembranous
colitis). We decided to measure the bone, hip capsule &
drain fluid conentrations achieved by parenteral cephradine.

Subjects & methods 14 patients (5 males & 7 females)
mean + SEM age (63.57 + 3.35 years), height (173.52 + 4.
01 cm) & weight (65.67 + 3.17 kg.) were studied. 12
patients had osteoarthrosis of the hip, 1 had rheumatoid
arthritis & 1 had avascular necrosis of the head of the
femur. These patients received one of the following
empirical parenteral regimes of prophylactic cephradine.

	Molecular weight	pKa	
		COO'	NH$_2$
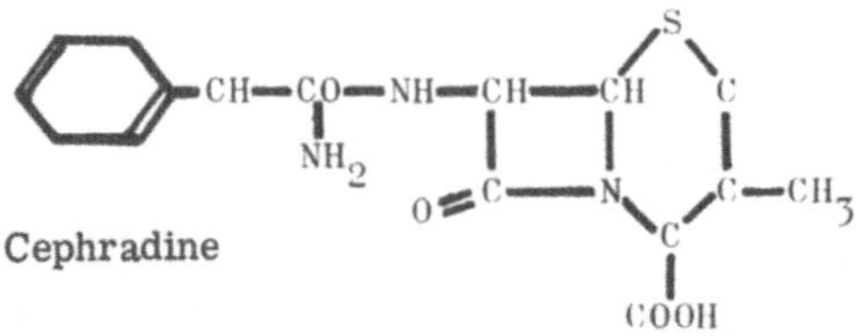 Cephradine	349.41	2.63	7.57
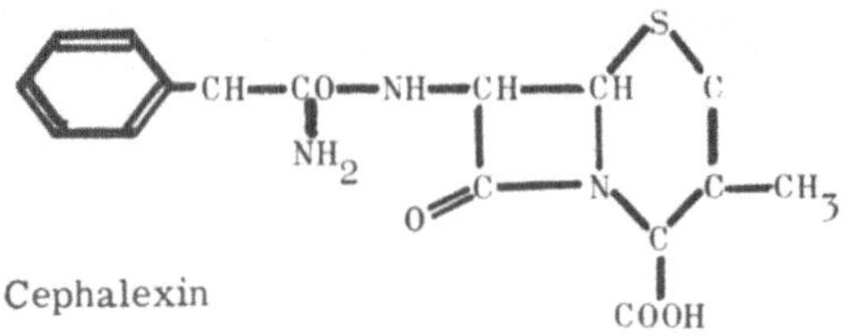 Cephalexin	347.7	5.2	7.3

FIGURE 1 : Chemical structure, molecular weight &
            pKas of cephalexin and cephradine.

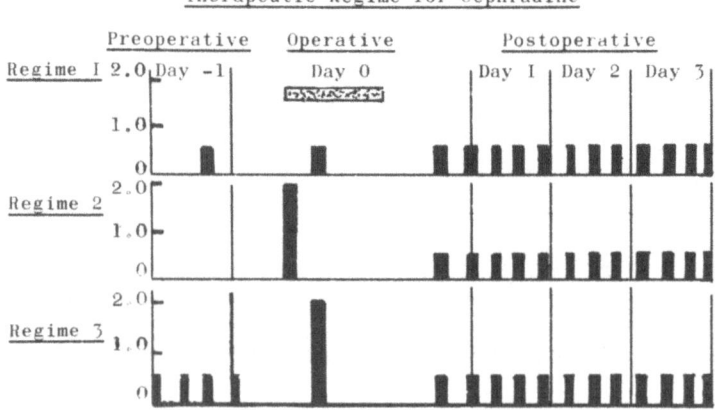

FIGURE 2 : Parenteral regimes of administration used
            for cephradine.

TABLE 1 : Pharmacological comparison of Lincomycin & cephradine.

ANTIBIOTIC	LINCOMYCIN	CEPHRADINE	
Molecular weight	443	349.41	
pKa	7.6	COO'	2.63
		NH_2^+	7.57
Protein binding	5-20%	10%	
Metabolism	+	o	
Excretion	Biliary + Renal	Renal	

TABLE 2 : Bone and Hip capsule concentrations of cephradine

Bone	Regime I		Regime 2		Regime 3	
	n	µg/g.	n	µg/g.	n	µg/g.
Cancellous	49	2.66±0.21	16	11.11±3.83	18	5.78±1.90
Cortical	-	----	2	0.00±0.00	-	-----
Cancellous & Cortical	2	2.15±0.42	27	8.44±1.05	-	-----
Pooled date (all bone samples)			95	4.88±0.54		
Hip capsule	13	2.59±0.25	-	-----	3	1.05±0.55

M.I.C. of CEPHRADINE against STAPH. AUREUS = 3.1 - 18.7 µg/ml

Regime I   Cephradine (1 g.) was given by intramuscular
injection 4 hours prior to operation.   An intravenous
infusion of 0.5 g. over 30 minutes was given at the time
the head of the femur was being removed.   Postoperatively,
cephradine (0.5 g. i.m. 6 hourly) was continued for up to
72 hours, until removal of the drains from the site of
operation.

Regime 2   The first dose of cephradine (2 g.) was given
by rapid i.v. infusion at the time of induction of
anaesthesia.   No infusion was given at the time of removal of the head of the femur.   Postoperatively, cephradine
(0.5 g. i.m. 6 hourly) was continued for up to 72 hours.

Regime 3   The same dose of cephradine that was given as
an infusion in Regime 2 (2 g.) was administered by intramuscular injection (0.5 g. 6 hourly) during the 24 hours
preoperatively.   The postoperative doses were identical
to those used in Regimes I & 2.

        Venous blood samples were collected prior to dosing,
immediately preoperatively & postoperatively, after the
infusion, and for up to 72 hours postoperatively.

        Samples of cortical, cancellous, mixed cortical-
cancellous bone, and hip capsule were collected during
the operation.   During regime 3, these samples were
collected prior to the infusion.

        The bone & capsule samples were agitated for up to
6 hours in a mixture of dipotassium hydrogen phosphate
$(11.7g. L^{-1})$ and dihydrogen potassium phosphate (4.5 g.
L^{-1}).   Adjacent bone samples were ground into a paste
with a pestle & mortar.

        The cephradine content of the samples was analysed
by small plate microbiological assay (3).   The concentra
tion range of the standard solutions of cephradine
monohydrate ranged from $0.0125 < 8$ µg/ml.   This enabled
the lowest limit of the assay to be below that for
lincomycin (2).

Results   The mean ± SEM plasma, bone, hip capsule &
drain concentrations of cephradine after each regime are
given in Tables II & III & IV.

        The mean ± SEM plasma cephradine ranged from 5.22 ±
0.57 (preinfusion) to 167.88 ± 54.87 µg/ml (immediately
postinfusion. Regime 2).   The latter concentration was
well in excess of the M.I.C. of cephradine against

TABLE III : Mean ($\overset{+}{-}$ SEM) Plasma concentrations of
Cephradine

Timing	Regime I µg/ml	Regime 2 µg/ml	Regime 3 µg/ml
Preoperative	8.01 ± 1.39	-----	6.67 ± 2.14
Preinfusion	5.22 ± 0.57	-----	------
Postinfusion	------	167.88 ± 54.87	138.63 ± 8.28
Postoperative	15.38 ± 2.50		

M.I.C. of Cephradine against Staph. aureus = 3.1 - 18.7 µg/ml.

TABLE 4 : Concentrations of cephradine in drain fluid
postoperatively.

Drain fluid	Regime I	Regime III	P
0-6 hours	6.42±1.74	11.95±5.55	NS
6-12 hours	3.30±0.62	9.92±4.09	NS
12-18 hours	3.43±0.79	7.03±1.13	<0.025
18-24 hours	2.87±0.81	6.43±0.99	<0.05

M.I.C. of Cephradine against Staph. aureus = 3.1 - 18.7

penicillinase producing Staph. aureus (18.7 µg/ml) (4).

Regime I The concentrations of cephradine in cortical &
cancellous bone were below the M.I.C. of cephradine
against penicillinase producing Staph. aureus (18.7 µg/ml)
(4).

Regime 2 The mean + SEM concentration of cephradine in
mixed cortical-cancellous bone (8.44 + 1.05 µg/g.) was
above the M.I.C. of some penicillin resistant, methicillin
sensitive strains of Staph. aureus (4.1 µg/ml), (4), but
below the M.I.C. of others (18.7 µg/ml.(4)). The cephradine concentration in cancellous bone (11.11 + 3.83 µg
/g.) was above the M.I.C. $_o$f 5 methicillin resistant
strains of Staph. aureus (9.0 µg/ml) (5).

Regime 3 The concentration of cephradine in cancellous
bone (5.78 + 1.90 µg/g.) was above the M.I.C. of non-
penicillinase producing Staph. aureus (3.1 µg/ml) (4),
and the mean M.I.C. of some penicillin resistant, methicillin sensitive Staph. aureus (mean M.I.C. = 4.1 µg/ml:
range 2.5 - 10.0 µg/ml).

The above comments about bone concentrations of
cephradine apply to the estimated results of the agitation
method. Figure 3 shows that although the correlation
between the results of the agitation & grinding methods
was good (r = 0.53, p <0.01), the regression line did not
extend back through the origin. This was due to lower
concentrations of cephradine being estimated by the
agitation method than were obtained from grinding adjacent
bone samples. The mean + SEM concentration of cephradine
in the ground samples was 42.57 + 6.85 µg/g. (range 2.04
- 90.63 µg/g.). Although there was considerable individual variation between the estimated concentrations in
each bone fragment, the mean + SEM concentration of
cephradine was well above the M.I.C. against penicillinase
producing Staph. aureus (18.7 µg/ml) (4).

The concentrations of cephradine in hip capsule
(1.05 < 2.59 µg/g.) were all well below the M.I.C. of
this antibiotic against non-penicillinase producing Staph.
aureus (3.1 µg/ml) (4).

The highest concentrations of cephradine in postoperative drain fluid were found during the first 6 hours
after operation in the patients receiving Regime 3
(11.95 + 5.55 µg/ml). Higher mean + SEM plasma conentrations of cephradine were maintained for 24 hours after
operation than during Regime I, this increase being

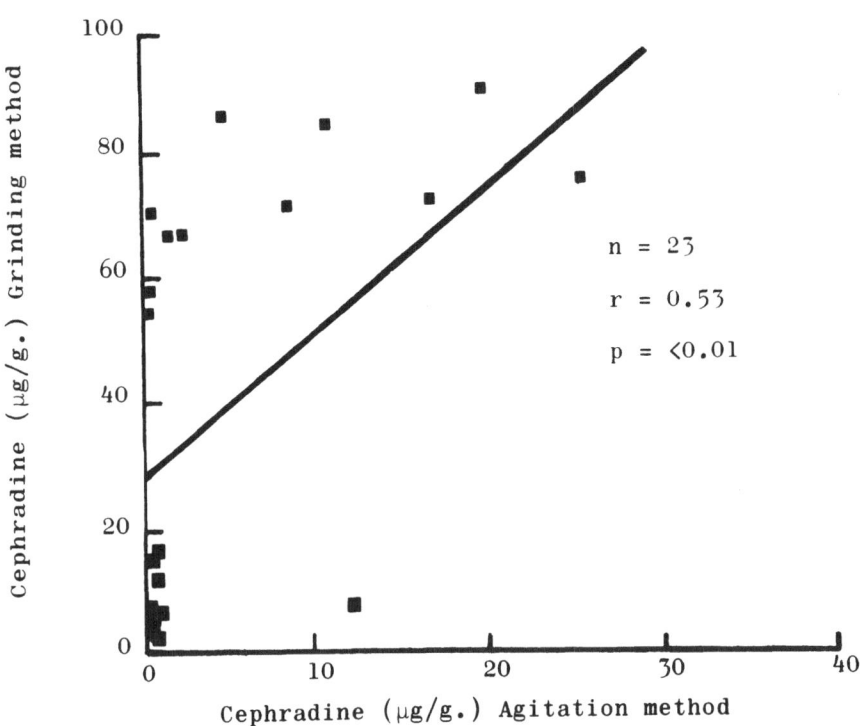

FIGURE 3: Correlation between Assayed Concentration of Cephradine in Bone Estimated by Grinding and Agitation Methods of Analysis

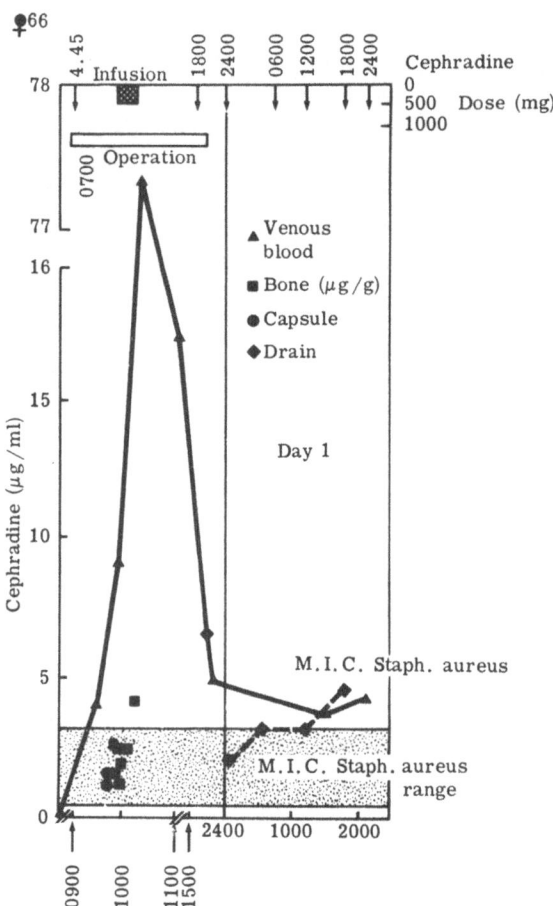

FIGURE 4:   Concentrations of Cephradine in Plasma, Bone,
Capsule and Drain Fluid in One of the Patients Receiving
Regime 1.

significant (P<0.025 - 0.05) after 12 hours. These
concentrations were all in excess of the mean M.I.C. of
cephradine against penicillin resistant, methicillin
sensitive Staph. aureus (4.1 μg/ml) but less than the
M.I.C. of methicillin resistant strains.(9.0 μg/ml).

Discussion Although the agitation method has proved a
reliable method for the analysis of bone concentrations
of lincomycin (2) & cephaloridine (7), our results
suggest that considerable amounts of cephradine remain
within the bone after the optimum period of agitation
(6 hours). This is surprising, since the protein binding
of cephradine is similar to lincomycin.

An alternative explanation is that the higher concentrations of cephradine estimated by the grinding
method represent cephradine situated within the vessels
of the Haversian system, in the intravascular compartment
of bone. Suspension of fresh bone samples taken from
patients who had not been exposed to antibiotics in solutions of the appropriate concentrations of cephradine,
as with lincomycin, did not show evidence of binding of
either drug to bone.

Grinding of bone samples confirmed that the mean ±
SEM concentration of cephradine (42.57 ± 6.85 μg/g.) in
the intravascular & extravascular compartments of bone
was well above the M.I.C. of the most resistant Staph.
aureus (18.7 μg/ml), (4) although some bone fragments
had lower concentrations.

This problem could not be resolved by dissolving
the bone in acid, since this would inactivate cephradine.

Regime 2 was used to assess the findings of other
workers (6.7), who had also measured the concentrations
of cephradine (6), cephalothin (6), & cephaloridine (7)
in bone. Effective concentrations of cephradine followed
4 g. given as a rapid i.v. bolus at the time of induction
of anaesthesia. These workers (6) had crushed the bone
fragments in liquid nitrogen before grinding them into a
paste. This probably accounts for the very much higher
concentrations of cephradine found in bone that were
obtained from the agitation method used in our study.

The design of the cephaloridine bone study (7) was
identical to ours. Bone fragments were taken from
patients undergoing THR and agitated in buffer for 6 hours
which was also found by these workers to be the optimum
period for agitation. By contrast to our study, there

was an excellent correlation between the bone concentrations of cephaloridine estimated by the two methods, the regression line passing through the origin. In our study, the position of the regression line (Fig. 3). suggests that the distribution of cephradine is into the intravascular compartment of bone, whilst that of cephaloridine appears to be extravascular.

We conclude that the administration of a rapid intravenous bolus of cephradine in a dose of 2 g. provides therapeutically effective concentrations of this drug against penicillin resistant Staph. aureus in plasma & some bone samples.

The discrepancy between the estimated concentrations of cephradine between adjacent bone fragments analysed by the two methods requires further elucidation. Although effective concentrations of cephradine are achieved in the intravascular compartment, cephradine does not appear to be as effective as lincomycin in penetrating the extravascular compartment of bone. It is however, a possible alternative to lincomycin in those patients in whom the latter drug is contraindicated.

References

(1) PARSONS, R.L., BEAVIS, J.P., HOSSACK, G.M. & PADDOCK, G.M. Lincomycin bone concentrations during total hip replacement. British Journal of Clinical Pharmac. 2, in press. (1975)

(2) PARSONS, R.L., BEAVIS, J.P., PADDOCK, G.M. & HOSSACK G.M. Lincomycin bone concentrations during Total hip replacement. Proceedings of the 9th International Congress of Chemotherapy. in press (1975).

(3) GROVE, D.C. & RANDALL, W.A. Assay methods of antibiotics: A Laboratory Manual. Medical Encyclopedia Inc., New York (1955).

(4) Eskacef Handbook. Smith, Kline & French Laboratories Ltd. (1975).

(5) Selwyn, S. Advertising of Antibiotics. Letter. British Medical Journal. 2, 239-240.

(6) Hierholzer, G., Lienzenmeier, G., Kleining, R., & Hoerster, G. Study of the Diffusion of various cephalosporins in the Bone tissue. Akt. Traumatologie, 4,

191 - 196. (1974)

(7) HUGHES, S.P.F., BENSON, M.K.D., & FIELD, C.A.
Penetration of Cephaloridine into Bone.
The Journal of Antimicrobial Chemotherapy. 1, in press.
(1975).

THIAMPHENICOL LEVELS IN HUMAN BILE IN THE PRESENCE OF BILIARY TRACT DISEASES

Yoshitaro Suzuki
Kiyohito Shibata, Jiro Yura, Michiteru Fujii,
Nagao Shinagawa, Toru Muramatsu
First Department of Surgery, Nagoya City University,
School of Medicine, Kawasumi 1, Mizuho, Nagoya, Japan

In the present study, the levels of thiamphenicol glycinate in bile and serum were determined in 37 patients following its intravenous administration in a dose of 1g.

Concentrations of thiamphenicol were determined by the thin-layer cup method, using Bacillus subtilis PCI 219 strain as the test microorganism. Serum and bile were diluted with a phosphate buffer of pH 7.0. The standard curve was plotted after dilution of samples with a phosphate buffer of pH 7.0.

Figure 1 summarizes the results of measurement obtained in 7 patients who had no disorders of the biliary tract (Group 1) and in 14 patients with cholelithiasis (Group 2). In Group 1, drug levels in common duct bile were generally higher in 2-hour bile samples than in 1-hour samples, averaging 65.3mcg/ml, and far higher than serum levels. In Group 2, the bile level of the drug averaged 48.6mcg/ml in 30-min bile, 47.8mcg/ml in 1-hour bile, but greatly varied from one individual to another. The bile level was far higher than its serum level in many of the patients of this group. Comparison of two groups revealed little difference in bile level in 1-hour bile samples, but showed higher drug levels for Group 1 in 2-hour samples.

In these 9 cholelithiasis (Group 3), total bile was collected continuously from a T-tube no less than 14 days after surgery when the bile flow became stabilized. The bile concentration of thiamphenicol showed a peak in 6 cases for 1-hour bile and in 3 cases for 3-hour bile. The average drug level in bile was 51.2mcg/ml in 1-hour bile, 39.2mcg/ml in 2-hour and 42.3mcg/ml in 3-hour. It decreased with increasing time. The serum level showed a peak in all the 30-min blood samples, averaging 44.8mcg /ml .

Concentration of Thiamphenicol in Human Bile (1g I.V.)
(Bile collected during Surgery)

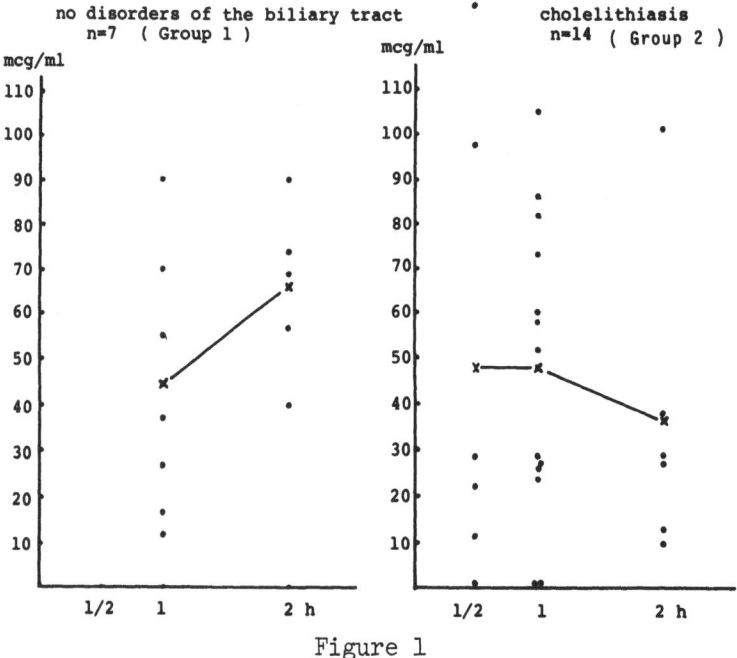

Figure 1

Group 3: Concentration of Thiamphenicol (1g I.V.) n=9
Bile collected from a T-tube

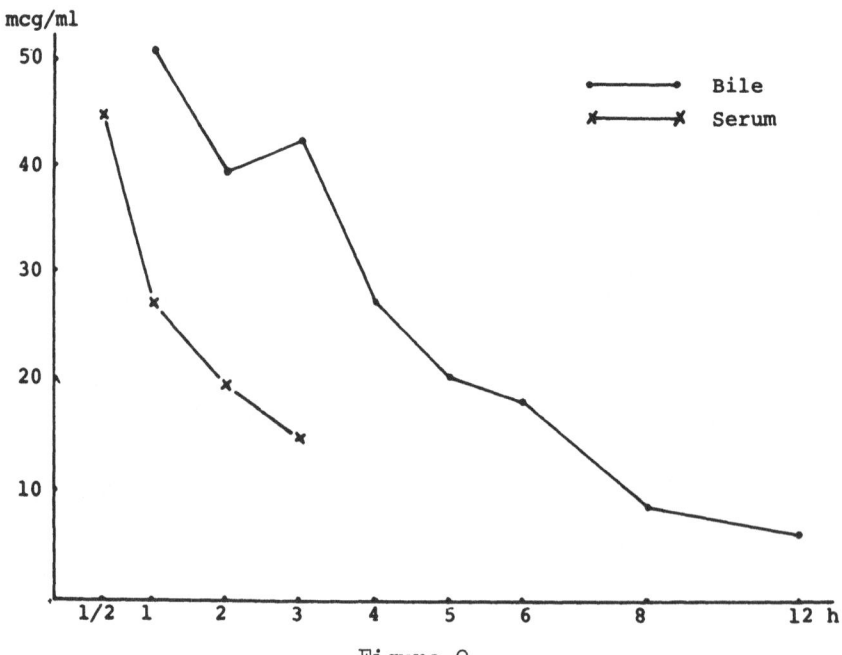

Figure 2

Table 1

Group 3: Recovery of Thiamphenicol from Bile
Bile collected from a T-tube

Case No.	hr 0	2 2	4 4	6 6	8 8	12	Recovery 0	12	Rate of Excretion	Remarks
1	2,893	600	nd	nd	nd		3,493		0.35%	Up to 3 hrs.
2	1,595	482	311	-	-		2,388		0.24%	
3	1,675	226	1,433	-	-		3,334		0.33%	
4	3,567	378	-	-	-		3,945		0.39%	
5	2,639	347	nd	nd	nd		2,986		0.30%	Up to 3 hrs.
6	1,068	388	835	nd	nd		2,291		0.23%	Up to 6 hrs.
7	864	2,447	824	735	1,138		6,008		0.60%	
8	1,029	1,879	1,480	672	nd		5,060		0.51%	2-hr. value unknown
9	5,489	3,170	1,055	443	1,303		11,460		1.15%	

(mcg)

Group 4: Bile Concentrations of Thiamphenicol in Patients
with Malignant Biliary Tumor n=7
(Bile collected from a Biliary Fistula)

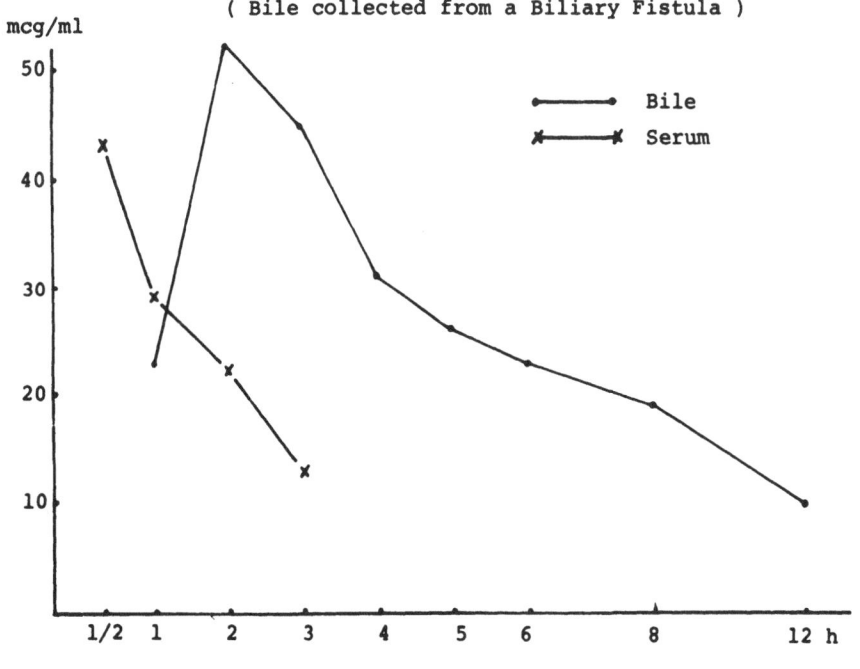

Figure 3

Table 2

Group 4 : Recovery of Thiamphenicol from Bile

Case No. \ h	0 ~ 2	2 ~ 4	4 ~ 6	6 ~ 8	8 ~ 12	Recovery 0 ~ 12	%
1	365	1,601	877	1,494	933	5,270	0.53
2	3,580	2,004	1,785	798	1,521	9,688	0.97
3	2,144	2,569	1,196	660	-	6,569	0.66
4	1,150	2,235	682	2,535	599	7,201	0.72
5	107	796	702	479	-	2,084	0.21
6	1,332	832	1,189	812	1,188	5,353	0.54
7	5,061	1,594	930	660	1,084	9,329	0.93

(mcg)

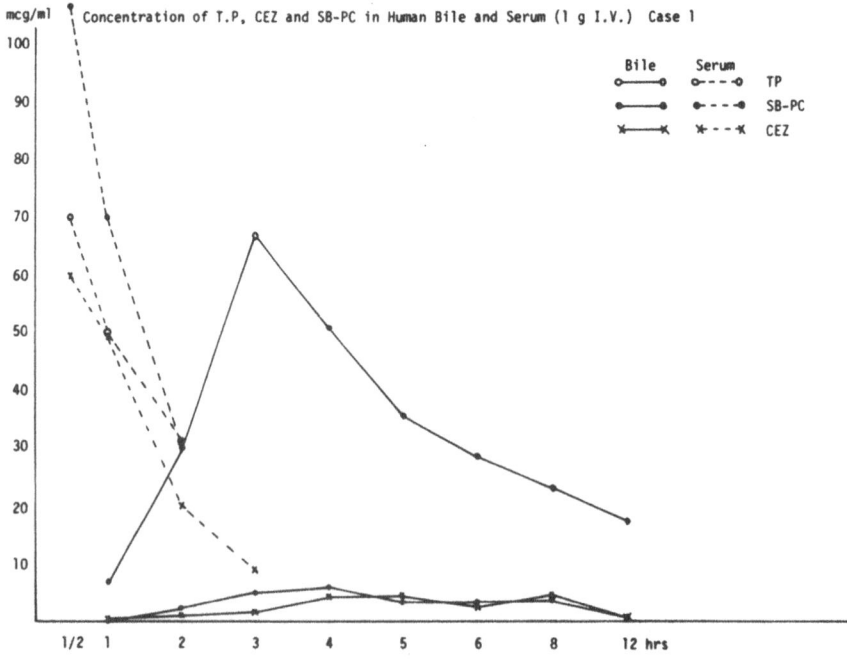

Concentration of T.P, CEZ and SB-PC in Human Bile and Serum (1 g I.V.) Case 1

The rate of drug recovery was lower than 0.5% in many of the cases. However, the actual rate of biliary excretion must have been higher than measured in those cases, because part of bile is assumed to have flowed into the duodenum.

In Group 4, the operation was limited to surgical preparation of a biliary fistula as a temporary expedient because of jaundice improvement, and it stands to reason to presume that all bile could be collected in the patients of this group. The drug level in bile varied to a considerable extent from one individual to another. The average drug concentration in bile reached a peak of 51.7mcg/ml in 2-hour bile, and the drug was found in bile at high concentrations for a long time.

Biliary excretion was rather high in all but one case, and an average of about 0.65% of the dose was recovered in 12 hours. Although Group 4 included a larger number of patients with advanced jaundice, drug level in bile were not far lower than in Group 3.

In 2 cases, a crossover test was carried out by intravenous administration of 1g of thiamphenicol, cefazolin and sulbenicillin. There was no big difference in liver function in the course of crossover test in each 2 cases.

Case 1: 66 year-old female, she was diagnosed as having cancer of the common bile duct and treated by cholecystostomy. Bile concentration reached a peak of 83mcg/ml in 3-hour bile for thiamphenichol and 3.6mcg/ml and 4.8mcg/ml in 4-hour bile for cefazolin and sulbenicillin,respectively. The rate of drug recovery up to 12 hrs. stood at 0.53% for thiamphenicol, 0.048% for cefazolin and 0.052% for sulbenicillin.

Case 2: 56 year-old female, she had a T-tube introduced into the common bile duct. The drug concentration in bile reached a peak of 49.3mcg/ml for thiamphenicol, 11mcg/ml for cefazolin and 8.9mcg/ml for sulbenicillin, all in 2-hour bile samples. The rate of drug recovery up to 12 hours stood at 0.97% for thiamphenicol, 0.12% for cefazolin and 0.11% for sulbenicillin.

In both cases, the bile concentration of thiamphenicol was about 5 to 10 times higher and recovery from bile was also about 10 times higher for thiamphenicol than for other two drugs. It was only thiamphenicol that was found in bile at a higher concentration than in serum.

A total of 16 patients of Group 3 and 4 were divided into those with normal liver function and those with liver disorders. The bile concentration was obviously lower in those with liver disorders. Generally speaking, the transport of chemotherapeutic agents to the liver is impaired in patients with liver disorders. In the present study, an attempt was made to clarify the relationship between the liver function and the bile concentration of thiamphenicol.

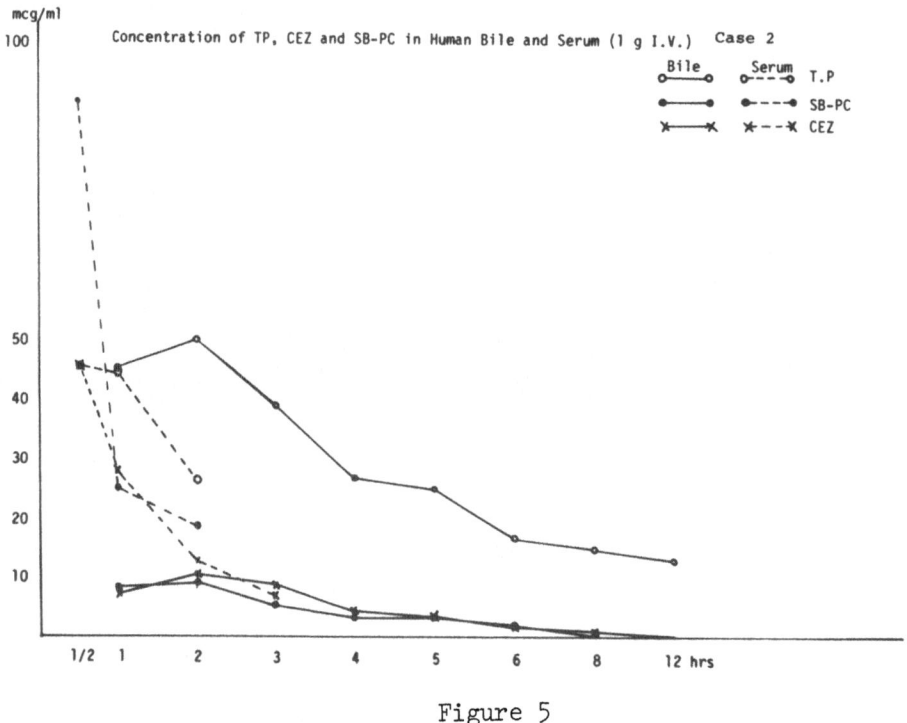

Figure 5

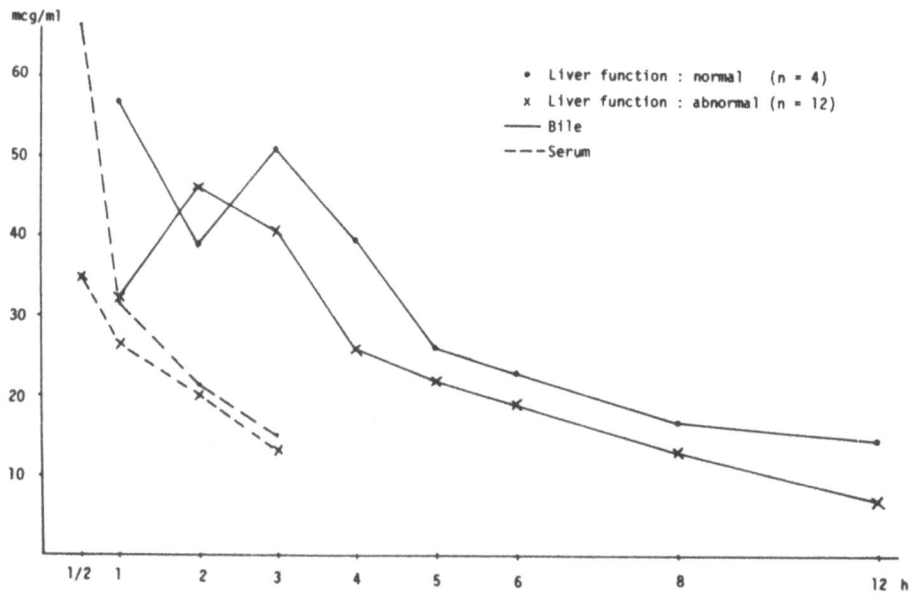

Figure 6

Concentration of Thiamphenicol in Human Bile and Al. Phos. (1 g I.V.)

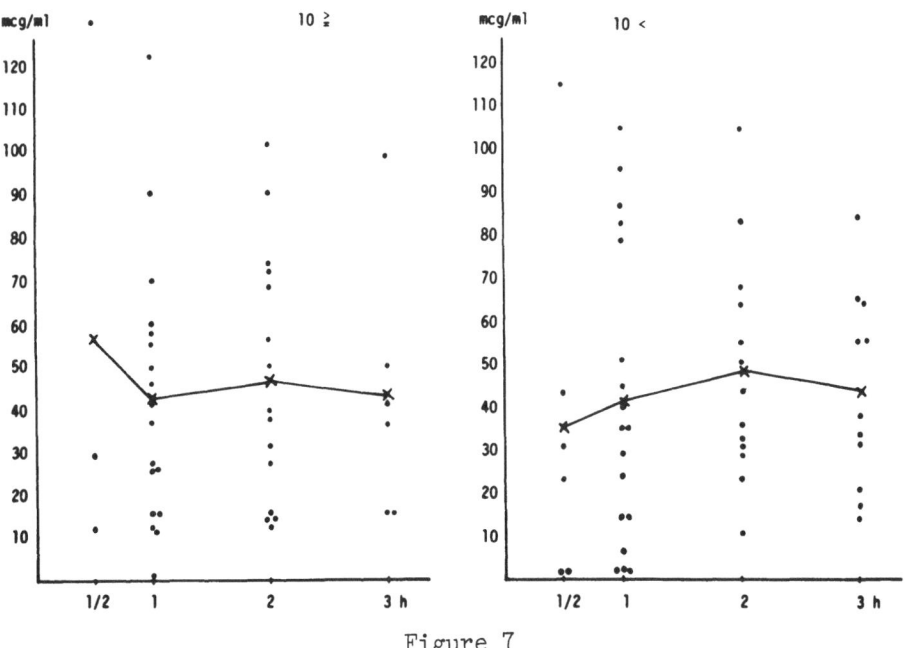

Figure 7

Concentration of Thiamphenicol in Human Bile and Total Bilirubin (1g I.V.)

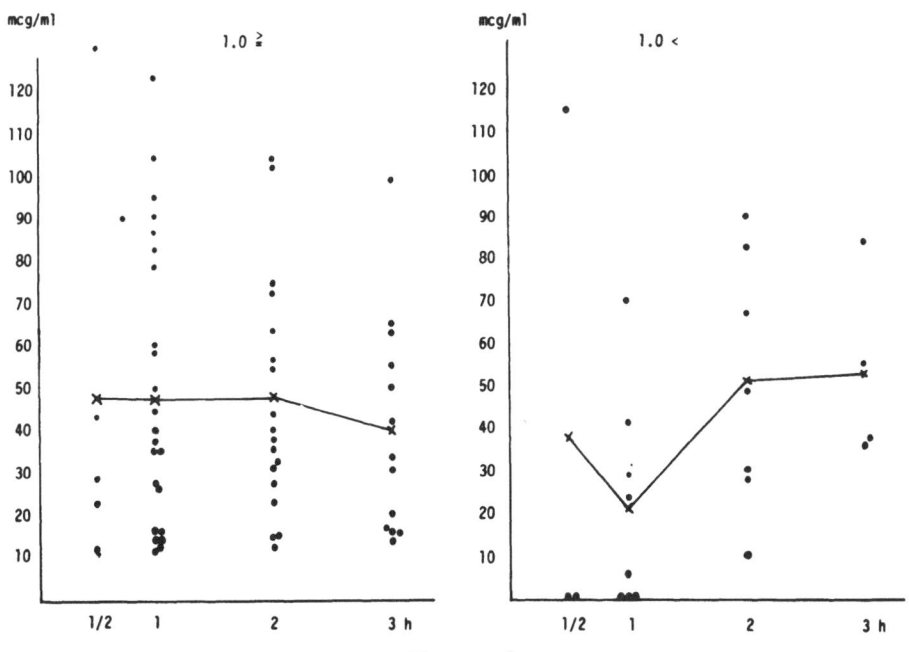

Figure 8

Concentration of Thaimphenicol in Human Bile and SGOT (1 g I.V.)

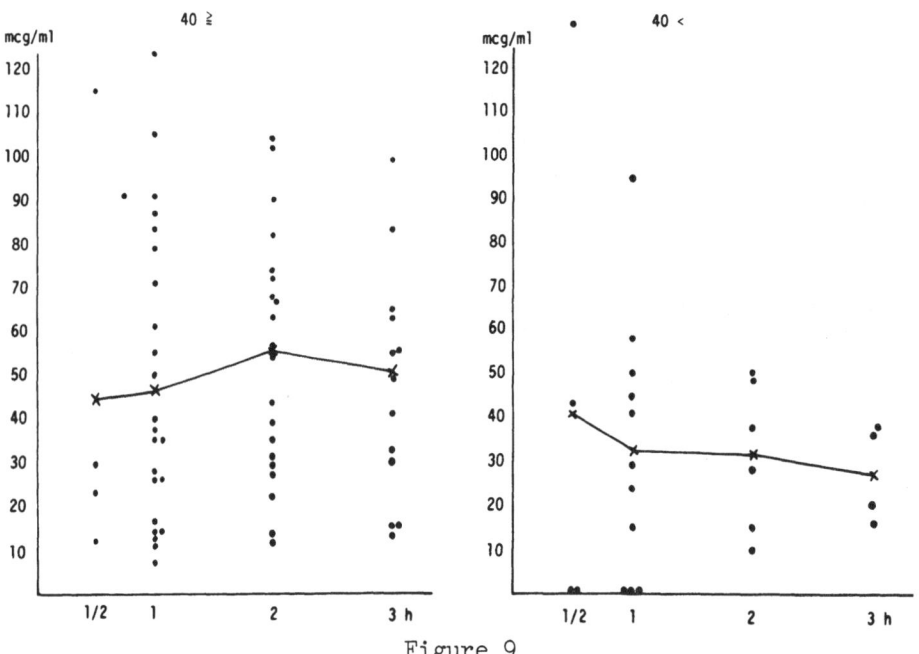

Figure 9

Concentration of Thaimphenicol in Human Bile and ZTT (1 g I.V.)

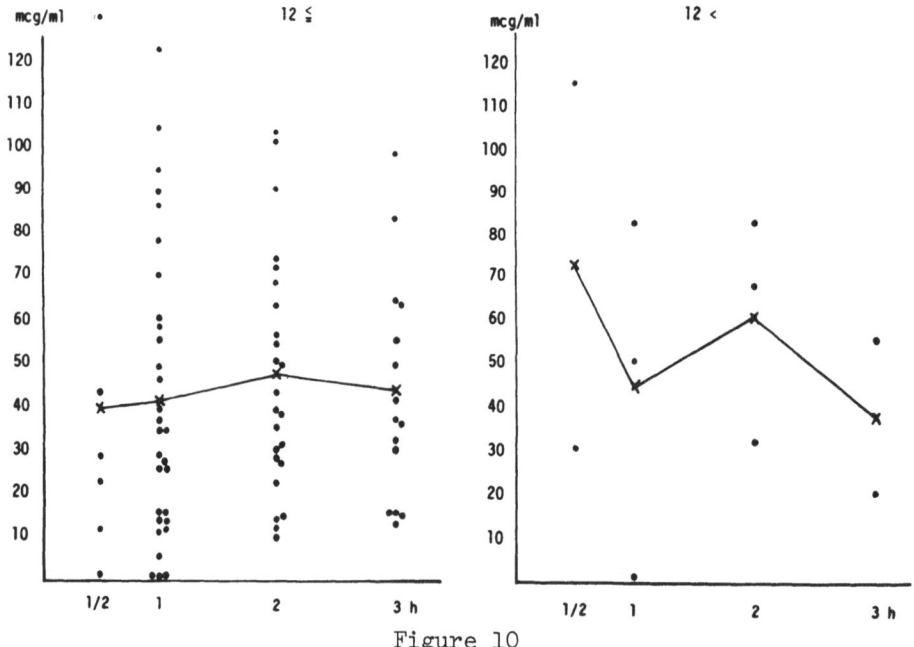

Figure 10

Examination revealed no relationship between the drug level in bile and alkaline phosphatase. A level of alkaline phosphatase did not seem to affect the bile level of thiamphenicol. It should be noted, however, that the investigated subjects did not include any patient with complete obstruction of the bile duct.

No relationship was noted either between total bilirubin and the bile concentration of thiamphenicol, even though the concentration of drug in 30- and 60-min bile seemed somewhat lower in those who showed an abnormal value of total bilirubin.

Bile concentrations of thiamphenicol appeared generally low in the subjects who showed an abnormal value of SGOT.

As for ZTT, its effect could not be made clear, because few patients showed an abnormal value of ZTT. As difficult it is to draw a definite conclusion from the results of the present study because the investigated subjects were small in number, it appeared that thiamphenicol had a closer relationship with SGOT than with total bilirubin and alkaline phosphatase.

Summary

The bile concentrations of thiamphenicol were higher than serum concentrations in all the investigated subjects, whether they had liver disorders or not, and rather high even in the patients with advanced jaundice. In Group 4 in which nearly all bile could be collected, the rate of thiamphenicol recovery from bile was as high as 0.65%. As regards the liver function, thiamphenicol showed a relatively distinct relationship with SGOT. However, the relationship between bile levels of drugs and the liver function may vary to some extent with each drugs, as suggested by Zaslow and Ayliffe et al, who reported that the bile concentration of ampicillin was affected by jaundice, that is, serum bilirubin. In short, it can be inferred from the results of the present study that the bile levels of drugs are affected not only by total bilirubin, alkaline phosphatase, SGOT and ZTT but also by the duration of jaundice and BSP.

REFERENCES

1. Schoenfield L. J.:Biliary excretion of antibiotics, New Eng. J. Med. 284: 1213-1214, 1971
2. Zaslow J., Rosenthal A.: The excretion and concentration of Terramycin in the abnormal human biliary tract, Ann. Surg. 139: 478-483, 1954
3. Ayliffe G.A.J. and Davies A.: Ampicillin levels in human bile, Brit. J. Pharmacol. 24: 189-193, 1965
4. Ideuchi H.: Metabolism of thiamphenicol and its biliary excretion, Chemotherapy 19: 51-56, 1971

BACTERIA IN BILE AND THEIR ROLE IN POSTOPERATIVE
INFLAMMATORY COMPLICATIONS IN BILIARY DISEASE

Nagao Shinagawa, Kiyohito Shibata, Jiro Yura,
Michiteru Fujii and Yoshitaro Suzuki
First Department of Surgery, Nagoya City
University, School of Medicine
Kawasumi 1, Mizuho, Nagoya, Japan

Some hypotheses have been proposed regarding
the mechanisms of development of postoperative
infections in cases of gallstone disese or malignant
disese of the bile duct. Infections are undoubtedly
related to the presence of bacteria in bile collected
during surgical procedures.

The frequency of positive bile cultures according
to the type of cases were investigated. Bacteria
could be cultured from 35 of 113 cases of gallbladder
stone, and from 37 of 43 cases of common bile duct
stone. Higher ratio of positive bile cultures was
found in intrahepatic stone. However, of 49 cases
of malignant disese of the bile duct, the ratio of
positive bile cultures was as low as 24.5 %.

TABLE 1: Frequency of Positive Bile Cultures According to
Type of Cases

Type of case	Number	Number of positive bile cultures (%)
Gallbladder stone	113	35 (30.9%)
Common bile duct stone	43	37 (86.0%)
Intrahepatic stone	21	19 (90.5%)
Malignant obstruction	49	12 (24.5%)

The postoperative infections according to the age
and bacteria in bile at operation were investigated.
Positive bile cultures were more frequently found in
older patients, with three-fourths of the positive
bile cultures obtained from patients over 60 years of
age. Postoperative infections were more frequently
encountered in cases showing a positive bile cultures,
that is, 13 out of 91 cases. In contrast, of 86 cases
in which cultures were negative, only 4 patients
subsequently developed bacerial infections.

TABLE 2: Postoperative Infections According to Age and Bacteria
in Bile at Operation (Gallstone Disease)

Age(yrs.)	Positive Bile Cultures		Negative Bile Cultures	
	No. of cases	No. of infections	No. of cases	No. of infections
< 30	3	1	7	0
30 ~ 39	8	1	18	2
40 ~ 49	20	3	25	1
50 ~ 59	28	3	26	1
60 ~ 69	25	3	8	0
>70	7	2	2	0
Total	91	13	86	4

TABLE 3: Postoperative Infections According to Location of
Gallstone and Bacteria in Bile at Operation (Gallstone Disease)

Location of Gallstone	Positive Bile Cultures		Negative Bile Cultures	
	No. of cases	No. of infections	No. of cases	No. of infections
In gallbladder	35	2	78	4
In common bile duct	37	6	6	0
Intrahepatic	19	5	2	0
Total	91	13	86	4

Postoperative infections according to location of gallstone and bacteria in bile at operation were investigated. Infections were noticed in 6 cases out of 37 of common bile duct stone with positive bile cultures, and in 5 cases out of 19 of intrahepatic stone with positive bile cultures. It may be concluded that postoperative infections would easily occure in the cases where gallstones are in common bile duct or liver, and bacteria in bile are positive.

The incidence of postoperative infections was investigated with regared to presence or absence of jaundice and the presence of bacteria in bile. They occurred in 10 cases out of 51 of jaundice with positive bile cultures. Thus, it is indicated that antibacterial prophylactic measures should be taken prior to surgery, and close attention should be paid in operation.

Postoperative infections were next studied with regared to the type of gallstone and the ratio of positive bile cultures. It is well known that in many cases of cholesterol stone, bacteria were not detecable in bile, but frequently detectable in bile in cases of bilirubinate stone. Postoperative infections also were found to be more frequent in cases of bilirubinate stone with positive bile cultures.

Table 4: Postoperative Infections Classified by Jaundice and Bacteria in Bile at Operation (Gallstone Disease)

Jaundice	Positive Bile Cultures		Nagative Bile Cultures	
	No. of cases	No. of infections	No. of cases	No. of infections
Jaundice	51	10	15	2
No jaundice	40	3	71	2
Total	91	13	86	4

TABLE 5: Postoperative Infections According to kind of Gallstone and Bacteria in Bile at Operation (Gallstone Disease)

Kind of Gallstone	Positive Bile Cultures		Negative Bile Cultures	
	No. of cases	No. of infections	No. of cases	No. of infections
Cholesterol stone	16	1	51	3
Bilirubinate stone	65	12	23	1
Others	10	0	12	0
Total	91	13	86	4

TABLE 6: Postoperative Courses in Relation to Bacteria in Bile at Operation (Gallstone Disease)

Bacteria \ Postoperative course	Mean days until defervesence	Re-pyrexia cases	Positive bacteria from postope. drain	Leucocytosis	
				10-20 days after operation	More than 20 days after operation
Negative Bile Cultures 86 cases	5.0 days	5 cases	3 cases	6 cases	2 cases
Positive Bile Cultures 91 cases	6.1 days	19 cases	33 cases	14 cases	7 cases

The postoperative course was studied comparing 86
cases with negative bile cultures with 91 cases of
positive cultures. No marked difference were noted in
mean days in which patients became aferbrile, 5.0 days
fore negative bile cultures and 6.1 days for positive
cultures. Differences were observed in re-pyrexia,
namely 5 cases in negative ones and 19 cases in
positive ones. Bacteria were frequently cultured from
postoperative drains. Positive cultures were obtained
in 33 cases. These cases included those in which
inflammatory complications occurred, as well as those
which may be explained merely as stained with bacteria.
In many positive bile cultures showed leucocytosis
after surgery.

Postoperative infections were noticed in 4 cases
out of 86 with negative bile cultures, while in 13
cases out of 91 with positive bile cultures.
Infections, which were frequently observed in the
positive bile cultures, included wound infections,
subphrenic abscess or septicemia. On the other hand,
postoperative infections were demonstrated in 25 of
58 cases with malignant diseases. In these cases,
the incidence of bacteria in bile was low in primary,
jaundice relieving operation. However, bacteria could
be cultured from the bile of such cases after 7 to 10
postoperative days and the ratio of postoperative
infections would be higher after secondary operation,
namely radical operation.

Relation was investigated between the bacteria in
bile and the postoperative causative bacteria in gallstone disease. Coincidence was noticed in 25 cases
out of 33, these numbers being numerous as there are
included the bacteria from postoperative drain (not
always a so-called infection). Coincidence was
observed with bacteria in bile in 5 cases out of 7 of
wound infection, 2 cases out of 3 of subphrenic
abscess, all 2 cases of acute cholangitis, and all 3
cases of septicemia.

Comparison was made between the bacteria in bile at
operation and the inflammatory causative bacteria
after operation. Among 7 cases of wound infection,
coincidence was noted in all 5 cases of acute or
supprative cholangitis and septicemia, though only 2
cases were not. Sensitivity pattern coincided with
these baceria, and it is presumed that they would be
the same bacteria. Attention should be paid that
there appeared after operation Pseudomonas and Proteus
which have been not proved in bile. This important
fact should be taken into consideration on the treatment of inflammatory complications.

TABLE 7:   Postoperative Infections in Relation to Bacteria in Bile at Operation.

Disease / Postoperative infection		Total of postope. infections (%)	Respiratory complication	Wound infection	Subphrenic abscess	Acute or suppurative cholangitis	Septicemia	Others
Gallstone Disease	Negative Bile Cultures 86 cases	4 (4.7%)	1	1	1	0	0	1
	Positive Bile Cultures 91 cases	13 (14.6%)	1	7	3	2	3	1
Malignant Obstruction 58 cases		25 (43.1%)	8	7	2	12	3	3

TABLE 8:   Postoperative Infections in Relation to Bacteria in Bile at Operation (Gallstone Disease).

Postope. infections	No.	Postoperative infection due to the same bacteria in bile No.	Percent
Bacteria from postoperative drain	33	25	75.8%
Wound infection	7	5	
Subphrenic abscess	3	2	
Acute or suppurative cholangitis	2	2	76.5%
Septicemia	3	3	
Others	2	1	
Total	50	38	76.0%

Bacterial cultures of bile and cultures taken from the postoperative patient were studied for purposes of treating infections associated with gall-stone disease. The organisms most frequently found in bile were E.coli, followed by Klebsiells and Enterobacter, Pseudomonas being only 4 strains. In contrast to this, After surgery the isolation rate of E.coli and Enterobacter decreased, the frequency of Klebsiella isolations was unchanged, but Pseudomonas isolation rates increased.

From the above results, it may be concluded that a prophylactic administration of antibiotic following bile duct surgery should take aim at bacteria in bile collected at operation. As several days are necessary until the completion of sensitivity measurement, an antibiotic in use should be checked up when the result will be obtained. It goes without saying, however, that an antibiotic may be chosen on the basis of bacteria in bile examined by duodenal tube before the operation. Attention should be paid on an every possibility that Klebsiella or Pseudomonas may be causative bacteria in the treatment of postoperative inflammatory complications with a prolonged course.

TABLE 9:   Bacteria in Gallstone Disease

Bacteria	Bacteria in bile at operation	Bacteria after operation
E. coli	42 strains	22 strains
Klebsiella	21	21
Enterobacter	14	5
Pseudomonas	4	12
Hafnia	4	3
Citrobacter	3	5
Proteus	2	3
Serratia	2	1
Other GNB	17	9
Enterococcus	8	5
Strept. viridans	5	2
Staphylococcus	3	1
Other GPC	7	1

REFERENCES
1. Keighley,M.R.B., et al.: Hazards of surgical treatment due to microorganisms in the bile, Surgery 75:578,
1974.
2. Kune,G.A., and Schutz,E.: Bacteria in the biliary
tract, a study of their frequency and type, Med.J.Aust.
1:255,1974.

CARINDACILLIN IN URINARY INFECTIONS OF OBSTETRICAL CONCERN

F. Concetti and F. Catizone

Obstetrical-Gynecological Department

Ospedale Civile, Cosenza, Italy

Prematurity, stillbirth and toxemia are frequent complications of mild and even inapparent urinary tract infections during pregnancy; according to Wren (1969), pyelonephritis carries during pregnancy a significant risk not only of premature delivery and toxemia but also perinatal death. On the other hand, the frequency of pyelonephritis in pregnancy is great (Boutros et al 1972), and a high incidence of radiologic abnormalities is also observed in these circumstances. Bladder infections usually do not seem to disturb the normal course of pregnancy (Wren 1969), but patients with bacteriuria of pregnancy are the only ones - or almost the only ones - in whom the conversion of bladder to kidney infections occurs, according to Fairley (1970).

In this framework, a general consensus exists on the necessity to always carry out an antimicrobial therapy, not only to prevent recurrent infections but also to decrease morbidity.

Because - both in our experience and in that of other Italian investigators (Sanna 1975) - E. coli, Proteus spp. and Pseudomonas aeruginosa are the germs responsible for 80-85% of the UTI in pregnancy, the chemoantibiotic treatment should be effected with drugs acting on these pathogens; the choice of the drug must be made by taking into consideration the potential toxic effects upon the fetus and the possible adverse effects on the mother, related, for instance, to the particular condition of her liver.

For these reasons, we generally prefer to treat the UTI during pregnancy with a nontoxic, broad-spectrum antibiotic having activity on Pseudomonas aeruginosa; for some months, carbenicillin (as both the disodium salt by parenteral route and the indanyl derivative by oral route) has been widely used. In fact, urinary levels obtained are, also with the oral administration of 1-2 grams daily, very high and superior to the average MIC for the usual germs involved in UTI.

MATERIALS AND METHODS

We wish to report on the clinical activity of the indanyl carbenicillin treatment of 32 cases suffering from UTI during pregnancy. In all the cases, the bacteriological examination of the urine revealed E. coli or Proteus spp. or Pseudomonas aeruginosa, with colony counts greater than 100,000/ml of urine and good in vitro sensitivity to carbenicillin.

From a clinical point of view, all the patients presented leukocyturia, erythrocyturia, pollakiuria, strangury and fever, and all the cases were classified as acute UTI. The treatment was carried out with 4 daily administrations of 1 g each of indanyl carbenicillin per os for 15 days.

RESULTS AND CONCLUSIONS

The results are reported in table 1 from a clinical viewpoint.

TABLE 1

Clinical results

Leukocyturia: positive results in 24 patients (75%)
Erythrocyturia: "   "   " 30   "   (95%)
Pollakiuria: "   "   " 26   "   (84%)
Strangury: "   "   " 26   "   (84%)
Fever: "   "   " 32   "   (100%)

The uroculture showed good bacteriological results in 60-75% of the cases according to the germs isolated.

The clinical tolerance of the drug was good. In a few cases, nausea was reported as a side effect.

According to our experience, indanyl carbenicillin should be used in UTI in pregnancy if the sensitivity tests show good _in vitro_ activity of the drug. In these cases, indanyl carbenicillin allows the oral administration of a safe drug able to obtain very satisfactory urinary levels.

REFERENCES

1. Boutros, P., Mourtada, H. and Ronald, A.R. (1972), Am. J. Obstet. Gynecol., 112, 379.
2. Fairley, K.F. (1970), in Renal Infection and Renal Scarring (edited by P. Kincaid-Smith); 107. Australia: Mercedes Publishing Services.
3. Sanna, A., "Microbiologia delle infezioni delle vie urinarie": paper read at the "Convegno di Chemioterapia – Tavola Rotonda su Chemioterapia delle infezioni Urinarie", Turin, June 19–20, 1975.
4. Wren, B.G. (1969), Med. J. Aust., 2, 596.

THE ACTIVITY OF EIGHT ANTIMICROBIAL COMPOUNDS, INCLUDING THREE

NITROIMIDAZOLE COMPOUNDS, AGAINST BACTEROIDES SP.

R. Wise, K.A. Bedford & Jennie Andrews

Department of Medical Microbiology

Dudley Road Hospital, Birmingham. B18 7QH.

SUMMARY

Eight antimicrobial agents were investigated for their in vitro activity against 40 strains of Bacteroides sp. Clindamycin was found to be highly active, but its activity affected by changes in inoculum size and the presence of serum. Metronidazole, nimorazole and tindazole were found to have a considerable degree of activity and less affected by inoculum and serum. Spectinomycin was moderately active. Mecillinam and two cephalosporins, cefazolin and cephaloridine, could not be considered to have a useful degree of activity.

INTRODUCTION

The increased awareness of the frequency of infections caused by the anaerobic organisms, in particular Bacteroides fragilis has stimulated interest in the search for effective antimicrobial agents.

The purpose of this study was to investigate the in vitro activity of a number of agents, in particular the nitroimidazole compounds, metronidazole, tindazole and nimorazole. We were also interested in assessing the possible effectiveness of spectinomycin a dibasic aminoglycoside antibiotic to which has recently been ascribed activity against the Bacteroides sp. by Phillips & Warren (1975).

MATERIALS AND METHODS

Forty recent clinical isolates of Bacteroides sp. were used
in this study. All were penicillin resistant, but were not
speciated further.

Eight antibiotics, mecillinam (FL1060), cephazolin,
cephaloridine, metronidazole, tindazole, nimorazole, clindamycin
and spectinomycin were investigated for their in vitro activity.
The minimum inhibitory concentration (MIC) of each antibiotic
against the 40 strains was ascertained by a routine agar plate
dilution method. The media employed was 'Oxoid D.S.T.' plus 10%
whole human lysed blood. The organisms were applied using a
'Denley Multipoint' inoculator at a concentration of approximately
1×10^5 organisms per ml and a 1 μl delivery. The plates were
then incubated overnight in Gas Pak jars (B.B.L.) at $37^{o}C$. The
MIC was defined as that concentration which inhibited 90% of the
original inoculum.

As mecillinam, cephazolin and cephaloridine had little
activity, further investigations were not performed using these
antibiotics. The effect of increasing the inoculum to approximately
1×10^8 organisms/ml was studied in 20 strains by the above method.
The effect on the minimum bacteriocidal concentration (MBC) of
increasing amounts of serum was investigated by performing doubling
broth ('Oxoid STB') dilutions in tubes. These tests, on 3 strains,
were performed in triplicate, one set containing 5% lysed human
blood, a second with 25% horse serum and the third containing 100%
horse serum and no broth. The inoculum was 1×10^5 organisms/ml.
The tubes were incubated as above and subcultured at 18 hrs on the
'Oxoid DST' agar with 10% lysed blood, and further incubated
anaerobically overnight.

We were particularly interested in the effect of different
anaerobic atmospheres upon the in vitro activity of spectinomycin.
The MIC of spectinomycin of the 20 strains of Bacteroides sp. was
performed by the agar plate dilution method as above, but the
plates were incubated in (a) Gas Pak, (b) Baird & Tatlock jar
containing H_2 plus 10% CO_2 , (c) similarly with pure H_2 , all at
$37^{o}C$. The results were read the next day.

RESULTS

In Table I the MICs of the 8 antimicrobial agents are
summarised. Mecillinam was the least active of all the agents
tested with MICs of 64 mg/l or greater. Cephaloridine and
cephazolin also exhibit little activity against these organisms
and would not be expected to be clinically useful.

TABLE I. Activity of eight antimicrobial agents against 40 isolates of Bacteroides sp. (10^5 organisms/ml)

	<0.06	0.06	0.12	0.25	0.5	1	2	4	8	16	32	64	128	256	>256
	concentration mg/l														
Clindamycin	40														
Cephaloridine								2	3	25	5		3		2
Cefazolin								2	12	20	2			1	3
Mecillinam												2	18	16	4
Nimorazole			13	25	2										
Tindazole		6	34	35											
Metronidazole			5												
Spectinomycin											40				

Clindamycin was found to be the most active drug, all the isolates being sensitive to less than 0.06 mg/l. There was little difference between the three nitroimidazole compounds, but tindazole was about twice as active as nimorazole or metronidazole. All the 40 isolates were uniformly sensitive to 32 mg/l of spectinomycin.

In Tables II - IV the effect of altering the conditions of the in vitro tests are shown. An increase in inoculum from 10^5 to 10^8 increases the MICs of the three nitroimidazole drugs by a factor of at least 8 to 16 fold. The MBCs of these three drugs are in the range of 0.5 - 1 mg/l except for nimorazole where they are higher, 8 - 16 mg/l, compared with an MIC of 0.12 - 0.25 mg/l. An increase in serum in the test tube from 25% - 100% results in an increase in the MBC of 2 - 4 fold.

The concentration of clindamycin necessary to kill the organisms was considerably higher (32 fold) than the concentration to inhibit them, but the presence of serum had a less marked effect upon the MBC. Spectinomycin was different in this respect, the MIC and MBC close together and the presence of serum had little effect upon the MBC.

There was little or no difference in the MIC of spectinomycin if 'Gas Pak' or 10% CO_2 plus H_2 were used as the anaerobic cultural atmosphere. It was interesting to note that if pure hydrogen was used no growth was obtained from the 20 strains tested. Inadvertent aerobiosis was ruled out by employing control organisms (Cl. tetani and Pseudomonas aeruginosa).

TABLE II. Effect of inoculum & serum on MIC/MBC of metronidazole

	No. tested	0.06	0.12	0.25	0.5	1	2	4	8	>16
MIC 10^5/ml	40		5	35						
10^8/ml	20				3	1	4	12		
MBC 10^5/ml										
5% L.H.B.	3				1	2				
100% Serum	3						1	2		
25% Serum	3			2	1					

TABLE III.   Effect of inoculum and serum on MIC/MBC of tindazole
and nimorazole against <u>Bacteroides sp.</u>

	No. tested	concentration mg/1								
		0.06	0.12	0.25	0.5	1	2	4	8	16
Tindazole										
MIC 10^5/ml	40	6	34							
10^8/ml	20						17	3		
MBC 10^5/ml										
5% L.H.B.	3				2	1				
100% Serum	3					2	1			
25% Serum	3			3						
Nimorazole										
MIC 10^5/ml	40		13	25	2					
10^8/ml	20						6	14		
MBC 10^5/ml										
5% L.H.B.	3								2	1
100% Serum	3						1	1	1	
25% Serum	3					2	1			

DISCUSSION

It is well recognised that clindamycin is one of the more
active drugs against <u>Bacteroides fragilis</u> (Bodner et al., 1972) and
this drug is considered by many to be the antibiotic of choice in
treating infections caused by this organism.   The more frequent
occurrence of severe side effects to this drug (Tedesco, Barton &
Alpers, 1974) has led to the search for further effective
antimicrobial agents.   Metronidazole has been noted to be active
against this group of pathogens (Whelan & Hale, 1973) and we
confirm this <u>in vitro</u> activity.   It is interesting to note that
tindazole consistently was twice as active as metronidazole.
Nimorazole had a similar activity to metronidazole.   The activity
of all three drugs was considerably affected by the size of inoculum
but only moderately affected by serum.

Although all the strains we investigated were remarkably

TABLE IV. Effect of inoculum and media on MIC/MBC of clindamycin and spectinomycin against Bacteroides sp.

Drug and inoculum	No. tested	concentration mg/l											
		<0.06	0.12	0.25	0.5	1	2	4	8	16	32	64	>64
Clindamycin													
MIC 10^5/ml	40	40											
10^8/ml	20		18	2									
MBC 10^5/ml	3												
5% L.H.B.	3						2					1	
100% Serum	3									1	1	1	
25% Serum	3								2			1	
Spectinomycin													
MIC 10^5/ml	40										40		
10^8/ml	20										5	13	2
MBC 10^5/ml	3												
5% L.H.B.	3											2	1
100% Serum	3											2	1
25% Serum	3											2	1

uniformly susceptible to 32 mg/l of spectinomycin and Philips and Warren showed there was a similar narrow range of antibiotic susceptibility. They noted that with serial subculture resistance to this drug emerged. Changes in inoculum size and the presence of serum had little effect on the MIC and MBC respectively.

Ferguson and Smith (1975) found the MIC to be 2 - 4 fold higher when employing a 10% carbon dioxide/hydrogen as the incubating atmosphere. We did not notice any significant alteration in MIC with changing from Gas Pak to 10% carbon dioxide/hydrogen. It is possible that the different media employed may affect the buffering capacity of the agar and so alter the apparent activity of the drug, although Philips' work in which four media were compared, did not suggest this. It was interesting to note that, in our hands, the Bacteroides isolates failed to grow in a pure hydrogen atmosphere

As it is possible to achieve blood levels of the nitroimidazole compounds and spectinomycin which are well above the minimum inhibitory concentrations, these antimicrobial agents may well merit clinical investigation in the treatment of Bacteroides infections.

ACKNOWLEDGEMENTS

We should like to thank both Dr. J.F.F. Rooney of Carlo Erba (U.K.) Ltd., for supporting this study and supplying the nimorazole, and Upjohn Ltd., for supplying the clindamycin and spectinomycin.

REFERENCES

Philips, I.& Warren, C. Susceptibility of Bacteroides fragilis to spectinomycin. Journal of Antimicrobial Chemotherapy 1: 91-95 (1975).

Bodner, S.J., Koenig, M.G., Treanor, L.L. & Goodman, J.S. Antibiotic susceptibility testing of Bacteroides. Antimicrobial Agents & Chemotherapy 2: 57-60 (1972).

Whelan, J.P.F., & Hale, J.H. Bactericidal activity of metronidazole against Bacteroides fragilis. Journal of Clinical Pathology 26: 393-395 (1973).

Tedesco, F.J., Barton, R.W. & Alpers, D.H. Clindamycin associated colitis: A prospective study. Annals of Internal Medicine 81: 429-433 (1974).

Ferguson, R.R. & Smith, L.L. Bacteroides fragilis and spectinomycin. Journal of Antimicrobial Chemotherapy 1: 245-246 (1975).

ACTIVITY OF FIVE NITROFURANS AGAINST NON-SPORING GRAM-NEGATIVE ANAEROBIC BACILLI

A.V. Reynolds, J.M.T. Hamilton-Miller and
W. Brumfitt
The Royal Free Hospital

Pond Street, Hampstead, London NW3 2QG

In a preliminary report (Brumfitt et al 1975) we showed that nifuratel was significantly more active than nitrofurantoin against 73 strains of Gram-negative anaerobic bacilli. We have now extended our investigations to cover a total of five nitrofurans (the clinically available nitrofurantoin, nifuratel, nitrofurazone and furazolidone and a compound under evaluation SQ 18,506), tested against 110 strains of Gram-negative anaerobic bacilli.

MATERIALS AND METHODS

Antimicrobial Compounds

Sodium nitrofurantoin (NFT), nifuratel (NFL), furazolidone (FZD), and SQ 18,506 (SQ), as pure substances, were kindly provided by Eaton Laboratories, The Wellcome Foundation, Smith, Kline & French Laboratories Ltd., and E.R. Squibb & Sons Inc., respectively. A commercially available solution (0.2%) was used as a source of nitrofurazone (NFZ).

Strains

A total of 110 Gram-negative anaerobic strains were tested. 43 strains were isolated from clinical material sent to the routine microbiology laboratory at this hospital. Dr S.M. Finegold kindly sent 9 strains, 8 of which had been isolated from clinical sources; all of these strains had been speciated. 18 strains were received from Dr A. Percival and 12 from Dr R.B. Sykes; these had also been isolated from clinical specimens. 5 strains were donated by Dr B.S. Drasar. Reference strains were obtained from the Center

for Disease Control (5), National Collection of Type Cultures (6),
Dr H. Beerens (8), and Dr M. Sebald (4).

Strains which had not been classified before receipt were
provisionally identified from their antibiograms (Finegold et al,
1967). Strains that were resistant to kanamycin (2 mg/ml),
polymyxin B (10 μg/ml), penicillin G (2 u/ml) and vancomycin
5 μg/ml) were identified as <u>Bacteroides fragilis.</u> Strains not
showing this pattern were labelled "unidentified Gram-negative
rods".

MIC

NFT was dissolved, and suitably diluted, in sterile distilled
water; NFZ was also diluted in water. NFL, FZD, and SQ were
dissolved, and diluted, in dimethylsulphoxide. 0.1 ml amounts of
the appropriate dilutions were added to bottles containing 25 ml
volumes of molten Brucella agar (BBL), supplemented with 5% lysed
defibrinated horse blood, 5 μg/ml haemin and 0.5 μg/ml menadione,
and two plates were poured from each bottle.

Strains were incubated anaerobically for 22 hours at 37C in
thioglycollate medium 135-C (BBL) supplemented with 0.5% yeast
extract (Difco), 5 μg/ml haemin and 0.5 μg/ml menadione. These
cultures were diluted 1/100 in 0.06 M, pH 7 phosphate buffer
containing 0.03% cysteine hydrochloride. 3 μl volumes of 25
suspensions were inoculated onto the plates using a multiple
inoculator (the inocumum size was c. 20,000 colony-forming units.
Plates were incubated anaerobically for 42 hours. Reproducibility
was controlled by including strain <u>B.fragilis</u> WAL 1 in each group
of organisms tested. Aerobic and anaerobic control plates were
included in each set. The GasPak system (95% H_2 + 5% CO_2) was
used throughout this study to obtain anaerobic conditions.

MIC was taken as the lowest concentration that prevented the
growth of no more than 3 colonies, that is 99.99% inhibition.

RESULTS

21 strains were received as <u>B.fragilis</u> and 11 as <u>Fusobacterium</u>
spp. 74 of the remaining strains were provisionally identified as
<u>B.fragilis</u> and 4 could not be identified on the basis of their
antibiograms.

The results of the MIC determinations are summarised in Table
1. NFL and FZD were the most active of the five agents, with
geometric mean MIC values of 0.30 μg/ml and 0.24 μg/ml respectively.
SQ had a mean MIC value of 1.69 μg/ml and NFZ 2.51 μg/ml.

Initial results with a broth dilution subculture method

Table 1. MIC's of 5 nitrofurans against non-sporing Gram-negative anaerobic bacilli.

	Number of strains inhibited at (μg/ml)									Geometric Mean MIC (μg/ml)
	0.062	0.125	0.25	0.5	1.0	2.0	4.0	8.0	16.0	
NFT						2	11	89	8	7.65
NFZ				1	4	63	42			2.51
SQ			6	9	20	49	23	3		1.69
NFL	2	30	27	41	10					0.30
FZD	5	29	42	33	1					0.24

indicate that all the compounds, except SQ, are bactericidal at 2 X MIC, giving >99.9% kill. SQ was bactericidal at 16 X MIC.

DISCUSSION

It is clear from the many reports currently appearing in the literature that the sensitivity patterns of anaerobic organisms are being actively investigated. Clindamycin is regarded by some as drug of choice for infections caused by anaerobic organisms where the sensitivity pattern of the infecting organism is unknown. However, resistant strains have been reported (Staneck and Washington 1974), and clindamycin may also cause pseudomembranous colitis (Editorial 1974). Chloramphenicol is uniformly active against anaerobic bacteria but clinicians are unwilling to use it because of its reputation for causing bone marrow toxicity. Metronidazole has been shown to be bactericidal against B.fragilis (Nastro and Finegold 1972) and initial clinical results so far seem promising (Tally et al 1972, 1975, Study Group 1974), but no parenteral preparation is presently available, and resistant strains of certain Gram-positive anaerobes have been isolated (Dornbusch and Nord 1974, Chow et al 1975). Thus, all the drugs currently used for the initial therapy of anaerobic infection have certain shortcomings.

Our studies suggest that compounds containing a primary nitro-group possess activity against anaerobic bacteria. We compared three nitroimidazoles, metronidazole, nimorazole and tinidazole (Reynolds et al 1975), and found tinidazole to be the most active. The nitrofurans also contain a primary nitro- group and the present study extends previous work (Finegold and Sutter 1972, Schoutens et al 1973) where NFT alone was tested and also shows that NFL and FZD are significantly more active than NFT against Gram-negative anaerobic bacilli.

Very little pharmacokinetic or toxicological data is available on the nitrofurans, so all the present results indicate is that further studies should be undertaken to ascertain whether this group of compounds may have a place in the therapy of systemic infections.

REFERENCES

Brumfitt, W., Reynolds, A.V. & Hamilton-Miller, J.M.T. 1975
    Lancet, $\underline{1}$, 460.
Chow, A.W., Patten, V. & Cuze, L.B. 1975 J.Infect.Dis., $\underline{131}$, 182.
Dornbusch, K. & Nord, C.E. 1974 Med.Microbiol.Immunol., $\underline{160}$, 265.
Editorial 1974 Brit.Med.J., $\underline{4}$, 65.
Finegold, S.M., Harada, N.E. & Miller, L.G. 1967 J.Bact. $\underline{94}$, 1443.
Finegold, S.M. & Sutter, V.L. 1972 p 275 in Host Resistance to Com-
    mensal Bacteria, MacPhee, T. Ed. Churchill Livingstone, Edinburgh.
Nastro, L.J. & Finegold, S.M. 1972 J.Infect.Dis., $\underline{126}$, 104.
Reynolds, A.V., Hamilton-Miller, J.M.T. & Brumfitt, W. 1975
    J.Clin.Path. In press.
Schoutens, E., Labbe, M., & Yourassowsky, E. 1973 Path.-Biol.
    $\underline{21}$, 349.
Staneck, J.L. & Washington, J.A. 1974 Antimicrob. Agents
    Chemother. $\underline{6}$, 311.
Study Group 1974 Lancet $\underline{2}$, 1540.
Tally, F.P., Sutter, V.L. & Finegold, S.M. 1972 Calif.Med.,
    $\underline{117}$, 22.
Tally, F.P., Sutter, V.L. & Finegold, S.M. 1975 Antimicrob.
    Agents Chemother. $\underline{7}$, 672.

THE SUSCEPTIBILITY OF BACTEROIDES FRAGILIS TO SPECTINOMYCIN

I.R.FERGUSON AND LYNDA L.SMITH

Public Health Laboratory Service

Public Health Laboratory, Luton and Dunstable
Hospital, Luton, Bedfordshire, England

SUMMARY

Minimum inhibitory concentrations (MICs) and minimum
bactericidal concentrations (MBCs) of spectinomycin were
determined for 90 clinical isolates of Bacteroides fragilis
Only 10% of strains tested were resistant to more than
80 ug/ml of spectinomycin. There was a marked diminution
of activity in acid media and the concentration of carbon
dioxide in the anaerobic atmosphere also affected the MICs.

INTRODUCTION

Spectinomycin was first described by Mason et al.
(1961), and during the same year Lewis and Clapp reported
its antimicrobial activity against a variety of Gram-
positive and Gram-negative organisms. Of the organisms
tested in vivo only Staphylococcus aureus developed
resistance to this new antibiotic; among the anaerobic
bacteria single strains only of Clostridium perfringens,
Cl.sporogenes and Cl.tetani were examined; no Bacteroides
species were included. In the preliminary experimental work
the sulphate salt was utilised, but in 1968 spectinomycin
was prepared as the dihydrochloride pentahydrate which is
now in clinical use. The antibiotic is a fused tricyclic
molecule including actinamin, a unique aminocyclitol
containing no aminosugar (Hoeksema et al., 1961). Thus,
like streptomycin, kanamycin and gentamicin, it is an
aminocyclitol antibiotic but it is not, as its name
suggests, a true aminoglycoside.

This antibiotic has been successfully used worldwide in the treatment of gonorrhoea, with high cure rates after single injections (Wilcox, 1962; Smithurst, 1972; Tuza and Hatos, 1973).

B.fragilis is universally resistant to the amino-glycosides; but since spectinomycin is devoid of an aminosugar moeity, it was felt that the susceptibility of B.fragilis should be tested against this antibiotic.

MATERIAL AND METHODS

Organisms

A total of 90 fresh clinical isolates of B.Fragilis from clinical material was tested. B.fragilis NCTC 9343 and NCTC 9344 were used as control organisms. All the organisms were identified as non-sporing Gram-negative obligate anaerobic bacilli showing typical volatile products of metabolism as determined by gas-liquid chromography, and standard biochemical reactions (Holdeman and Moore, 1972).

Sensitivity Medium

The antibiotic medium (Sensitest, Oxoid CM 409) was prepared as directed by the manufacturer. It was dispensed in 19 ml volumes prior to autoclaving. When required the agar was melted by steaming, and cooled to 56°C. The appropiate antibiotic solution was then added together with 0.2 ml of a stock filter sterilized haemin-menadione solution to give a final concentration of 5 ug/ml and 0.5 ug/ml respectively (Sutter et al., 1972)

In one series of plates, using both diagnostic sensitivity test agar (DST) and sensitest agar, the pH of the media was adjusted to pH6, 7 and 8 as determined with a pH meter.

Preparation of Spectinomycin Plates

The antibiotic dilutions of spectinomycin were made in normal sterile saline to give final concentrations in the medium over the range 20 ug/ml to 100 ug/ml. These

dilutions were dispensed in small aliquots and stored at
-20°C. When required 1 ml of each solution was added to
19 ml of sensitest agar at 56°C and the molten agar poured
into 9 cm Petri dishes on a level surface. The plates were
stored overnight at 4°C, and prior to use were dried for
2 hours at 37°C. Although there is increased oxygen
absorption into the medium at refrigerator temperatures
this does not adversely affect the growth of B.fragilis.

Inoculation of Plates

Colonies of the test organisms from 48 hour-old
cultures on horse blood agar plates were emulsified in
2 ml nutrient broth to produce a faint turbidity. This,
made up to 10 ml with broth (Ingham et al., 1968), gave
a density of approximately 10^6 organisms/ml as determined
by surface viable counts (Miles and Misra, 1938). The
suspensions of test organisms were inoculated onto the
antibiotic plates, and onto control antibiotic-free plates
using a phage typing apparatus which delivered 0.02 ml.
The two control organisms were included on each plate. The
inoculated plates were immediately incubated for 18-24
hours at 37°C in an atmosphere of 92.5% hydrogen and 7.5%
carbon dioxide in GasPak 150 vented jars(BBL), employing
the evacuation-replacement technique. In one series, two
different anaerobic techniques were used in parallel, the
evacuation-replacement and GasPak System.

Reading Results

The MIC of spectinomycin was defined as the lowest
concentration producing absence of bacterial growth. The
MBC was determined by replica plating all MIC plates on
which growth was absent onto antibiotic-free horse blood
agar plates (Elek and Hilson, 1954). These plates were
incubated anaerobically for 18-24 hours, and the end-
point was read as growth of more than 20 colonies.

RESULTS

The MICs and MBCs of spectinomycin for the 90 strains
tested are shown in table I. Control organisms NCTC 9343
and NCTC 9344 gave MIC and MBC levels of 60 ug/ml. As is
clear from the Table, 81 strains (90%) were inhibited by
80 ug/ml of less, and 75 strains (82%) were killed over
the same range of spectinomycin.

Table I   MICs and MBCs of spectinomycin for 90 strains
            of Bacteroides fragilis

					ug/ml					
	20	30	40	50	60	70	80	90	100	>100
MIC	–	4	7	4	27	20	19	6	2	1
MBC	–	1	6	6	25	18	19	7	4	4

Table II shows that the MICs for 33 strains were
diminished at high pH and markedly increased at low pH.
There was little significant difference in the MICs when
DST and sensitest agars were employed in the study.

Table II   Effect of pH and medium on MICS of spectino-
            mycin for 33 strains of Bacteroides fragilis

				MIC ug/ml							
Medium	pH	20	30	40	50	60	70	80	90	100	>100
Sensitest	8	–	3	17	5	8	–	–	–	–	–
DST	8	4	11	8	10	–	–	–	–	–	–
Sensitest	7	–	–	–	–	6	6	20	1	–	–
DST	7	–	–	–	–	2	14	17	–	–	–
Sensitest	6	–	–	–	–	–	–	–	–	3	30
DST	6	–	–	–	–	–	–	–	–	9	24

In Table III the effect of the difference in carbon
dioxide concentrations in the anaerobic atmosphere on the
MICs of 32 strains is demonstated. With relatively low
concentrations when using the GasPak System the MICs were
10 to 20 ug/ml lower than when using 7.5% carbon dioxide.

Table III   Effect of carbon dioxide on MICs of spectino-
            mycin for 32 strains of Bacteroides fragilis

			MIC ug/ml						
	30	40	50	60	70	80	90	100	CO_2 conc.
Replacement	–	1	6	7	14	3	1	–	7.5%
GasPak	–	2	19	9	2	–	–	–	Variable (0.5 – 2.7%)

DISCUSSION

Clindamycin and lincomycin, which are bacteriostatic
antibiotics, have become established as the drugs of
choice in the treatment of infections due to B.fragilis.
Recent adverse reports of the side effects (Leading
article, 1974), which we have not encounted, may prompt
some clinicians to seek an alternative therapeutic agent.
Tetracycline resistance occurs in approximately 50% of
B.fragilis, so that it has limitations in clinical use.
Phillips and Warren (1974) and Okubadejo (1974) reported
that co-trimoxazole is active against most strains of
B.fragilis, but this has been challanged by Rosenblatt
and Stewart (1974).

Little data has been published on the serum levels
obtained following administration of spectinomycin. In a
limited study, Novak et al., (1974) reported serum levels
in the range 144-210 ug/ml (mean 176 ug/ml) in patients
receiving 2 g intravenously over a 2 hour period; these
levels were determined at the end of the infusion. In
their study no ototoxicity, hepatotoxicity, nephrotoxicity
or local reaction was shown. Earlier, Wagner et al.,
(1968) reported peak serum levels averaging 138 ug/ml
after one hour in patients receiving 2 g by intramuscular
injection; 4 hours after injection the mean serum level
was 62.8 ug/ml, and after 5 hours was 39.8 ug/ml. When
these in vivo results are related to the in vitro MIC
levels determined in the present study, it is clear that
by the 4th post-injectional hour the serum levels have
become ineffective against some strains (48 of 90); by
the 5th hour the level is ineffective against most strains
(79 of 90).

The MIC results in this study appear to be at
variance with those reported by Phillips and Warren (1975).
Using diagnostic sensitivity test agar and the GasPak
System, they found that 93% of their strains of B.fragilis
were inhibited by 16 ug/ml. They also demonstated some
variation in the MIC when different media were employed.
On Wellcotest agar and Isotonic Sensitest agar most strains
had MICs of 32 ug/ml and on Mueller-Hinton base, 50% of
strains had MICs of 64 ug/ml.

The inhibitory effect of acidity on the activity of
spectinomycin, first noted by Phillips and Warren, was
confirmed in the present study. A similar effect on the
activity of lincomycin and erythromycin against B.fragilis
was reported by Ingham et al., (1970), who noted that the

presence of carbon dioxide in the anaerobic atmosphere greatly reduced the activity of these antibiotics. Recent work in this laboratory, (Ferguson et al., 1975) has demonstrated that the GasPak envelopes give a marked variation in carbon dioxide concentrations in the anaerobic atmosphere ranging from 0.5% to 2.7%. Thus spectinomycin activity is also influenced by carbon dioxide concentrations.

These differences between MICs of B.fragilis To spectinomycin once again highlight the continuing problem of achieving uniformity in methodology between laboratories when testing antibiotic susceptibility of anaerobic bacteria. Since the growth of many anaerobes is greatly enhanced by carbon dioxide, it is clearly important that the carbon dioxide is accurately defined, if results from different workers are to be meaningfully compared.

Undoubtedly spectinomycin has a place in the treatment of gonorrhoea. It now seems clear that this antibiotic may find a place in the treatment of infections due to B.fragilis, as chemotherapy with a bactericidal antibiotic is often preferable to treatment with a bacteriostatic one.

This matter can be resolved only by a prospective clinical trial. Adjustment of the parentral dose, and the interval between doses may yield more acceptable serum levels. The reported absence of toxicity favours an increased dosage regime. It may also be preferable to combine spectinomycin with a second bactericidal drug such as metronidazole (Flagyl) which is highly effective against B.fragilis infections (Preliminary Communication, 1974).

ACKNOWLEDGEMENTS

We are indedted to Dr.A.T.Willis for encouragement and support, to Mrs Kathleen Williams for able technical assistance, and to the Upjohn Company for supplies of spectinomycin and for a generous grant towards the cost of the study.

REFERENCES

Elek,S.D. and Hilson,G.R.F.(1954),Journal of Clinical Pathology,7,37.

Ferguson,I.R.,Phillips,K.D. and Tearle,P.V.(1975), Journal of Applied Bacteriology, in the press.

Hoeksema,H.A.,Argedoulis,A.D. and Wiley,P.(1962), Journal of the American Chemical Society,84,3212.

Holdeman,L.V. and Moore,W.E.C.(1972), Anaerobic laboratory manual.Virginia Polytechnic Institute and State University; Blacksburg.

Ingham,H.R.,Selkon,J.B.,Codd,A.A. and Hale,J.H. (1968),Journal of Clinical Pathology,21,432.

Ingham,H.R.,Selkon,J.B.,Codd,A.A. and Hale,J.H. (1970),Journal of Clinical Pathology,23,254.

Leading article.(1974),British Medical Journal,4,65.

Lewis,C. and Clapp,H.W.(1961),Antibiotics and Chemotherapy,11,127.

Mason,D.J. Smith,R.M. and Dietz,A.(1961),Antibiotics and Chemotherapy,11,118.

Miles,A.A. and Misra,S.S.(1938),Journal of Hygiene, Cambridge,38,732.

Novak,E.,Schlagel,C.A.,LeZotte,L.A. and Pfeifer,R.T. (1974),Journal of Clinical Pharmacology,14,442.

Okubadejo,O.A.(1974),Lancet,1,1061.

Phillips,I. and Warren,C.(1974),Lancet,1,827.

Phillips,I. and Warren,C.(1975),Journal of Antimicrobial Chemotherapy,1,91.

Preliminary communication.(1974),Lancet,2,1540.

Rosenblatt,J.E. and Stewart,P.R.(1974),Antimicrobial Agents and Chemotherapy,6,93.

Smithurst,B.A.(1972),New Zealand Medical Journal, 75,82.

Sutter,V.L.,Kwok,Y-Y. and Finegold,S.M.(1972), Applied Microbiology,23,268.

Tuza,F.L.C. and Hatos,G.(1973),Medical Journal of Australia,2,1090.

Wagner,J.G.,Novak,E.,Leslie,L.G. and Metzler,C.M.
(1968),International Journal of Clinical Pharmacology,
1,261.

Wilcox,R.R.(1962),British Journal of Venereal
Diseases,38,150.

CHLORAMPHENICOL AND THIAMPHENICOL IN INFECTIONS BY ANAEROBIC GRAM NEGATIVE BACILLI

GARCIA, J.A. ; SAENZ, M.C. ; MARTIN, F. ; PRIETO, J.

Department of Microbiology. Faculty of Medicine

University of Salamanca. Fonseca, 2 (SPAIN)

The increase of infections through anaerobic germs, the improvements in the present techniques of diagnosis, and the resistance to antibiotics by a greater number of strains, have brought about increase in publications on this subject at the present time.

Most authors agree that Gram negative anaerobic bacilli are responsible for the most serious and frequent clinical cases, ocurring either isolated from or together with another flora, without clearly explaining their role in the process from which they were isolated.

In general, the processes caused by most Gram negative bacilli establish therapeutic problems due to the resistance to antibiotics by these bacteria, and sometimes, to the lack of knowledge of their sensitivity to certain antibiotics, Werner and Pulvever (1971). We have therefore considered it important to study a phase of this subject, which although new in our country, has already been analyzed by other authors, Bodner et al (1972), Martin et al (1972) and Van Beers et al (1975).

We have studied the behaviour of 200 strains of Gram negative anaerobic bacilli against Chloramphenicol and Thiamphenicol. The former is undoubtedly, the most active antibiotic against all types of anaerobic germs and few strains are resistant to it. The semisinthetic antibiotic, derived from Chloramphenicol has not as yet been proved harmful to the bone marrow.

Table I : Sensitivity of B. fragilis to Chloramphenicol and Thiamphenicol.

Bacteroides	Chloramphenicol					
	0.8	1.6	3.1	6.2	12.5	25
B. vulgatus	1	13	6	2		
B. thetaiotaomicron	2	3	18	3		
B. fragilis	2	10	54	4		
B. distasonis		3	13	1		
B. ovatus			4	1		
TOTAL	5	29	95	11		

Bacteroides	Thiamphenicol					
	0.8	1.6	3.1	6.2	12.5	25
B. vulgatus			4	14	4	
B. thetaiotaomicron				9	16	1
B. fragilis			4	48	18	
B. distasonis				8	9	
B. ovatus				1	4	
TOTAL			8	80	51	1

MATERIAL AND METHODS

We have studied 191 strains isolated from various pathological products. Out of these, 134 were identified as B. fragilis, and 57 as Fusobacterium (Sphaerophorus). Nine collection strains were included, as controls, in our investigation.

The identification of the genus was done according to the behaviour of these Gram negative bacilli in media containing bile, Polymyxin, Brilliant Green, Phosphomycin, Penicillin and Treonine. As orientation fact we considered the morphological aspects, Werner and Pulverer (1971), and Finegold et al (1974).

The identification of species or subspecies was done according to the fermentation of sugars, and other biochemical tests : Dowell and Hawkins (1972).

The antibiotics tested were : Levorotatory Chloramphenicol with a biological activity of 977 μg/ml., provided by Carlo Erba Laboratories, and Levorotatory Thiamphenicol biological activity of 1040 μg/ml. provided by Zambon Laboratories (Spain).

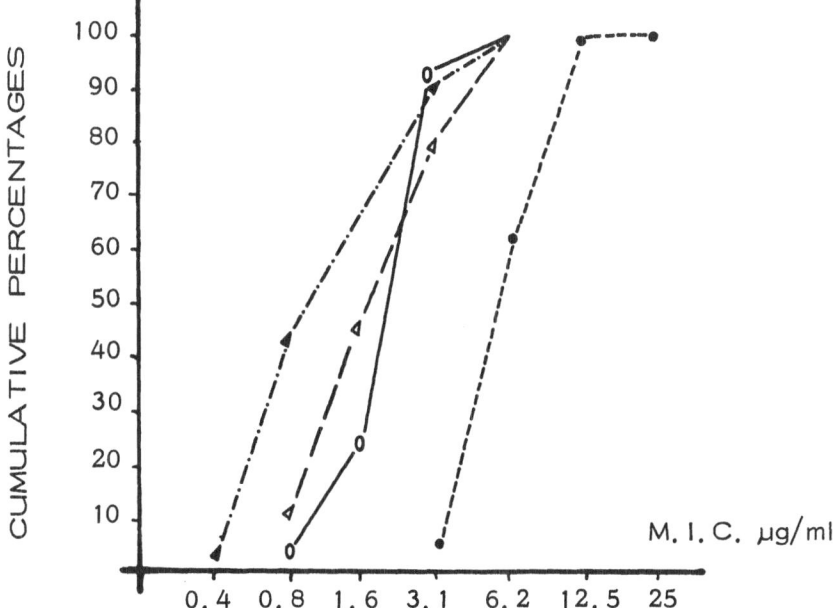

Fig. 1 : Comparative activity of Chloramphenicol and Thiamphenicol against Bacteroides and Sphaerophorus.
► Sphaerophorus (Thiamphenicol). ► Sphaerophorus (Chloramphenicol)
o B. fragilis (Chloramphenicol).   • B. fragilis (Thiamphenicol).

The sensitivity tests for the M. I. C. were performed through
the method of progressive dilutions in solid medium, smearing on
the surface a suspension of 10^5 ger/ml. , with a calibrated loop,
Garcia Rodriguez et al. (1974) and Van Beers et al (1975).

Table II : Sensitivity of Sphaerophorus to Chloramphenicol and
        Thiamphenicol.

Antitiotic	Species	μg/ml.				
		0.4	0.8	1.6	3.1	6.2
Chloramphenicol	necrophorus			3	1	
	varius		2	12	11	7
	freundii		5	8	7	4
	TOTAL		7	23	19	11
Thiamphenicol	necrophorus				2	2
	varius		14	9	7	2
	freundii	2	10	7	4	1
	TOTAL	2	24	16	13	5

RESULTS

The results were different when Chloramphenicol and Thiamphenicol were studied.

As for Chloramphenicol, all the strains tested were inhibited by a concentration lower than 6.2 µg/ml. (Table I).

The activity of this antibiotic against Sphaerophorus and Bacteroides was quite similar (Fig. 1), both showing the same median M.I.C.,which was 2.9 .

Thiamphenicol behaved differently. We found a strain of B. fragilis which was only inhibited with a concentration of 25 µg/ml.. Furthermore 36% of the Bacteroides studied needed a concentration of 12 µg/ml. for their inhibition (Table I) Summarizing, it was much less effective than Chloramphenicol against B. fragilis (M.I.C. of 8.4), but it surpassed Chloramphenicol in activity when it was tested against the genus Sphaerophorus (Median M.I.C. of 1.9), all strains being sensitive to concentrations below 6.2µg/ml. (Table II).

DISCUSSION

The Chloramphenicol M.I.C.'s against Bacteroides which we found coincide in their minimum values, 0.8µg/ml., with those obtained by other authors. Nevertheless, the median M.I.C. of our strains, 2.9 µg/ml. is one of the lowest, in comparison with Sutter's 5.4, and Garrod's 7.8. Most of Bodner's results are between 3.1 and 6.2, and Thornton et al (1970) indicate a median M.I.C. of 12.5µg/ml.

When Thiamphenicol was tested against Bacteroides, we obtained similar results to those found by Van Beers et al. although we did not observe any strain with a sensitivity below 3.1 µg/ml. Curiously, and unlike Chloramphenicol, Thiamphenicol behaved differently against Sphaerophorus, since its activity ranged between concentrations of 0.4 and 6.2 µg/ml., and with a M.I.C. of 1.9µg/ml. Thus, it was much more active against Sphaerophorus than against Bacteroides, and its behaviour against Sphaerophorus was superior to that of Chloramphenicol. One must assume that the varied nature of the results is due to the defective solubility of Thiamphenicol, which necessitated the utilization of Dimethylformamide as a solvent.

In general, Chloramphenicol is very active, Kislak (1972), and Monif and Baer (1974), and has a greater diffusion power than Thiamphenicol but is potentially much more toxic. On the other hand, Thiamphenicol is active against 99.5% of the strains, at therapeutic concentrations is more effective against Sphaerophorus, and does not have toxic effects, for which its clinical utilization is more advisable.

REFERENCES

BODNER, S. J.; KOENING, M. G.; TREANOR, L. L. and GOODMAN, J. S. (1972). - "Antibiotic Susceptibility Testing of Bacteroides". - Antimicrob. Ag. Chemother. 2 : 57.

DOWELL, V. R. and HAWKINS, T. M. (1972). - "Laboratory Methods in Anaerobic Bacteriology, CDS Laboratory Manual". - Center for Disease Control Atlanta, Georgia

FINEGOLD, S. M.; SUTTER, V. L.; ATTEBERY, H. R. (1974) "Isolation of Anaerobic Bacteria: 365. Manual of Clinica Microbiology 2nd. Ed. Edite by. LENNETTE, SPAULDING y TRANT. American. Society for Microbiology. Washinton, D. C.

GARCIA RODRIGUEZ, J. A.; PRIETO PRIETO, J. y GARCIA SANCHEZ, J. E. (1974). - "Los Bacilos Anaerobios Gram negativos, como responsables de Infecciones : Su sensibilidad frente a 7 Cefalosporinas Diferentes". - Rev. de Quimiot. 1 : 143.

GARROD, L. P. (1955). - "Sensibility of Four Species of Bacteroides to Antibiotics". - Brit. Med. J. 2 : 1529.

INGHAM, H. R.; SELKON, J. B.; CODD, A. A. and HALE, J. H. (1970). - "The Effect of Carbon Dioxide on the Sensitivity of Bacteroides fragilis to Certain Antibiotics in Vitro". - J. Clin. Pathol. 23 : 254.

KISLAK, J. W. (1972). - "The Susceptibility of Bacteroides fragilis to 24 Antibiotics". - J. Infect. Dis. 125 : 295.

MARTIN, W. J.; GADNER, M., and WASHIGTON, J. A. (1972) "In Vitro Antimicrobial Susceptibility of Anaerobic Bacteria Isolated from Clinical Specimens". - Antimicrob. Ag. Chemother. 2 : 148.

MONIF, G.R.G. and BAER, H. (1974).- "In Vitro Susceptibility of Bacteroides Strains to Tetracycline, Chloramphenicol,
Doxicycline and Clindamycin". - Obst. and Gynecol. 43 : 211.

SUTTER, V.L.; and WASHINGTON, J.A. (1974).- "Susceptibility Testing of Anaerobes" : 435. Manual of Clinical Microbiology 2nd. Ed. Edit. by LENNETTE, SAPULDING and TRUANT
American Society for Microbiology. Washington, D.C.

THORNTON, G.F.; and CRAMER, J.A. (1970).- "Antibiotic Susceptibility of Bacteroides Species". - Antimicrob. Ag. Chemother. 509.

VAN BEERS, B.; SCHOUTENS, E.; VANDERLINDEN, M.P.
and YOURASSWSKY, E. (1975).- "Comparative in Vitro Activity
of Chloramphenicol and Thiamphenicol on Common Aerobic and Anaerobic Gram negative Bacilli (Salmonella and Shigella excluded)"
Chemother. 21 : 73.

WERNER, H., and PULVERER, G. (1971).- "Häufigkeit
und Medizinische Bedeutung der Eitererregenden. Bacteroides und
Sphaerophorus-Aten". - Dtsche. Med. Wschr. 96 : 1325.

THE EFFECT OF ANTIMICROBIAL AGENTS ON ANAEROBES IN

FECAL FLORA

KEIU NINOMIYA, KUNITOMO WATANABE, SHUNRO KOBATA
HIROMU IMAMURA, IZUMI MOCHIZUKI, TOSHIO MIWA
YASUO SHIMIZU, KAZUE UENO AND SHOICHRO SUZUKI
Department of Bacteriology, Gifu University,
School of Medicine, Japan
Tsukasa-machi, Gifu-shi, Gifu-ken, Japan

INTRODUCTION

In recent years, many investigators, ourselves included, have examined the effect of antimicrobial agents on anaerobes in human fecal flora of healthy adults and patients. Dr. Finegold's laboratory has been engaging in this subjects to report on excellent studies. At the same time, Dr. Ueno and his associates were studying same subjects, especially changes of Bacteroides using selective isolation media which they had formulated. In this study, we would like to report on the effect of antimicrobial agents on the anaerobes in fecal flora of Japanese residing in Japan. Additionally, the fecal anaerobic bacteria in patients with urogenital deseases was examined after treatment of various antimicrobial agents for a certain period.

MATERIALS and METHODS

Antimicrobial agents were administered to 8 healty volunteer subjects and 4 patients for certain period, to study the changes in number of bacteria and anaerobic species in the feces. The feces was collected before, during and after administration. Fresh feces from sub- jects was collected in large petri dishes for process- ing immediately after arrival in the laboratory. About one gram of feces was measured out and under an O_2 free CO_2 gas enviroment, using our special diluent for feces, the specimens were diluted by 10 fold dilutions. 0.1 ml of each dilution was inoculated to each medium.

The steel wool method with an atmosphere of 90 %
nitrogen and 10 % carbon dioxide was used throughout
this study.

After incubation period of 4 days, colonies were
picked from each media and each strain was identified.
Anaerobes isolated were identified according to the VPI
manual, the WVA manual, the CDC manual and our own manual.

Lincomycin, clindamycin, doxycycline and metronidazole were administered to healthy volunteer and gentamycin, kanamycin, colistin, amikacin, rifampicin, p-amino
salicylic acid and isonicotinic acid hydrazide were
given to patients. the dosage of each drug is shown on
each table.

RESULTS

In the case with administration of 0.8 g of lincomycin per day for 7 days, B. fragilis ss. thetaiotaomicron was predominant throughout this examination.
Fusobacterium sp. found with the level of 10^6 per gram
of feces diminished to less than 10^2 viable cell by
this drugs.

The results with another case of lincomycin are
shown in Table 1. Among the largest comprnents in fecal
flora, before the administration of this drug, B. fragilis
ss. distasonis was predominant throughout this experiment. B. fragilis ss. thetaiotaomicron was decreased,
extremely, during , 1st and 7th day after administration. And B. fragilis ss. vulgatus showed a decrease
as much as B. fragilis ss. thetaiotaomicron after administration. On the other hand , B. fragilis ss. fragilis increased to be predominant the 7th day after administration of it, for the first time.

Table 1   Effect of lincomycin on B. fragilis group
           in fecal flora

organism	before	during	after	
			1st	7th
B. fragilis				
ss. distasonis	10^*	9	9	10
ss. vulgatus	10	9	-**	-
ss. thetaiota-				
omicron	10	-	-	-
ss. fragilis	-	-	-	9

* : Results are expressed as bacterial count (1/log of
    bacteria per gram of feces)
** : below the level of 10^8 per gram of feces

B. fragilis ss. thetaiotaomicron, ss. distasonis
and ss. vulgatus were cultured predominantly before the
administration of 0.6g of clindamycin per day for 7 days.
Among them, B. fragilis ss. thetaiotaomicron and ss.
distasonis were diminished midway and recovered after
administration. And B. fragilis ss. vulgatus was firstly
decreased after administration of clindamycin.
Fusobacterium showed the change like to B. fragilis ss.
thetaiotaomicron.

Table 2 shows the results with another case given
this drug. It was found that the most predominant organisms were changed throughout this experiments. Namely,
B. fragilis ss. vulgatus, ss. distasonis, ss. thetaiotaomicron and Bacteroides sp. was individually predominant
on each point of the examination. Fusobacterium and C.
perfringens,which have not been isolated , increased
the 7th day after administration of clindamycin.

The effect of 0.2 g of doxycycline per day for 7
days on anaerobes in fecal flora was as follows. Before
the administration of this drug, the largest components
in fecal flora consisted of three kinds of B. fragilis.
Of them, B. fragilis ss. vulgatus was remaining through
the examination but B. fragilis ss. thetaiotaomicron
was diminished during and recovered after administration.
B. fragilis ss. fragilis continued to be decreased since
the begining of the administration. The other hand, B.
fragilis ss. distasonis increased to be predominant
after the administration of doxycycline.

Table 2   Effect of clindamycin on anaerobes in
           fecal flora

organism	before	during	after 1st	7th
B. fragilis ss. vulgatus	10^*	$-^{**}$	-	-
B. fragilis ssp.	9	-	-	-
B. fragilis ss. distasonis	-	10	-	-
B. fragilis ss. thetaiotaomicron	-	-	9	-
Bacteroides sp.	-	-	-	9
Fusobacterium sp.	-	-	-	8
C. perfringens	-	-	-	4

*: Results are expressed as bacterial count (1/log of
   bacteria per gram of feces)
**: below the level of 10^6(Bacteroides) or 10 (Fuso-
    bacterium and C. perfringens) per gram of feces

Table 3   Effect of doxycycline on anaerobes
           in fecal flora

organism	before	during	after
B. fragilis ss. distasonis	10*	-**	-
B. fragilis ssp.	8	-	-
Bacteroides sp.	10	9	-
Fusobacterium sp.	8	6	-
B. fragilis ss. vulgatus	-	8	. 9

*: Results are expressed as bacterial count (1/log of
   bacteria per gram of feces).

**: below the level of 10^6 (Bacteroides) or 10 (Fusobac-
terium)

        The results with administration of this drug to
another case is presented in Table 3. Among Bacteroides
being predominant in fecal flora before administration,
B. fragilis ss. distasonis and B. fragilis ssp. were
diminished and Bacteroides sp. was unchanged during
that, which was also decreased after. On the contrary,
B. fragilis ss. vulgatus showed increases during and
remained predominantly after administration of doxycycline. Fusobacterium exhibited such changes as Bacteroides sp.
        Table 4 shows the results with administration of
metronidazole, which has strong antibacterial effect
against anaerobes,especially, B. fragilis. B. fragilis
ss. vulgatus was unchanged but B. fragilis ss. distasonis
B. fragilis ssp. were isolated only before the administration of this drug. B. fragilis ss. fragilis and ss.

Table 4   Effect of metronidazole on anaerobes
           in fecal flora

organism	before	during	after
B. fragilis ss. vulgatus	9*	9**	10
B. fragilis ss. distasonis	9	-	-
B. fragilis ssp.	9	-	-
B. fragilis ss. fragilis	-	-	9
B. fragilis ss. thetaiota- micron	-	-	10
Fusobacterium sp.	8	-	-
C. perfringens	-	-	5

*,** : see Table 2.

Table 5   Organism isolated from fecal flora of
          patients treated antimicrobial agents

case	chemothrapy	organism	bacterial count/g
1	gentamycin 80 mg per day, for 5 days	B. fragilis ss. fragilis	10^{*}
		B. fragilis ss vulgatus	10
		Fusobacterium	9
		total aerobes	8
2	kanamycin 3 g and colistin 0.6g per day, for 3 days	B. fragilis ss. distasonis	9
		total aerobes	5
3	amikacin 0.6g per day, for 3 days	B. fragilis ssp.	9
		total aerobes	9
4	rifampicin 0.6 g, PAS** 10g and INAH*** 0.3 g per day, for 10 days	B. fragilis ssp.	10
		total aerobes	9

* : Results are expressed as 1/log of bacteria
    per gram of feces
** : p-aminosalicylic acid
*** : isonicotinic acid hydrazide

thetaiotaomicron and C. perfringens increased for the
first time after administration of metronidazole.
    In another case of this drug, there were little
changes of a number of bacteria and organisms consis-
ting, in fecal flora , throughout this experiment.
    Details on antimicrobial agents, dosage of these
drugs, duration of therapy, a number of bacteria and
anaerobic bacterial species are presented in Table 5.
A number of total anaerobes was not or little changed.
This finding may be suggested because these organisms
were little susceptible to drugs ,excluding rifampicin,
used. However a number of aerobes susceptible to that
was not decreased exception of case 2. Dosage of drugs
used may be slightly effective on bacteria in intestinal
flora. As these antimicrobial agents were treated on
purpose to decrease intestinal bacteria of patients,
this results may remain as future problem.

SUMMARY

The effect of lincomycin, clindamycin, doxycycline and metronidazole on anaerobes in fecal flora of
healthy volunteer subjects was studied.

In many of cases, a number of anaerobic bacteria
especially, Bacteroides fragilis group, was unchanged
or little changed. However , the changes of predominant
organisms in fecal flora were found remarkably among
B. fragilis group.

For instance, in the case of administration of
clindamycin, the results are as follows. Before administration of this drug, B. fragilis ss. vulgatus has
been predominant organisms. This organisms was decreased
below the level of 10^6 per gram of feces and B. fragilis
ss. distasonis increased to be predominant during administration of this drug. The first day after administration of it, this organisms was also diminished such
as B. fragilis ss. vulgatus and B. fragilis ss. thetaiotaomicron increased, which was decreased as same as
organisms previously described 7th day after administration of clindamycin.

Additionally, fecal flora of patients with urogenital deseases were studied after treatment of various antimicrobial agents for a certain period. Although
aerobic bacteria were generally susceptible to drugs
treated in this experiments, a number of these organisms was unchanged or little changed excluding case 2.
Anaerobic bacteria little susceptible to drugs used,
exception of rifampicin, showed no decrease in all
cases. B. fragilis group were always most predominant
in fecal flora. Because these drugs were treated on
purpose to expel microorganisms from intestine or bowel
of patients, our findings may remain as future problems.
Indeed, dosage of drugs treated may be little in comparison with that in foreign country.

INCIDENCE AND SIGNIFICANCE OF ANAEROBES IN THE ABDOMEN

H. H. Stone, M.D. and L. D. Kolb, B.S.

Department of Surgery, Emory University School of Medicine

69 Butler Street, S.E., Atlanta, Georgia 30303 U.S.A.

Since the thorough literature review by Altemeier and his documentation that both anaerobic as well as aerobic species are responsible for the bacterial peritonitis in perforated appendicitis, seldom have reports cited anaerobes as being involved in infections developing after peritoneal, pelvic, or perineal contamination by intestinal contents (1,3,4,6,7). Recently, however, Gorbach and associates have repeatedly stressed an almost routine soilage of the peritoneal cavity by anaerobes whenever gastrointestinal perforation has occurred as a result of disease or trauma (4,7). Subsequent infections following such contamination have also been due primarily to a multiplicity of bacterial species having both anaerobic as well as aerobic culture requirements. This synergistic combination of aerobes and anaerobes has appeared to offer a valid argument for the polymicrobial basis, not a single species, as the cause of the majority of infections developing on a surgical ward (4,6).

CLINICAL STUDY

During a seven month period, all patients undergoing emergency laparotomy for trauma or acute abdominal disease at Grady Memorial Hospital had anaerobic as well as aerobic cultures taken immediately upon peritoneal entry. After aspirating 1 or 2 ml of peritoneal fluid, the specimen was injected directly into a tube of supplemented peptone broth. A sterile venting unit was then inserted; and the entire culture unit was placed in a special incubator located within the operating room suite itself. By this means, incubation within 2 minutes was assured.

Several of the patients had peritoneal cultures repeated at

half hour or hourly intervals throughout the course of operation.
Identical methods were also used for culture of all postoperative
wound and intra-abdominal infections. In addition, any patient with
signs or symptoms of an associated bacteremia had both aerobic and
anaerobic blood cultures drawn.

Bacteriology

Within 24 hours of inoculation, broth cultures were processed
for both aerobic and anaerobic growth. Aerobic bacterial species
were isolated and identified according to standard laboratory
methods, while antibiotic sensitivity testing was done according to
the technique of Bauer, et al. (2).

Anaerobic isolates were confirmed as being true anaerobes and
then further identified as to genus by simple bacteriologic tests
and gas chromatography. Methods generally conformed to those described by Holdeman and Moore (5). Although speciation of all
bacterial isolates was routine, it became obvious that, except for
Clostridia and Bacteroides fragilis, determination of exact anaerobic
species was of no practical value in clinical practice. Tests of
susceptibility to both clindamycin and cephalothin were later run on
all anaerobic isolates by agar-dilution techniques.

Antibiotic Therapy

During the initial three months, cephalothin was administered
to all patients prior to, during, and for five days after operation.
The usual dose was 2 gm given intravenously every six hours. Randomization of antibiotics was then begun and continued during the
last four months of the study. Patients with even hospital numbers
received identical doses of cephalothin at the same time intervals.
If the hospital number was odd, however, clindamycin was given intravenously according to the same schedule but at 300 mg per dose. If
sepsis worsened or developed, an aminoglycoside (gentamicin or
tobramycin) was added to the antibiotic regimen.

Data Analysis

Results were correlated on the basis of aerobic and/or anaerobic
bacteria isolated, individual bacterial species, antibiotic sensitivities, disease process producing the initial contamination, incidence of wound and peritoneal infection, species and incidence of
complicating bacteremias, and antibiotic administered. Comparisons
between initial contaminants and bacteria responsible for subsequent
infection were made as were benefits and complications from use of
each study antibiotic. Finally, prevalence as well as importance of

anaerobic bacteria contaminating the peritoneal cavity was determined.

RESULTS

During the study period, 512 patients underwent emergency laparotomy and provided the basic material for culture analysis (Table
1). There were 202 patients in the initial three months when cephalothin was the routine agent. During randomization, an additional
163 received cephalothin, while 147 were given clindamycin. No
differences were noted between types of cases or incidence of infectious complication with respect to the different antibiotics.
However, the initial group of consecutive patients receiving cephalothin had a significantly greater incidence of both wound and
intra-abdominal sepsis than did either randomized group. This discrepancy was believed due to greater attention being paid to operative technique and wound care as well as a marked reduction in
frequency of colon injuries during the latter months.

Complications of antibiotic administration were relatively
common. Phlebitis developed in 18% of patients receiving cephalothin. Clindamycin, on the other hand, had produced such a severe
enteritis in 7% and so pronounced a rash in another 14% that the
antibiotic accordingly was discontinued. Overall, the rate of
adverse reaction to each antibiotic therapy regimen was not significantly different between the two groups.

Aerobic Bacteria

Approximately half of the 512 patients had at least one species
of aerobic bacteria contaminating the peritoneum at the time of
operation, an incidence of 47.7%. There were 460 aerobic isolates
from these 244 patients, thereby giving an average of 1.89 different
species per patient.

TABLE 1

INCIDENCE OF INFECTION AFTER EMERGENCY LAPAROTOMY

POSTOPERATIVE INFECTION

	Pat.	Wound	Abdominal
Routine Cephalothin	202	53	16
Random Cephalothin	163	24	5
Random Clindamycin	147	21	4
TOTAL	512	98	25

The most commonly grown organism was E. coli, which represented
a third of all aerobic isolates (Table 3). The remaining gram-
negative rods made up 43% of the aerobic flora. Of the gram-positive
species, Enterococcus was by far the single most frequently encountered isolate.

Antibiotic susceptibility of the aerobes demonstrated a consistent superiority of the aminoglycosides, only fair activity by
cephalothin, and essentially no benefit from clindamycin, that is
except against species of Staphylococcus (Table 2).

Anaerobic Bacteria

At least one species of anaerobic bacteria was recovered from
the peritoneal cavity of 159 patients, an incidence of 31.1%. The
382 anaerobic isolates averaged 2.4 per patient, with one to nine
different species per patient.

There was considerable variation as to anaerobic genera, although Bacteroides was the largest group and represented more than
35% (Table 3). Bacteroides fragilis alone accounted for 14%.
Eubacteria was the next most frequently encountered genus, although
such a designation often became a catch-all for unspecified gram-
positive rods. Clostridia were noted in only 7%.

Antimicrobial sensitivity was tested only to cephalothin and
clindamycin. Clindamycin was uniformly superior and was most impressive against isolates of Bacteroides fragilis.

TABLE 2

DISC SENSITIVITIES OF AEROBIC BACTERIAL ISOLATES
Percent of 428 Isolates Sensitive to Various Antibiotics

	Isol	ANTIBIOTIC DISC CONCENTRATION (mcg)				
		Gen. 10	Carb. 50	Cep. 30	Chl. 30	Clin. 2
E. coli	164	99	89	65	95	0
Kleb-Ent.	78	100	27	41	95	0
Proteus	69	91	67	67	58	0
Ps. aerug.	20	95	80	0	0	0
Misc. G-neg.rods	29	97	79	52	90	0
Staph.	13	100	85	100	−	100
Entero.	55	80	100	0	−	13

TABLE 3

ANAEROBES CULTURED FROM THE PERITONEAL CAVITY
- 382 Isolates from 159 Patients -

GRAM POSITIVE COCCI		GRAM NEGATIVE COCCI	
Peptostreptococcus	22	Megasphaera	1
Peptococcus	18	Veillonella	15
Ruminoccccus	1	Acidaminococcus	4
Sarcina	1		
Gaffkya	1		

GRAM POSITIVE RODS		GRAM NEGATIVE RODS	
Clostridium	29	Bacteroides	136
Bifidobacterium	11	(sp. fragilis	54)
Lactobacillus	10	Fusobacterium	13
Lachnospira	1	Leptotrichia	9
Eubacterium	75	Succinivibrio	1
Propionibacterium	34		

Incidence of Anaerobes

The progression of appendicitis from a simple erythematous
process, through suppuration and gangrene, to its final stage of
perforation was reflected in the change in incidence of aerobic and
anaerobic cultures. Going from simple to suppurative appendicitis,
there was a gradual increase in the frequency of culturable aerobic
species. Anaerobes were almost never present until gangrene of the
appendiceal wall had developed. On gross perforation, anaerobes
became the dominant microbial flora. Other types of peritonitis
had variable frequencies of anaerobic participation.

In abdominal trauma, perforating wounds of the colon and rectum
uniformly contaminated the peritoneal cavity with both anaerobic
as well as aerobic species. Perforations of the stomach and small
bowel produced minimal soilage, which paralleled exactly what had
been noted for rupture of gastric and duodenal ulcers. Enterolysis
without inadvertent enterotomy for the relief of mechanical intestinal obstruction had no growth on culture of the peritoneum.
However, the spill of obstructed small bowel contents produced a
contamination equalling what resulted when intestine was already
gangrenous and required resection.

Exposure to Air

Prolonged exposure of the abdomen, a wound, or even an abscess

to atmospheric oxygen significantly reduced the chances of isolating
an anaerobe. For example, in perforative gastrointestinal trauma,
the ability to isolate anaerobic bacteria from peritoneal fluid
diminished as the time of exposure to air increased. Although all
patients with colon wounds had initial contamination by anaerobes,
such species could be detected in only 10% one hour after the abdomen had been opened. Similar reductions in recoverability of
anaerobes were noted in cases of gastric and small bowel perforation.

Even anaerobic bacteria actively participating in an established peritonitis were susceptible to kill by atmospheric oxygen. Although almost every specimen from patients with perforated appendicitis contained anaerobes if taken immediately upon surgical entry
to the abdomen, the incidence of such fell to 30% by the end of one
hour.

Bacteriology of Infections

Irrespective as to the site of postoperative infection — wound
or intra-abdominal — the incidence of anaerobe involvement was
always less than its relative population in the initial contaminant.
This reduction in frequency of anaerobic participation averaged 28%.
Merely exposing of the wound or peritoneal cavity to atmospheric
oxygen appeared to be the main factor responsible for such a difference.

Complicating bacteremias developed in 21 patients (Table 4).
Blood cultures grew 69 different bacterial isolates, of which 21 or
30% were anaerobes. It was also noted that Enterococcus was more
commonly recovered from the blood than was Bacteroides.

TABLE 4

COMPLICATING BACTEREMIAS
Positive Blood Cultures in 21 Patients

	Patients
Gram neg. rods	11
Enterococcus	7
Bacteroides	6
Eubacterium	4
Peptostreptococcus	4
Clostridium	2
Candida	1
Other	3
TOTAL	21

Finally, no significant difference was found between the two randomized treatment groups with respect to frequency of aerobic or anaerobic bacterial participation in postoperative wound and intra-abdominal infections.

DISCUSSION

Based upon the present study as well as previous reports, the evidence is irrefutable that not only aerobic, but also anaerobic, bacteria routinely contaminate the abdomen whenever perforation of the colon or rectum has occurred (1,4,6,7). Also, since intraluminal flora of obstructed small intestine parallels that of the colon, spill of such contents soils the peritoneum with the same bacteria (6). Postoperative wound and intraperitoneal infections likewise harbor anaerobic as well as aerobic species (4,6,7).

Anaerobes exist and propagate only when the local oxidation-reduction potential has been significantly reduced. Such a diminished oxygen tension is provided by necrotic tissue and marked local ischemia. However, the most common infections evolve as a synergism between aerobic and anaerobic bacteria (4,6). Growing in symbiosis, bacteria with opposite oxygen requirements can so alter local environment by their metabolic end-products that conditions become conducive to survival and even proliferation of each partner. The present study has shown that the majority of wound and intra-abdominal infections complicating disease, trauma, or surgery of the gastrointestinal tract are based upon this symbiotic relationship. Indeed, strict anaerobe sepsis is uncommon (6,7).

Principles of treatment revolve around two basic considerations: 1) alterations in local environment so as to impair or even kill the infecting anaerobes, and 2) administration of antimicrobial agents with specific activity against anaerobic species (6). One way to change local environment is the excision of all necrotic tissue and conversion of the infectious process to an open wound. Redox potentials are significantly increased by exposure to atmospheric concentrations of oxygen. Nevertheless, anaerobes may persist if aerobic species in the immediate vicinity maintain a local, yet considerably decreased, oxidation-reduction potential. This dependency of anaerobic species on aerobic counterparts probably explains the response, even though transient, of mixed infections in non-gangrenous tissues, such as the peritoneal cavity, to therapy with antibiotics active only against aerobic pathogens (6).

Ischemic or frankly gangrenous tissues have been deprived of an adequate blood supply and therefore never acquire bactericidal concentrations of parenterally administered antibiotics. Thus,

administration of antibiotic active against anaerobic species is of
value primarily when anaerobic bacteremia has complicated either a
pure or mixed infection (6). Although the patient may improve
dramatically following such antibiotic therapy, recurrence of sepsis
is a certainty unless gangrenous tissues are debrided and the infection is converted to an open wound. There can be no substitute;
it is the mainstay of definitive therapy for anaerobic infections.

SUMMARY

To amplify recent interest in anaerobic infections following
abdominal disease, trauma, or surgery, 512 consecutive patients subjected to emergency celiotomy had both aerobic and anaerobic cultures
taken of peritoneal fluid as well as all complicating wound and
intra-abdominal infections. During four of the seven study months,
patients had antibiotic therapy randomized between clindamycin or
cephalothin.

Results demonstrated that anaerobes uniformly contaminate the
peritoneal cavity whenever distal or obstructed intestine has been
perforated, irrespective of the cause. Although all but one of the
123 complicating wound and intra-abdominal infections were due solely
or at least in part to aerobic pathogens, 2/3 of such infections also
contained one or more different anaerobic species acting in synergism
with the aerobes. No significant difference in incidence of post-
operative infection or in infecting bacteria could be found with
respect to antibiotic administered or etiology of perforation. Indeed, duration of bacterial exposure to atmospheric oxygen was the
most critical factor influencing culture recoverability of anaerobic
organisms, likelihood of ensuing wound or peritoneal sepsis partici-
pated in by an anaerobe, and success in control of established infections harboring anaerobes.

REFERENCES

1. Altemeier, W.A.: The Bacterial Flora of Acute Perforated Ap-
        pendicitis with Peritonitis. Ann. Surg., 107:517, 1938.

2. Bauer, A.W., Kirby, W.M.M., Sherris, J.C., and Tuck, M.: Anti-
        biotic Susceptibility Testing By a Standardized Single
        Disc Method. Am. J. Clin. Pathol., 45:493, 1966.

3. Beazley, R.M., Polakavetz, S.H., and Miller, R.M.: Bacteroides
        Infections on a University Surgical Service. Surg.,
        Gynec., & Obstet., 135:742, 1972.

4. Gorbach, S.L., and Bartlett, J.G.: Anaerobic Infections. New

Eng. J. Med., 290:1177, 1237 & 1269, 1974.

5. Holdeman, L.V., and Moore, W.E.C.: Anaerobe Laboratory Manual.
     VPI Anaerobe Laboratory, Blacksburg, Va., 1972.

6. Stone, H.H., Kolb, L.D., and Geheber, C.E.: Incidence and
     Significance of Intraperitoneal Anaerobic Bacteria. Ann.
     Surg., 181:705, 1975.

7. Thadepalli, H., Gorbach, S.W., Broido, P.W., Norsen, J., and
     Nyhus, L.: Abdominal Trauma, Anaerobes, and Antibiotics.
     Surg., Gynec., & Obstet., 137:270, 1973.

METRONIDAZOLE IN THE TREATMENT OF ANAEROBIC INFECTION IN MAN

J.B. SELKON*, J.H. HALE and H.R. INGHAM

PUBLIC HEALTH LABORATORY, NEWCASTLE GENERAL HOSPITAL

WESTGATE ROAD, NEWCASTLE UPON TYNE

In recent years there has been a growing awareness of the importance of B. fragilis as a cause of human infections, in particular abdominal sepsis and cerebral abscess (Gillespie and Guy 1956; Ingham et al.1968; Pearson and Anderson 1970; Okubadejo et al.1973). B. fragilis, in contrast to other anaerobic bacteria, is relatively resistant to penicillin and ampicillin, and in recent years an increasing proportion have been found to be resistant also to tetracycline. B. fragilis is invariably sensitive to chloramphenicol, clindamycin and lincomycin and the latter two antibiotics have been recommended for the treatment of these infections (Ingham et al. 1968; Kislak 1972; Bartlett et al. 1972). Recently metronidazole has been shown to possess a high degree of activity against B. fragilis, in vitro, with minimal bactericidal concentrations of 0.16 μg per ml to 2.5 μg per ml (Whelan and Hale 1973).

In view of metronidazole's lack of toxicity, we have studied its role in the treatment of infections with B. fragilis in man and have recently published three case histories which demonstrate that it is highly effective (Ingham et al. 1975). These case histories demonstrated three particular aspects of the use of metronidazole in the treatment of B. fragilis infections. As shown in Table 1, the first patient, who had a cerebral abscess, had previously, on two occasions, undergone surgical drainage and received a full course of chemotherapy. In one instance, the chemotherapy was penicillin, chloramphenicol and cotrimoxazole for 6 weeks, and in the other it was lincomycin for 4 weeks. Some months after both these courses of treatment the patient relapsed. On the third admission, after surgical drainage, he received metronidazole, 600 mg 8-hourly for 6 weeks, and since then there has been no further relapse. This highly effective eradication of the B. fragilis, B. oralis and

TABLE 1

THREE PATIENTS TREATED WITH METRONIDAZOLE

DIAGNOSIS	BACTERIOLOGICAL AGENT	PREVIOUS UNSUCCESSFUL CHEMOTHERAPY	
CEREBRAL ABSCESS	B. fragilis B. oralis Anaerobic Streptococcus	1) PENICILLIN CHLORAMPHENICOL COTRIMOXAZOLE	6 weeks
		2) LINCOMYCIN	4 weeks
SEPTICAEMIA	B. fragilis	GENTAMICIN	
SEPTICAEMIA	B. fragilis	GENTAMICIN	

anaerobic Streptococcus responsible for this abscess, indicates that its action in vivo was clearly bactericidal and that the abscess cavity was sterilised.

The second patient (Figure 1) had a severe septicaemia due to pyelonephritis resulting from a vesico-colic fistula and this patient demonstrated a very rapid decrease of pyrexia after metronidazole was started, the temperature falling to normal and the blood cultures becoming sterile within 24 hours.

The third patient (Figure 2) had a B. fragilis septicaemia resulting from peritonitis which followed the removal of a rejected transplanted kidney. Again the salient feature of this case was the rapid fall in temperature following initiating treatment with metronidazole. An additional feature, was the need to adjust the dosage of metronidazole because the patient had no renal function and was being haemodialysed. It was shown that for this purpose that the microbiological assay of metronidazole was more suitable than the polarographic method since the latter method measured, in addition to the microbiologically active substance, inactive meta- bolides which accumulate in the absence of normal renal function. With haemodialysis every 2 days, a dosage of 600 mg of metronidazole

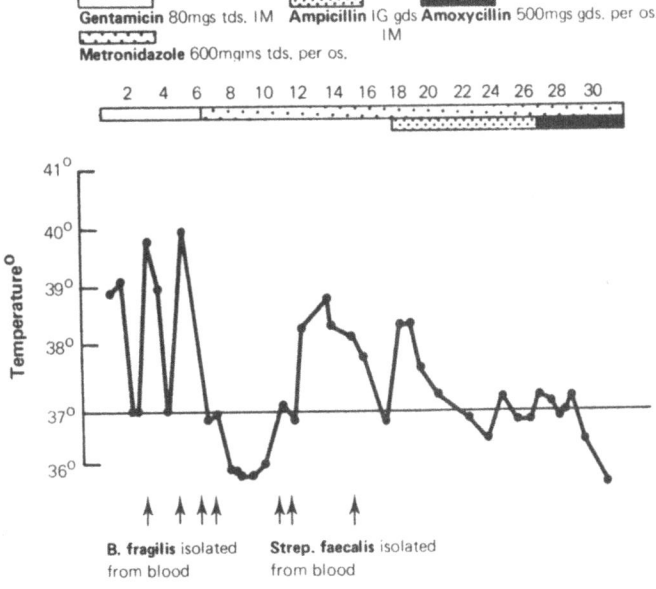

FIGURE 1 — CASE 2

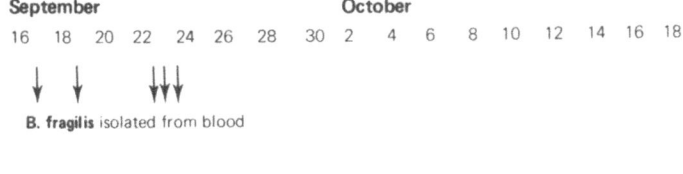

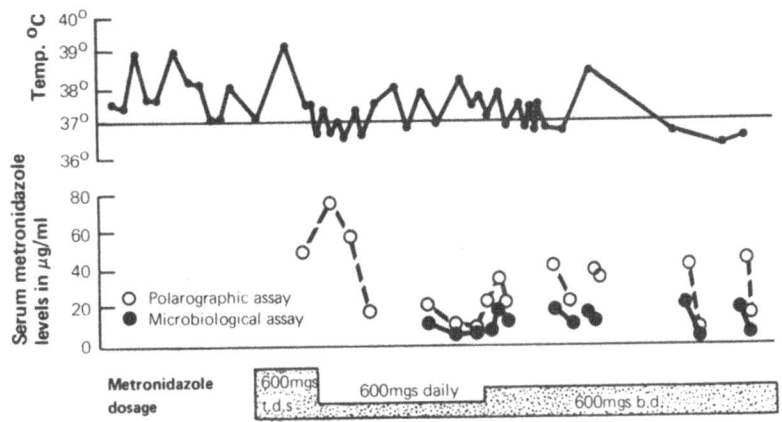

FIGURE 2 — CASE 3

daily, was unsatisfactory in terms of clinical response, and this
had to be increased to 600 mg 12-hourly. With this dosage eradication of the infection was achieved.

We have used metronidazole in a large number of other patients
with infections due to B. fragilis or anaerobic Streptococci and in
all instances with successful results. In our experience the dominant feature has been the rapidity with which these organisms have
been eradicated from the lesions. However, a major limiting factor
of metronidazole was the need to give it orally since it is usually
required for patients in whom this route for administration is not
possible or not appropriate, such as those with ileus, on gastric
suction or in bacteraemic shock. We have therefore studied the
use of metronidazole intravenously. Metronidazole powder was dissolved in a phosphate citric acid buffer at pH 6.0, to give a
0.5% w/v solution and sterilised by autoclaving at $115^{\circ}C$ for 30
minutes. The solution was given as an intravenous infusion over
20 minutes to administer a dose of 600 mg of metronidazole. The
metronidazole was usually administered as part of a mixed regimen,
the other agents being ampicillin and colistin or gentamycin. To
date, we have administered metronidazole intravenously to 49 patients,
usually for one week but with a range of 4 days to 3 weeks. Table 2
shows the results of serial serum assay results at 1 hour, 4 hours
and 8 hours after the infusion. The average concentration at 1
hour was 35.2 μg/ml (range 20.7 to 48.2 μg/ml); at 4 hours it was
33.9 μg/ml (range 16.3 to 48.9 μg/ml) and at 8 hours it was 23.7
μg/ml (range 16.5 to 27.5 μg/ml).   These concentrations are well
above even the highest MBC for B. fragilis, 2.5 μg/ml.

TABLE 2

SERUM LEVELS AFTER I.V. ADMINISTRATION OF 600 mg METRONIDAZOLE

	TIME AFTER INFUSION: CONCENTRATION μg/ml		
	1 to $1\frac{1}{2}$ hours	4 hours	8 hours
Mean	35.2	33.9	23.7
n	11	9	5
Range	20.7 to 48.2	16.3 to 48.9	16.5 to 27.5

TABLE 3

LIVER FUNCTION TESTS, ELECTROLYTES AND BLOOD UREA AFTER A
COURSE OF METRONIDAZOLE 600 mgs 6-HOURLY I.V.

	LIVER FUNCTION TESTS	UREA	ELECTROLYTES
Number of Patients	11	29	29
Abnormal Results	0	0	0

We have carried out tests for toxicity in 34 patients and
Table 3 summarises the findings obtained with a battery of liver
function tests, blood urea and serum electrolytes. No abnormal
results have been encountered so far. In addition, the blood
white cell count has been followed and no instances of neutro-
paenia have occurred.

The intravenous administration of metronidazole has proved as
effective as the oral preparation in the treatment of established
infections with B. fragilis and anaerobic Streptococci.

REFERENCES

Bartlett, J.G., Sutter, V.L. and Finegold, S.M. (1972), New
    England Journal of Medicine, 287, 1006-1010.
Gillespie, W.A. and Guy, J. (1956), Lancet, 1, 1039-1042.
Ingham, H.R., Selkon, J.B., Codd, A.A. and Hale, J.H. (1968),
    Journal of Clinical Pathology, 21, 432-436.
Kislak, J.W. (1972), Journal of Infectious Diseases, 125, 295-299.
Okubadejo, O.A., Green, P.J. and Payne, D.J.H. (1973), British
    Medical Journal, 2, 212-214.
Pearson, H.E. and Anderson, G.V. (1970), Obstetrics and
    Gynaecology, 35, 31-36.
Whelan, J.P.F. and Hale, J.H. (1973), Journal of Clinical
    Pathology, 26, 393-395.
Ingham, H.R., Rich, G.E., Selkon, J.B., Hale, J.H., Roxby, C.M.,
    Betty, M.J., Johnson, R.W.G. and Uldall, P.R. (1975),
    Journal of Antimicrobial Chemotherapy, 1, 235-242.

THE USE OF PROPHYLACTIC CEPHALOTHIN IN WOMEN UNDERGOING EMERGENCY CESAREAN SECTION

Bruce Work, M.D.* and Williams J. Ledger, M.D.**
*University of Michigan
**LAC-USC Medical Center, Women's Hospital, Room 5K36
1240 North Mission Road, Los Angeles, California 90033

INTRODUCTION

Previous surveillance studies of infectious morbidity in Obstetrics showed an increased incidence of serious post partum pelvic infections in women, who during labor required a cesarean section. Because a previous study had demonstrated a reduction in the number of post-operative pelvic infections when prophylactic antibiotics were used in non-pregnant pre-menopausal women undergoing vaginal hysterectomy,[1] a similar prophylactic antibiotic regimen was employed in women in labor undergoing cesarean section.

MATERIALS AND METHODS

All patients in labor requiring an emergency cesarean section, were eligible for the study. Patients with a history of penicillin allergy were not used. The study was double blind, with the assignment of placebo or cephalothin based upon a random table of numbers. Eligible patients either received an intravenous two gram dose of cephalothin when the decision was made to do a cesarean section and two subsequent two gram doses at six hour intervals or a similar appearing inactive placebo with the same schedule of administration. Eighty patients were studied, of whom forty received cephalothin and forty received placebo.

RESULTS

There were differences noted in the clinical responses to the two regimens. These are noted in Table I.

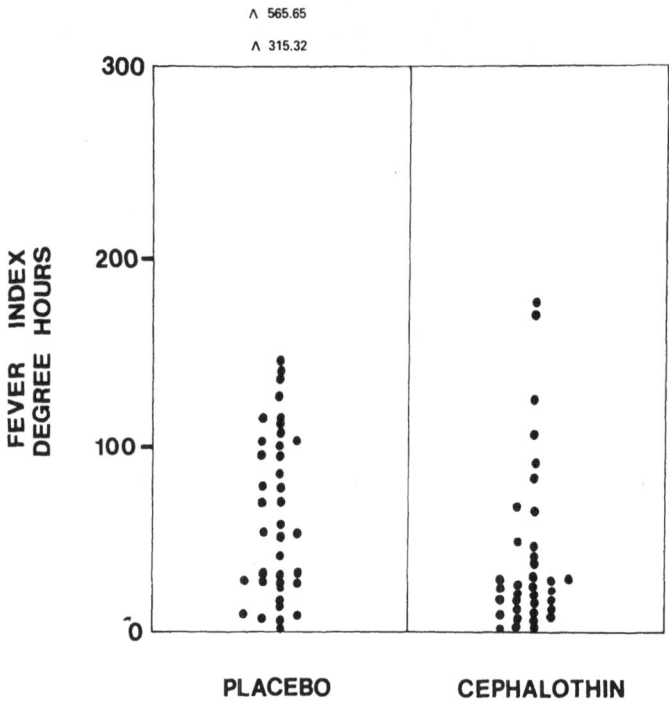

FIGURE 1 : The use of Phrophylactic
              Cephalothin

TABLE I

Postpartum Soft Tissue Infections

	Cephalothin	Placebo
No postpartum evidence of infection	26	13
Abdominal wound infection	3	2
Endomyometritis	6	13
Endomyometritis and septic pelvic thrombophlebitis	2	2
Postpartum adnexal abscess	0	1

In addition to this direct evaluation of post-partum infection, an indirect measure, the fever index calculated in degree
hours was calculated in these two groups of women. There was a
wide scatter of values, (see Figure One) but the number of degree
hours was significantly less in patients receiving cephalothin.
(Note - the temperature record of one patient who received
cephalothin and developed a post-partum endomyometritis was not
available for analysis.)

DISCUSSION
    There was a favorable response to the use of prophylactic
cephalothin in a group of women at high risk for infection following cesarean section. This study had the advantage of evaluating
a relatively uniform group of patients. This selection process
excluded women undergoing elective repeat cesarean section, who
have a lower incidence of post-partum infection, and avoids the
difficulty of a study group with a varying degree of risk.[2] In
this high risk population, the group receiving cephalothin had
more patients with no post-partum evidence of infection and
significantly fewer degree hours of fever. Of more clinical sig-
nifiance was the lowered incidence of post-partum endomyometritis
in patients receiving prophylaxis. These are the types of post-
partum infections that antibiotic prophylaxis should prevent.
These results were achieved without any serious maternal or fetal
reactions to the prophylactic antibiotic regimen. This is a
favorable clinical response to systemic antibiotics. If the only
goal of therapy was a reduction infectious morbidity, prophylactic antibiotics would be considered successful agents in women
undergoing cesarean section.

Despite these favorable responses, this prophylactic regimen failed to prevent the serious infectious complications following cesarean section. The most serious post-partum infections following this emergency operative procedure are those which require anticoagulants for suspected septic pelvic thrombophlebitis and those in which operative intervention for the care of a pelvic abscess is needed. The relative numbers of patients with these serious problems was similar, three received placebo and two cephalothin, whether or not prophylactic antibiotics were used. In each of the women receiving prophylactic cephalothin who had a serious post-operative pelvic infection, Bacteroides was recovered from cultures from the infection site. This organism was not recovered from those women with serious post-operative pelvic infections, who received placebo.

These results suggest that prophylactic cephalothin alone is not the best therapeutic approach to high risk pregnancy patients undergoing cesarean section. The number of serious infections following this regimen was not significantly reduced and in those women with serious infections following this regimen the troublesome anaerobe, Bacteroides was recovered. In view of these results, a number of alternative regimens need to be evaluated by prospective study. These include the use of another additional prophylactic antibiotic effective against <u>Bacteroides fragilis</u>, or the prompt use of such an antibiotic in patients who become febrile after the use of prophylactic cephalosporin on the day of operation, or the elimination of prophylactic antibiotics with the use of a combination of therapeutic antibiotics only in symptomatic postpartum patients. Future studies should clarify the relative benefits of these different regimens.

REFERENCES

1. Ledger, W.J., Sweet, R.L., and Headington, J.T., "Prophylactic cephaloridine in the prevention of post-operative pelvic infections in pre-menopausal women undergoing vaginal hysterectomy." Amer J. Obstet. Gynec. 115:766, 1973.

2. Gibbs, R.S., DeCherney, A.H., and Schwartz, R.H., "Prophylactic antibiotics in cesarean section: A double-blind study." Amer J. Obstet. Gynec. 114:1048, 1972.

CLINDAMYCIN PROPHYLAXIS IN APPENDICECTOMY WOUND INFECTIONS

O.A. OKUBADEJO, T.N.D. PEET, D.T.L. TURNER

PUBLIC HEALTH LABORATORY, PORTSMOUTH and
ROYAL HOSPITAL, PORTSMOUTH

SUMMARY

In a trial using clindamycin for the prevention of wound
sepsis in appendicectomy, a hundred patients were studied. 48
patients received clindamycin and 52 served as controls. 8 of the
48 treated (16.7%) and 15 of 52 untreated (29%) patients had post-
operative wound infection; the difference was not statistically
significant.   The majority of infected wounds had a mixture of
bacteroides strains and organisms of the family enterobacteriaceae,
and bacteroides were three times more common than any other
bacteria in the peritoneal swabs.   The untreated patients also had
bacteroides in their wounds approximately four times more often
than the treated patients. Therefore clindamycin was effective in
stopping the growth of bacteroides in wounds, but did not reduce
the incidence of wound sepsis to a satisfactory level.

INTRODUCTION

Post-operative wound sepsis occurs in 10% to 60% of patients
following appendicectomy, the highest incidence being found in
those with pre-operative conditions such as peritonitis, perforation,
appendix abscess or gangrene. (Lancet 1971, Gilmore and Martin 1974,
Leigh et al 1974). Recent evidence indicates that the patients'
intestinal flora, especially bacteroides strains, are a major
cause of the wound infections. (Leigh 1974, Leigh et al 1974),
and it is known that the strains can be killed in vitro with
clindamycin. Therefore we decided to see whether clindamycin
would reduce the incidence of the wound infections to a satisfactory level.

A clinical trial with 100 patients who had emergency appendicectomy was made to determine the value of the drug in controlling
wound sepsis, and the results are presented in this paper.

METHOD

Patients were randomly divided using numbers from Fisher's
Tables (Fisher and Yates 1949), into two groups of which one received clindamycin, and the other group served as control. The
dose of clindamycin given was 150mgms. t.i.d. for adults, and
75mgms. t.i.d. for children below the age of 8 years. The drug
was started on the first post-operative day and given for 7 days.
At operation, intraperitoneal swabs were taken from the appendix
wall and fossa before resection, and were sent to the laboratory
immediately for culture. Pre-operative conditions such as abscess,
perforation, peritonitis and gangrene were noted and recorded on
a proforma. Appendicectomies with these pre-operative conditions
were classified as "complicated", and the others "uncomplicated".
The wounds were inspected by the surgical team in hospital, and
the patients' general practitioners were requested by letter to
help with further inspection for two weeks after dishcarge from
hospital. Wound infection was defined as an abscess or purulent
discharge with pain and inflammation. Swabs were taken from all
infected wounds for bacteriological investigation.

All swabs were cultured on blood and MacConkey agar plates
aerobically, and Diagnostic Sensitivity Agar (DST Oxoid),containing
10% lysed horse blood and 100μg/ml gentamicin anaerobically. Cooked
meat medium prepared in the laboratory was also inoculated. All
cultures were incubated at 37^{0}C for 48 hours, and the cooked meat
was subcultured on to blood and DST agar as mentioned above.
Anaerobiosis was secured with Baird-Tatlock jars containing 95%
hydrogen and 5% CO_2. The organisms isolated were identified by
using standard methods. (Cowan and Steel 1966, Sutter et al 1971).

RESULTS

Of the 100 patients in the trial, 48 were given clindamycin
and 52 were controls.

Wound Infections

Post-operative wound infections were seen in 23% of all
patients, 8 in the clindamycin group and 15 in the controls. A
significantly high rate of infection was found among patients after
"complicated" appendicectomies. Thus 18 of 30 patients (60%)
with complications were infected compared with 5 of 70 (7.1%) after

Table 1.   Number of Patients in Clindamycin and Control Groups,
           their Complications and Wound Infections

	Clindamycin Group		Control Group		Total
	WOUNDS		WOUNDS		
	Infected	Not infected	Infected	Not infected	
Complicated appendicitis	6	7	12	5	30
Uncomplicated appendicitis	2	33	3	32	70
TOTAL	8	40	15	37	100

Table 2.   Number of Patients with Bacteroides in Peritoneal Swabs,
           and Wound Infections.

Bacteria in Peritoneum	Clindamycin Group				Control Group				TOTAL
	WOUNDS				WOUNDS				
	Infected		Not infected		Infected		Not infected		
	*c.	uc.	c.	uc.	c.	uc.	c.	uc.	
Bacteroides with or without other bacteria	1	1	4	4	6	2	1	3	22
+Other bacteria no bacteroides	1	1	1	4	2	0	1	0	10
No growth	4	0	2	25	4	1	3	29	68
TOTAL	6	2	7	33	12	3	5	32	100

* c = Complicated appendicitis;   uc = Uncomplicated appendicitis

+ Other bacteria include E. coli, Klebsiella species, Proteus species,
  Pseudomonas aeruginosa, Staphylococcus albus, Streptococcus faecalis,
  anaerobic and microaerophilic streptococci, and Lancefield Group B.
  streptococci.

"uncomplicated" operations. (Table 1). X^2 = 30.8, p<0.005. The results also showed that post-operative wound infections often occurred in patients whose peritoneal swabs gave a growth of bacteroides on culture. Ten of 23 patients with wound infections had bacteroides in peritoneal swabs, compared with 9 who had no growth, and 4 with bacteria other than bacteroides. 8 of 48 patients (16.7%) in the clindamycin group had post-operative wound infection compared with 15 of 52 patients (29%) in the control group, but the difference was not statistically significant. X^2 = 1.48 p>0.5.

Bacteriological Findings (Table 2)

Peritoneal swabs. Only 32 of the 100 peritoneal swabs taken gave a bacterial growth, and 22 of these had bacteroides strains. Bacteroides were not cultured from the remaining 10 swabs which gave growths of other bacteria such as Escherichia coli, Staphylococcus albus, Streptococcus faecalis, microaerophilic and anaerobic streptococci, and Lancefield Group B streptococci.

Wound swabs. Nineteen of 23 swabs (82.6%) taken from the infected wounds grew bacteroides, and the majority, 15 of 19, (78.1%) were in the control group. Therefore clindamycin had some success in stopping the growth of bacteroides strains.

Length of Stay in Hospital. (Fig. 1)

The majority of patients with "uncomplicated" appendicectomies were discharged from hospital by the 6th day after operation. This contrasts with the 15th day in patients who had "complicated" operations and wound infections. The results suggest that clindamycin reduced the length of stay in hospital in patients with "complicated" appendicectomies, but this did not reach a statistically significant level.

Side Effects of Clindamycin

Four patients who received clindamycin developed diarrhoea and evidence of pseudomembranous colitis was found in one, a woman of 90 who died from pulmonary oedema and bronchopneumonia on the 26th day after operation.

Post-operative Chest Infections

Four patients in the control group had a post-operative bronchopneumonia which was successfully treated with ampicillin.

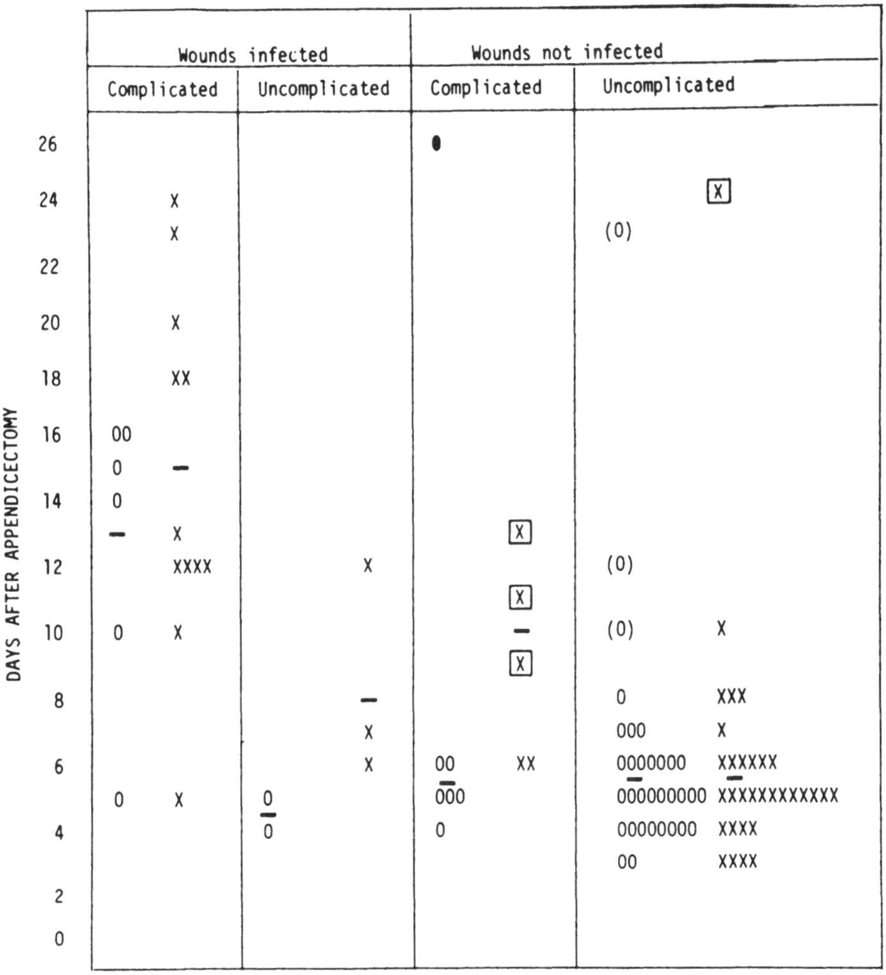

Key:-

0 = Patient in clindamycin group.
X = Patient in control group
▬ = Average number of days in a group. The 3 outliers are excluded.
● = Pseudomembranous colitis
(0) = Diarrhoea
☐ = Chest infection

Fig. 1. Length of Stay in Hospital

The infection contributed to a prolonged length of stay in hospital.

DISCUSSION

In this trial, the incidence of wound infection increased significantly among patients with "complicated" appendicitis, and this confirms the findings of other workers. (Crossfill et al 1969; Gilmore et al 1973; Leigh et al 1974). This finding is probably related to delay in operation which may be inevitable in some patients; for example, with mild symptoms, the general practitioner or surgeon may not be consulted early. The results show that operation wounds are contaminated with intestinal bacteria which given rise to post-operative wound infections, and the organisms are usually a mixture of bacteroides and members of the enterobacteriaceae. This confirms the old report of Veillon and Zuber (1898) and the recent ones of Leigh (1974) and Leigh et al (1974). We confirm the findings of Leigh et al (1974) that bacteroides strains are isolated more often than other bacteria from the appendix fossa and appendix wounds in perforated appendicitis. Nevertheless, clindamycin as given in this trial did not reduce the incidence of wound infections to a significantly low level, and this finding differs from the suggestions and retrospective findings of Leigh et al (1974). Many workers oppose the use of systemic antibiotic-prophylaxis in surgery. Margarey et al (1971) and Longland et al (1971) have shown that systemic penicillin, ampicillin, streptomycin or tetracycline are not effective, and Price and Sleigh (1970) reported a reduction in the rate of infection when antibiotic-prophylaxis was abandoned. Although our findings with respect to the mixed infections are consistent with those of the authors mentioned above, it is possible that a different method of prophylaxis would be successful. For example, a recent report by Stokes et al (1974) indicated that short-term prophylaxis with tobramycin or gentamcin plus linco-mycin, achieved a significant reduction in wound infection in patients who had had intestinal resections, a similar regimen incorporating clindamycin might be useful in appendicectomies.

Acknowledgments

We are grateful to Mr. B.L. Williams, Surgeon, Royal Portsmouth Hospital for his help with these studies and for permission to report on his patients, and to Dr. D.J.H. Payne, Director, Public Health Laboratory, St. Mary's General Hospital, Portsmouth for advice, and to Upjohn Ltd., for a grant and generous supply of the clindamycin used in this trial.

REFERENCES

1. Cowan, S.T., and Steel, K.J. (1966). Manual for the Identification of Medical Bacteria. London Cambridge University Press.
2. Crossfill, M., Hall, R., and London, D. (1969). British Journal of Surgery, 56, 906.
3. Fisher, R.A., and Yates, F. (1949). Statistical Tables for Biological, Agricultural and Medical Research. Oliver & Boyd, London.
4. Gilmore, O.J.A., Martin, T.D.M., and Fletcher, B.N. (1973) Lancet, 1, 220.
5. Gilmore, O.J.A., and Martin, T.D.M., (1974). British Journal of Surgery, 61, 281.
6. Lancet (1971) Editorial. 2, 195.
7. Leigh, D.A. (1974). British Medical Journal, 3, 225.
8. Leigh, D.A., Simmons, K., and Norman, E., (1974). Journal of Clinical Pathology, 27, 997.
9. Longland, C.J., Gray, J.G., Lees, W., and Garrett, J.A.M., (1971). British Journal of Surgery, 58, 117.
10. Margarey, C.J., Chant, A.D.B., Rickford, C.R.K., and Margarey, J.R. (1971). Lancet, 2, 179.
11. Price, J.D.E., and Sleigh, J.D., (1970). Lancet, 2, 1213.
12. Stokes, E.J., Waterworth, P.M., Franks, V., Watson, B., and Clark, C.G., (1974). British Journal of Surgery, 61, 739.
13. Sutter, V.L., Atterby, H.R., Rosenblatt, J.E., Bricknell, K.S., and Finegold, S.M. Anaerobic Bacteriology Manual, Department of Continuing Education in Health Sciences University Extension, and The School of Medicine UCLA (1972).
14. Veillon, A., and Zuber, A., (1898). Archives de Medicine Experimentale et d'Anatomie Pathologique, 20, 517.

PROPHYLACTIC USE OF BACTRIM IN SURGICAL GYNAECOLOGY

A COMPARATIVE STUDY

Doctor Claude LECART, Dr. J.A. BERBEN,
Dr. A. LUYX, Dr. R. SEMOULIN
Gynaecology & Obstetrics Department
Hôpital St Pierre, rue de Bruxelles, 69
3000   LEUVEN

The bactericidal combination sulfamethoxazole-trimethroprim today
remains one of the very rare examples of true synergy in antibiotherapy for bacterial infections. By synergy, is to be understood
the potenttiation of one component by the other, verified in this
instance by in vivo and in vitro measurements of the minimum inhibiting concentrations (M.I.C.).
With regards to a series of microorganisms, these M.I.C. are reduced to an often important extent when both drugs are present
(tables 1 and 2). If one takes as example the curative dose (C.D.)
that curing 50% of the animals experimentally infected with
Haemophilus influenzae, one finds that although this reaches 70,6
mg/kg for sulfamethoxazole and 149 mg/kg for trimethoprime when
the drugs are used separately, when they are combined it falls to
3,66 and 0,73 mg/kg respectively.
If the potentiation is expressed by the ratio C.D. 50 single drug/
C.D. 50 drug in combination, one obtains the factors 19 for the
sulfonamide and 204 for trimethoprime, which is certainly considerable.
Oral co-trimoxazole has been subject to clinical study in many
types of infection (pulmonary, urinary, E.N.T., gastro-intestinal,
skin, etc.), where its efficacy, wide spectrum of activity and
good clinical and biological tolerance have earned for it a useful rating among the antibiotics. It is the clinical trials concerning surgical infection (3-6), and also those in both obstetrics and gynaecology (7) that have especially attracted our attention.

Generic term : co-trimoxazole-Trade name : Bactrim, Roche Products

In the last mentionned study, the authors registered excellent
results in 80% of 60 cases, and gave their preference to co-
trimoxazole most particlarly in urinary infections following
various surgical procedures on the female genital tract.
We have recently had the opportunity of pursuing a clinical study
of parenteral co-trimoxazole of composition identical to that of
the tablets : to the ampoule, 400 mg of sulfamethoxazole + 80 mg
of trimethoprim (for a volume of 5 ml).
We chose to use it for prophylaxis in a series of gynaecological
operations for which we were accustomed to providing preventive
antibiotic treatment.

Table 1 - Potentiation of sulfamethoxazole and trimethoprim in
vitro (1)

Microorganisms	Minimum inhibiting concentration (M.I.C.)ug/ml			
	Sulfamethoxazole (SMZ)		Trimethoprim (TMP)	
	Alone	with TMP	Alone	with TMP
Haemophilus influenzae	10	0,3	1	0,015
Pneumococcus	30	2	2	0,1

Table 2 - Potentiation of sulfamethoxazole and trimethoprim in
the mouse (2)

Microorganisms	C.D. 50 (Curative Dose 50%) mg/kg			
	Sulfamethoxazole (SMZ)		Trimethoprim (TMP)	
	Alone	with TMP	Alone	with TMP
Haemophilus influenzae	70,6	3,66	149	0,73
Pneumococcus	217,4	98,8	335,5	19,8

Method

To interpret the results of anti-infective prophylaxis in a single
series of patients, however numerous, must be illusory unless
there is a comparable control group, either treated with another
known evaluated antibiotic, or receiving no prophylactic treatment.

Preferring not to make an exception to our routine of providing
anti-infective prophylaxis, we decided to carry out a comparative
study between Bactrim and tetracycline, i.e. with 2 series receiving treatment.
The patients were divided according to a random table into 2
groups, the one receiving co-trimoxazole, the other the control
drug. Posology was as follows (starting on the day of operation) :

- Bactrim : 2 ampoules twice daily by infusion for 2 days, follow-
            ed by 2 tablets twice daily for about one week ;

- Tetracycline : Reverin 150 mg twice daily by infusion for 2 days
                 followed by Terra SF, 2 capsules of 250 mg thrice
                 daily for about one week.

Prophylaxis was considered to have failed in the event of any pulmonary, urinary or other infection occuring during the period of
anti-infective protection.

Results

Our series comprised 93 cases, 47 in the Bactrim and 46 in the
tetracyline group.
Breakdown according to age (table 3) and type of operation, by
abdominal or vaginal approach (table 4) shows the two groups to be
quantitatively and qualitatively comparable, an essential condition for the validity of any judgement concerning the two drugs.
The results (table 5) are divided into 2 categories, protection
or failure, according to the absence or presence of infective
complications arising during and in spite of anti-infective prophylactic treatment.

Table 4 - Breakdown according to type of approach

	BACTRIM	TETRACYCLINE
Abdominal	34	39
Vaginal	13	7
Total	47	46

Table 4 - <u>Breakdown according to age</u>

	BACTRIM	TETRACYCLINE
< 20 years	-	1
21-30 "	5	7
31-40 "	12	9
41-50 "	16	14
51-60 "	6	5
61-70 "	4	7
> 70 "	4	3
Total	47	46

Table 5 - <u>Results</u>

	BACTRIM	TETRACYCLINE
Protection	44	37
Failure	3	9
Cause :		
urinary inf.	2 °	9 °
Pulmonary inf.	1	-
Total of cases	47	46

° p   0,05

The infective complications were all urinary, except for one of bronchitis in the Bactrim group, promptly controlled without change of treatment. On the basis of a count of the bacterial colonies in the urine ($>$ 100.000 organisms/ml = infection) they were found to differ in the 2 series : 2 for Bactrim and 9 for the tetracycline, this difference having statsitical significance in favour of Bactrim.

The organisms concerned are shown in table 6.
Except for Enterococci they were all Gram-negative, as is usually
the case with urinary infections. In decreasing order of frequency, the findings for the two groups were :

	Bactrim	Tetracycl.
Colibacillus & coliform microorg.	1x	6x
Enterococcus	-	4x
Pseudomonas	1x	2x
Proteus	-	2x

All these organisms were resistant to the antibiotics administered. The correlation is therefore excellent between clinical
and laboratory findings, which is not always the case as regards
antibiograms.

Tolerance

Administration of the drugs by perfusion did not give rise to
local sign of intolerance, except for one patient of the Reverin
group.
For both means of administration, general tolerance was on the
whole good and without s-gnificant difference between the two
groups. However, the relatively frequent incidence of skin manifestations of an allergic nature (rash, pruritis, erythema)
should not be overlooked ; these were somewhat more frequent in
the patients treated with Bactrim (table 7).

As regards blood tolerance, the serial blood counts effected
before operation and during the post-operative period did in-
dead show a fall in the red corpuscles, haemoglobin rate and
haematocrit, without notable difference between the two groups,
but this may be considered as a consequence of the surgery itself
since there was a rapid return to normal values by the end of
hospitalization. No abnormality was seen as regards with cells.

Commentary

The excellent activity of co-trimoxazole in the treatement of
urinary infections was demonstrated in a series of controlled
studies, where the chemo-therapeutic combination proved frequently to be better than the control antibiotic, wheter this
was ampicillin (8), chloramphenicol (9), doxycycline(10-11),
demethylchlortetracycline (12-13) or nitrofurantoin (14-15).
It is therefore scarcely surprising that in preventive therapy
co-trimoxazole is found to be superior to tetracycline for urinary tract infections, the frequency of which in surgical gynaecology can be explained by the proximity of the anal area and
by the manipulation generally required for pre-operative

investigation (cystography, cystometry etc.) which tend to promote the proliferation of microorganisms. To these factors should
be added the almost routine use of a urethral catheter in the
early post-operative period, which inevitably short-circuits
the natural defences and so leads to bacterial proliferation in
the urine.

For these reasons we systematically practise antibiotherapy,
despite the opinion of the bacteriologists who, not illogically
advise against the prophylactic use of antibiotics in order to
avoid selection of resistant and perticularly dangerous strains,
able to overcome all the defences of the body and the therapeutic means available at the present day. There are nevertheless
circumstances, as in the great majority of gynaecological-and
urological- operations, where anti-infective protection seems to
offer advantages outweighing the above-mentionned risk.
Need we add that the protection provided by an antibiotic can in
no way be a reason for dispensing with the requirements for asep-
sis and correct operative technique.

Summary

Anti-infective prophylaxis was used in two comparable series of
patients undergoing gynaecological surgery, the one group being
treated by Bactrim, the other by tetracycline.
These 2 antibiotics were administrated parentarally for 2 to 3
days, beginning ont the day of operation, and thereafter orally
during 5 to 6 days.
Bactrim was found to be significantly better than the tetracycline for the prevention of urinary infections.

REFERENCES

1. Barnett, M., Bushby, M. (1970) Trimethoprim and the sulpho-
      namides. Vet.Record, 87, 2, 43-51.

2. Bohni, E. (1969) Vergleichende bakteriologische Untersuchungen
      mit der Kombination Trimethoprim/Sulfamethoxazole in vitro
      and in vivo. Chemotherapy, Suppl. 14, 1-21.

3. Briozzo, C.A. (1970) Bactrim en cirugia. Dia Med. Urug.,
      36, 444, 671-677.

4. Craven, J.L., Pugsley, D.J., Blowers, R. (1970) Trimethoprim
      -sulphamethoxazole in acute osteomyelitis due to penicillin-
      resistant Snaphylococci in Uganda. Brit.med.J., 3, 201-203.

5. Hernandez Carbajal, B. (1969) Treatment of chronic osteomyelitis with Bactrim and the ambulatory method (first
   report) 6th International Congress of Chemotherapy,
   Tokyo, 10-15 August 1969.

6. Burkhardt, S., Weber, M.J., Jakob, R., Stirnemann, H.
   Doppenblindversuch mit sulfamethoxazol + trimethoprim
   (Bactrim) versus doxycyclin bei prae- und postoperativen
   infektionen. V. Internationalen Kongress fur Infektions-
   krankheiten, Wien, 318 - 5.9/1970.

7. Chong, D.K., Lean, T.H. (1970) Obstetrical and gynaecological
   infections. Use of trimethoprim-sulphamethoxazole. Proc.
   Obstetr.Gynaecol.Soc.Singapore, 1, 1, 42-47.

8. Reeves, D.S., Faiers, M.C., Pursell, R.E., Brumfitt, W. (1969)
   Trimethoprim-Sulphamethoxazole : Comparative study in
   urinary infection in hospital. Brit.med.J. I, 541-544.

9. Ganthaler, F., Bohni, E., Huber, F. (1971) Etude comparative
   du Bactrim et du chloramphenicol dans les infections
   urinaires chroniques. Schweiz. Med.Wschr., 101, 832-838.

10. Van Belle, F., Vergisson, R. (1974) Klinische studie van de
    parenterale en orale toediening van co-trimoxazol in
    vergelijking met doxycycline. Folia St. Jan 15, 32-37.

11. Derluyn, J., Verduyn, H. (1974) Etude comparative du co-
    trimoxazole et de la doxycycline injectables en chirurgie
    urologique. Acta.urol.belg., 42, 4, 485-491.

12. Derluyn, J., de Jaegher, K., Vereecken, R., Verduyn, H. (1973)
    Le co-trimoxazole dans les infections urinaires : une
    etude comparative avec un antibiotique en double aveugle.
    Acta.urol.Belg., 41, 3, 449-458.

13. Kraytman, M., Schoutens, E., Yourassowsky, E. (1972) Comparaison
    en double anonymat du sulfamethoxazole + trimethoprime
    et de la demethylchlortetracycline dans le traitement des
    infections urinaires. Acta clin.belg., 27, 1-2, 435-441.

14. Meert, M., Leemans, J. (1973) Etude comparative de l'association
    sulfamethoxazole'trimethoprime dans les infections urinaires.
    Ars Medici 28, no.special.

15. de Leval, J. (1972) Evaluation selon la methode du double
    anonymat d'un nouveau bactericide dans les infections
    urinaires. Rev.med.Liege, 27, 15, 500-505.

CARBENICILLIN THERAPY FOR ANAEROBIC INFECTIONS

Haragopal Thadepalli, M.D., Jong T. Huang, M.D.
Dennis G. Hooper, M.S. and Albert H. Niden, M.D.
Department of Internal Medicine, Martin Luther King, Jr.
Gen. Hosp. & Charles R. Drew Postgrad. Med. School
Los Angeles, California, U.S.A.

Summary

Thirty-two patients with anaerobic infections of the chest, abdomen, pelvis, and soft tissue were treated with intravenous carbenicillin alone. Thirty were cured. The microbiologic and clinical results indicate that carbenicillin could be used as a single agent in anaerobic infections.

Introduction

Carbenicillin, primarily introduced for the treatment of gram-negative infections, pseudomonas in particular, has been found to have good spectrum of activity against anaerobic bacteria in vitro (Blazevic and Matsen, 1974). The clinical efficacy of this drug was not established. For this reason, we evaluated carbenicillin in clinical anaerobic infections.

MATERIALS AND METHODS

Thirty-two adults with anaerobic infections were treated with I.V. carbenicillin. Included were 12 pleuro-pulmonary and 9 pelvic infections and 6 intra-abdominal abscess. The other five had soft tissue infections. Fourteen patients had previously failed on other antibiotics. The culture specimens were obtained by transtracheal aspiration in lung infections, thoracentesis in empyema, surgical aspirates of pus from abdominal and pelvic abscess, and direct needle aspirates from subcutaneous abscess. In one patient blood culture was the only source. Specimens were collected in sealed bottles or rubber stoppered glass tubes filled with oxygen-free carbon dioxide. Freshly prepared blood agar plates and roll-tubes were used for initial isolation. The final identification of anaerobic bacteria were made by biochemical reactions in pre-reduced media and gas-liquid chromatography. In vitro sensitivity testing for anaerobes was performed by agar dilution method.

303

Serum carbenicillin levels were measured by microtitre technique
against a susceptible strain of Escherichia coli.

RESULTS

There were 1 to 6 isolates (1 to 3 aerobes and 1 to 4 anaerobes) per specimen. Anaerobes were found in pure culture in 15
patients. Seventeen patients had aerobes as well. They were
gamma-streptococcus (str.) not group D (7), Escherichia coli (7)
alpha str. (4), group D str. (4), proteus (3), and one each of
lactobacillus, klebsiella, micro-aerophilic str., beta hemolytic
str. gr. A., Mycobacterium tuberculosis, Pseudomonas (Ps) aerugo-
nosa, Ps. maltophilia and Citrobacter fruendii.

Fifty-eight anaerobic isolates were recovered from 32 patients
(see table). The minimal inhibitory concentration (MIC) of the
anaerobes were 32 mcg/ml of carbenicillin with the exception of
Bacteroides fragilis s.s. distasonis (MIC=64 mcg/ml). Serum carbenicillin levels in 5 patients at the end of the first, second
and fourth hour after infusing 6 grams of carbenicillin I.V., were
125 to 250 mcg/ml after one hour, 62 to 125 mcg after two hours
and 31 mcg/ml after four hours.

ANAEROBES ISOLATED FROM 32 PATIENTS TREATED WITH CARBENICILLIN

Peptostreptococci(P)	Number of patients	Clostridium(C)	Number of patients
P. intermedius	10	C. ramosum	4
P. anaerobius	2	C. glycolyticum	1
P. productus	1	C. cochlearum	1
P. asaccharolyticus	1		
		Bacteroides(B)	
Peptococci (Pc)		B. fragilis s.s. fragilis	4
Pc. prevotii	4	B. fragilis s.s. distasonis	3
Pc. variabilis	3	B. fragilis s.s. theta-	
Pc. magnus	2	iotaomicron	1
Pc. constellatus	1	B. fragilis s.s. other	1
		B. melaninogenicus s.s.	
Gaffkya anaerobia	1	asaccharolyticus	1
		B. capillosus	3
Eubacterium(E)		B. oralis	1
E. lentum	4	B. putredinis	1
E. aerofaciens	1	B. ocharaseus	1
E. tenue	1		
		Fusobacterium varium	1
Lactobacillus species	1	Unidentified gram	
		negative rod	1
Actinomyces naeslundii	2		

The clinical response was good in 30 patients and poor in 2 because of persistent sepsis secondary to iatrogenic enterovesical fistula in one and pulmonary tuberculosis in the other. The majority of patients became afebrile in two days. Roentgenographic improvement of the parenchymal lesions of the lung were noted in 7 to 10 days. Oral therapy was initiated (2 tablets thrice a day for 14 days) when the clinical status improved.

DISCUSSION

Bacteroides fragilis, a frequent isolate in anaerobic infections is resistant to penicillin (Hoogendijk,1965) and tetracycline (Bodner and Koenig, 1966). Cephalosporins are equally ineffective (Thadepalli et al 1973). Chloramphenicol has excellent in vitro activity, but therapeutic failures might occur with susceptible organisms (Thadepalli et al 1973). Clindamycin, on the other hand, has good in vitro and in vivo efficacy (Gorbach and Thadepalli, 1974, Chow et al 1974).
Carbenicillin has a good spectrum of activity against anaerobes in vitro, with the exception of a few strains of Bacteroides (B) fragilis (Blazevic and Matsen, 1974). In our study all but one strain of 58 anaerobic isolates were susceptible to carbenicillin. Nine patients were infected with bacteroides of which eight had B. fragilis at the infected site, and all were cured·with carbenicillin. There were two patients that failed because of unrelated complications. The overall therapeutic efficacy of carbenicillin was excellent.
In view of the good clinical response, the observed serum levels of the antibiotic and the in vitro susceptibility of anaerobes, it is concluded that carbenicillin is effective in the treatment of anaerobic infections.

REFERENCES

Blazevic, D.J. and Matsen, J.N. (1974). Antimicrob. Agents & Chemother. 5, 462.
Bodner, S.J. and Koenig, M.G. (1966). Ann. Int. Med. 251. 428.
Chow, A.W., Montgomerie, J.Z. and Guze, L.B. (1974). Arch. Int. Med.134, 78.
Gorbach, S.L. and Thadepalli (1974) Arch. Int. Med. 134, 87.
Hoogendijk, J.L. (1965), Antonie van Leewenhoek 31, 383.
Martin. W.J., Gardner, M. and Washington, J.A., (1972) Antimicrob. Agents & Chemother. 1, 148.
Thadepalli, H., Gorbach, S.L., Broido, P., Norsen, J., and Nyhus, L. (1973) Surgery, Gyn & Obst. 137, 270.
Thadepalli, H., Gorbach, S.L. and Bartlett (1973) Proceedings Interscience Conf. Antimicrob. Agents & Chemother., Washington, D.C.

"A COMPARISON OF CLINDAMYCIN OR CHLORAMPHENICOL IN OBSTETRIC-GYNECOLOGIC INFECTIONS"

William J. Ledger, M.D.
LAC-USC Medical Center
Women's Hospital, Room 5K36
1240 North Mission Road
Los Angeles, California 90033
C.L. Gee and W.P. Lewis

INTRODUCTION

Information is needed to determine the relative effectiveness of clindamycin and chloramphenicol in the treatment of serious soft tissue pelvic infections in women. Recent advances in anaerobic technology indicate anaerobes can be recovered from a majority of soft tissue pelvic infections. Of more significance is the observation that the most serious infections currently seen on the Obstetric-Gynecologic service of the Los Angeles County-University of Southern California Medical Center (LAC-USC) are those in which Bacteroides fragilis is recovered. This gram negative rod has unique antimicrobial susceptibilities. Of the currently approved antimicrobial agents, clindamycin and chloramphenicol have the most effectiveness, based upon laboratory susceptibility testing. Each has the potential for serious toxicity, life threatening suppression of the bone marrow with chloramphenicol and life threatening pseudomembranous enterocolitis with clindamycin. In an attempt to determine the relative effectiveness of these two agents, a comparative study was done in Obstetric-Gynecologic patients who on clinical grounds were thought to have serious soft tissue pelvic infections.

MATERIALS AND METHODS

The fifty patients in this study, were seriously ill, with a high probability for an anaerobic infection. Based upon a random series of numbers, patients were assigned either clindamycin or chloramphenicol. Other antibiotics were employed, including penicillin or a penicillin like antibiotic and an aminoglycoside. In addition, operative intervention in the form of abscess removal or drainage, was performed as needed. The clinical diagnosis of the primary site of infection in the two groups is noted in Table I.

TABLE I

Type of Soft Tissue Pelvic Infection

	Clindamycin	Chloramphenicol
I. Community Acquired		
Infected Abortion	7	7
Pelvic Inflammatory Disease	13	14
II. Hospital Acquired		
Post delivery pelvic infection	4	4
Post operative pelvic infection	1	0

RESULTS

Anaerobes were recovered from 41 of 50 or 82% of the initial cultures. Bacteroides fragilis or a fusiform gram negative rod was recovered from 21 (42%) of the patients. Six of the patients (12%) had a bacteremia and three bacteremias were anaerobic. Direct culture of pelvic abscess contents obtained at operation; in patients with pre-operative exposure to antibiotics had a lower yield of anaerobes for only six of fourteen (42.8%) grew anaerobes.

The clinical response to the two regimens was similar. There were no deaths in this series. Operative intervention in addition to the antibiotics was needed in 27 women, (54%) 15 of the patients receiving clindamycin and 12 receiving chloramphenicol. The types of operative intervention are noted in Table II. None of the patients requiring operative intervention had organisms recovered from the infection site, which were resistant in the laboratory to the antibiotics employed. One patient receiving clindamycin developed diarrhea and one patient receiving chloramphenicol had a generalized rash. Both had prompt cessation of symptomatology when these drugs were discontinued.

An analysis of the fever index, a quantitative indirect measure of morbidity revealed no differences between the two groups, Figure one. The range of response in degree hours of these patients requiring operative intervention is noted in Figure two and Figure three.

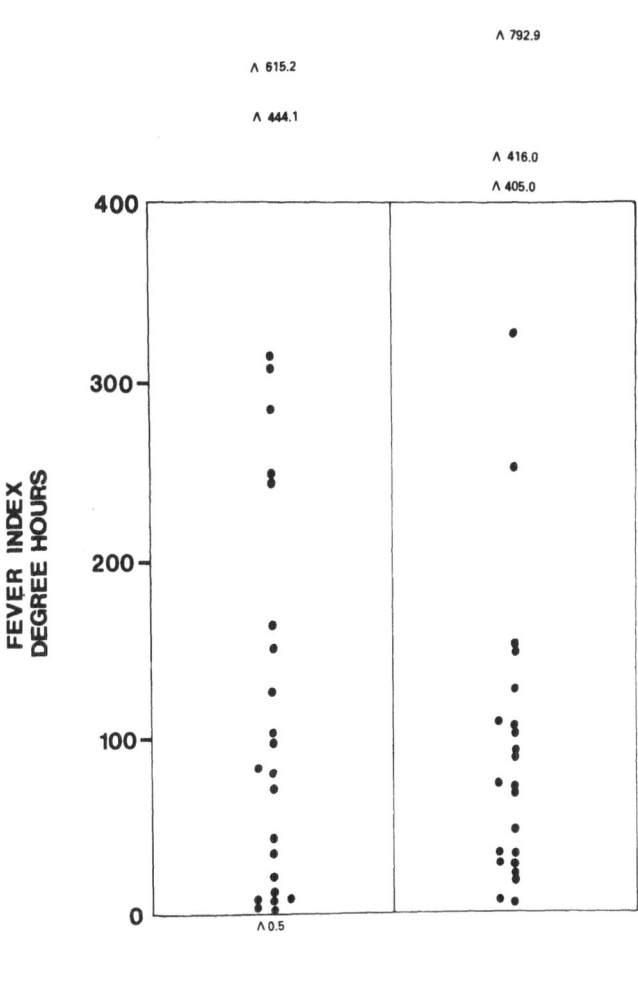

Figure 1

TABLE II

Operations Performed

	Clindamycin	Chloramphenicol
D&C	7	5
Culpotomy drainage of pelvic abscess	4	1
Laparotomy and removal of pelvic abscess	4	6
	15	12

DISCUSSION

A combination of three antibiotics used in this study, was employed to provide coverage against the most frequently encountered organisms in soft tissue pelvic infections. A previous study, comparing either penicillin or clindamycin in combination with an aminoglycoside showed no difference in the clinical results.[1] There were therapeutic failures in patients receiving penicillin in whom Bacteroides fragilis was recovered and failures in patients receiving clindamycin in whom an enterococcus was recovered. The use of triple regimen provided coverage against the enterococcus, making the use of clindamycin or chloramphenicol the only variable in the study.

This study could not demonstrate any clinical superiority to either of these two regimens. Utilizing triple antibiotic coverage in seriously ill, urban poor patients, a number of interesting antibiotic-host relationships was seen. These powerful antibiotic combinations did not eliminate the necessity of operative intervention, for this was required for cure in the majority of patients. In fact, Figure two demonstrates the critical importance of operation, in the cure of these serious soft tissue pelvic infections, for previously febrile patients rapidly became afebrile after drainage. The fact that no resistant organisms were recovered from the abscesses, illustrates the unsolved problem of delivering active antibiotic to the site of infection. A similar range of minor toxicity to these two antibiotics was seen, with the incidence of diarrhea and enterocolitis with clindamycin, far less than has been reported by Tedasco.[2]

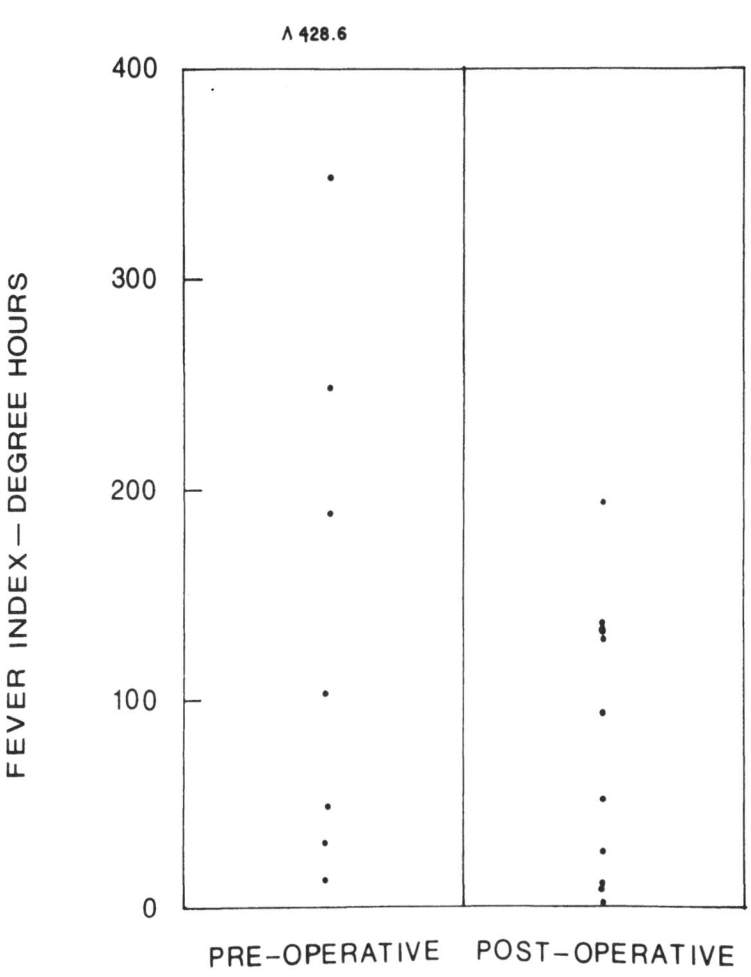

Figure 2

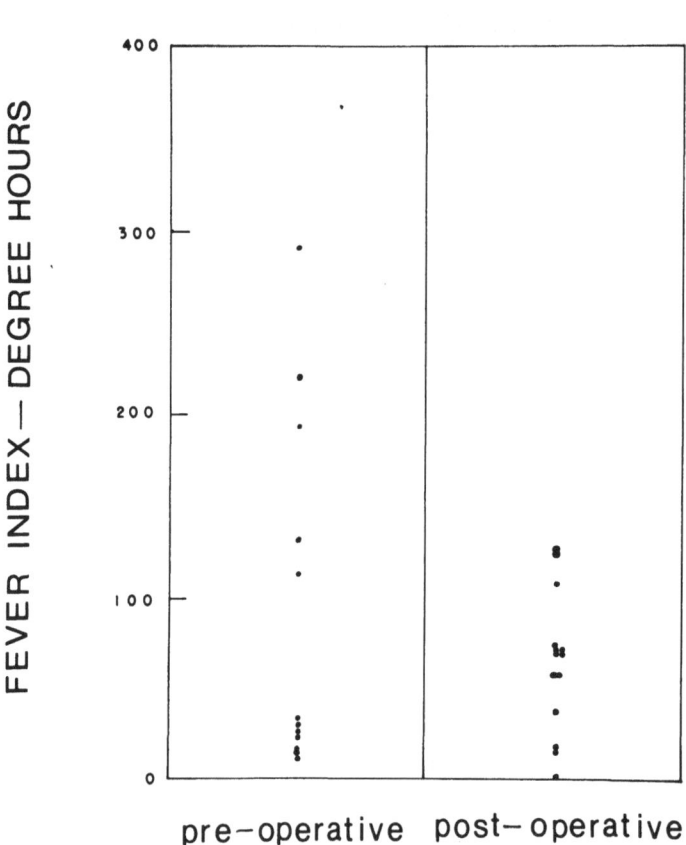

CLINDAMYCIN

Figure 3

A recurring problem in the evaluation of soft tissue pelvic infections in women is the evaluation of the microbiologic data. The judgement to use triple antibiotics was empirical and made before any laboratory results were available. <u>Bacteroides fragilis</u> was not isolated in the majority of women in this comparison of clindamycin and chloramphenicol, but the study accurately reflects the realities of clinical decision making. In addition, there is the difficulty of obtaining cultures directly from the site of infection. Our anaerobic cultures were plated on reduced media by clinicians and immediately incubated in an anaerobic jar. This system of clinical anaerobic microbiology is capable of recovering anaerobes from the majority of genital tract specimens. It is sensitive enough to make mucous membrane contamination a major problem of analysis. We prefer transvaginal peritoneal aspiration for anaerobic culture, but was not employed in many patients because of concern about the intraperitoneal rupture of a pelvic abscess during these diagnostic attempts. Positive blood cultures are a distinct help in these seriously ill patients, but our yield of positives was only 12%.

These results suggest a number of important clinical applications in the future care of Obstetric-Gynecologic patients with serious soft tissue pelvic infections. The early use of powerful antibiotics has not eliminated the necessity for operative intervention and the failure of patient response to powerful antibiotics should indicate the need for operative intervention rather than consideration of possible resistant organisms. Most important in a prospective clinical study, no difference in either the clinical effectiveness or the toxicity of these two agents was noted. If they are equivalent drugs a decision about the primary agent of choice can be made, based upon the individual physicians concern about the toxicity of these agents.

REFERENCES

1. Ledger, W.J., Kriewall, T.J., Sweet, R.L., and Fekety, F.R.,Jr. "The use of parenteral clindamycin in the treatment of Obstetric-Gynecologic patients with severe infection" Obstet-Gynec, 43:490, 1974.

2. Tedasco, F.J., Barton, R.W. and Alpers, D.H., "Clindamycin associated colitis. A prospective study." Ann Intern Med. 81:429, 1974.

TREATMENT OF ANAEROBIC LUNG INFECTIONS

Carbenicillin Compared to Clindamycin and Gentamicin

Haragopal Thadepalli, M.D. and Albert Niden, M.D.
Department of Internal Medicine, Martin Luther King,
Jr. General Hospital and Charles R. Drew Postgraduate
Medical School, Los Angeles, California U.S.A.

SUMMARY

Twenty-three patients (pts) with anaerobic lung infections
were treated with either carbenicillin (12 pts) or clindamycin and
gentamicin (11 pts). Anaerobes were recovered from all specimens.
Fifteen pts. had aerobic bacteria as well. No significant difference was noted in clinical or bacteriologic response between
the two antibiotic groups suggesting that carbenicillin alone is
effective in the treatment of anaerobic lung infections.

Introduction

Anaerobic infections are often polymicrobial and associated
with aerobic bacteria (Gorbach and Bartlett, 1974). Modified anaerobic techniques and cultures of transtracheal aspirates increased
the recognition of anaerobic lung infections (Bartlett, et al 1973).
Modern practice to 'cover-all' bacteria lead to the current use of
clindamycin and gentamicin. Carbenicillin has good activity against
anaerobes in vitro (Blazevic and Matsen, 1974), but its effect in
vivo is unknown.

METHODS AND RESULTS

Twenty-three patients with anaerobic lung infections received
either carbenicillin (24G/day) or clindamycin (1.8G/day) and gentamicin (160 mg/day). The clinical and roentgenographic findings of
the chest were the basis of diagnoses. Included were lung abscess
(6), aspiration pneumonia (6), empyema (6) and necrotizing pneumonia
(5). Cultures were obtained by transtracheal aspiration (17 pts.)
and thoracentesis (6 pts.). Eight pts. had anaerobes in pure cul-

315

TABLE I   AEROBIC ISOLATES

	Carbenicillin	Clindamycin Gentamicin
Streptococci	5	4
Enterococci	5	2
Neisseria	1	1
Klebsiella	0	1
Citrobacter	1	0
Pseudomonas	1	0
Mycobacterium Tuberculosis +	1	1
Nocardia	0	1
Total aerobes per group	14	10

+ received antituberculous therapy

TABLE II   ANAEROBIC ISOLATES

	Carbenicillin	Clindamycin Gentamicin
Peptostreptococcus	7	5
Peptococcus	5	7
Bacteroides	4	4
Fusobacterium	1	0
Eubacterium	0	1
Clostridium	2	1
Actinomyces	2	0
Total isolates per group	21	18

ture. Fifteen had aerobes as well (see Table I). No significant difference in the total number of aerobic (11 and 12) or anaerobic isolates (18 and 22) was noted between the two groups.

Anaerobic isolates (Table II) were identified by their re- actions in pre-reduced media and gas-chromatography. Peptococci predominated in both groups followed by bacteroides and clostridia. Majority of anaerobes were susceptible to less than 32 mcg/ml of carbenicillin and 2.34 mcg/ml of clindamycin by agar dilution tech- nique. Carbenicillin levels at the end of one hour were 125 to 250 mcg/ml and 64 to 125 at the end of two hours by microtitre method.

Overall clinical response in both groups was excellent. Fever subsided in a period of 1.5 to 2 days, intravenous therapy was dis- continued after 13 to 14 days and remarkable improvement in roentgeno- graphic appearance of the chest was noted in 10 days. There were no adverse effects in either antibiotic group.

DISCUSSION

Aspiration pneumonia, lung abscess and empyema are often due to anaerobic bacteria (Bartlett & Finegold, 1974). Since aerobes are found in mixture with anaerobes, antibiotic combination such as clindamycin and gentamicin has been advocated. Whether they could be cured with clindamycin alone (Gorbach and Thadepalli,1974) needs further verification. Carbenicillin in vitro was found to have good antimicrobial effect on anaerobes (Blazevic and Matsen, 1974). In this study clindamycin and gentamicin combined therapy was compared to carbenicillin alone. The clinical response in both anti-biotic groups was excellent. They defervesced rapidly and the serial roentgenograms showed significant improvement in 2 weeks followed by total resolution in 4 to 6 weeks in both groups. The most common anaerobe in anaerobic infections are gram positive cocci and negative rods. The latter are frequently resistant to penicillin. Either clindamycin or chloramphenicol is commonly used with gentamicin in initial therapy. Our study suggests that carbenicillin obviates the need for polyantibiotic therapy. All antibiotics have adverse effects of their own. Pseudo-membranous colitis associated with clindamycin (Tadesco et al, 1974) bone marrow suppression secondary to chloramphenicol (Woodward and Wisserman, 1958) and carbenicillin produced hemostatic defects (Brown et al, 1974) are the potential adverse effects of these drugs.

In conclusion, clindamycin and gentamicin combined therapy or carbenicillin alone provide good coverage for anaerobic lung infections. The serum antibiotic levels, in vitro susceptibility of anaerobes and the observed clinical response suggests that carbenicillin alone could be used in the treatment of anaerobic lung infections.

References

Bartlett, J.G., Rosenblatt, J.E. and Finegold, S.M. (1973), Ann Int. Med. 79, 535

Bartlett, J.G. and Finegold, S.M., (1974), Amer. Rev. Resp. Dis. 110, 56

Blazevic, D.J. and Matsen, J.M. (1974). Antimicrob. Agents 5, 462

Brown, C.M., Natelson, E.A., Bradshaw, M.W., Williams, Jr., T.W. and Alfrey, Jr., C.P. (1974) New Eng. J. Med. 291, 265.

Gorbach, S.L. and Bartlett, J.G. (1974) New Eng. J. Med. 920, 1117, 1237, 1289.

Gorbach, S.L. and Thadepalli, H. (1974) Arch. Int. Med. 134, 87.

Tadesco, F.J., Barton, R. Ward Alpers, D.H. (1974) Ann Int Med 81, 429.

Woodward, T.E., and Wisserman, C.L., Jr., (1958 Chloromycetin Chloramphenicol) Antibiotic Monograph, 1, No. 8. Med. Encyclo-pedia, Inc. New York, Lib. Cong. No. 58-12394.

THE ACTION OF ERYTHROMYCIN AND PENICILLIN ON THE

BACTERIAL FLORA IN TONSIL TISSUE

J. C. GOULD

Central Microbiological Laboratories

Western General Hospital, Edinburgh

INTRODUCTION

One of the reasons for tonsillectomy is the removal of infected tissue to reduce recurrent upper respiratory tract infection. This report is part of an investigation to provide bacteriological support for this procedure, to measure the effect of systemic antibacterial agents on the microflora found and to examine the possible relationship of this flora to other disease. This paper refers to the first two objects only.

MATERIAL AND METHODS

The patients examined were children referred for tonsillectomy at an ear nose and throat clinic and had clinical evidence of chronic infection and hypertrophy of the tonsillar gland.

The tonsils were swabbed in 478 such patients presenting sequentially at the clinic in whom there was no history of current chemotherapy. These swabs were immediately plated onto suitable culture media and examined for pathogenic bacteria after incubation.

Initial Group

One hundred and thirty-three children from this series at random and their excised tonsil tissue was placed in clean sterile containers and sent for detailed bacteriological examination within two hours. In the laboratory the tissue was weighed and washed repeatedly

with sterile water and the washings examined quantitatively for bacteria.   Following this the capsule was
stripped from the gland and approximately one gram of
the remaining tissue was taken and disintegrated in a
tissue blender in a known volume of sterile distilled
water.   Decimal dilutions of this homogenate were now
prepared and 0.1 ml aliquots of each dilution were
uniformly spread over the surface of blood-agar and
heated blood-agar culture plates (one containing 10 units
per ml of Bacitracin) and these were incubated for 48
hours aerobically, anaerobically and in carbon dioxide
at 37°C.   Colony counts were made and differentiation
and identification of the main kinds of bacteria followed.
Sub-cultures of specimen colonies were prepared for sensitivity tests to antibacterial agents and Streptococci
were grouped by Lancefield's method and Haemophilus
tested for 'X' and 'V' factor requirements.   Other
pathogens such as the pneumococcus, N.meningitidis and
Staphylococcus pyogenes were identified by appropriate
tests.

Antibiotic Treatment

A number of children to have tonsillectomy were
selected at random after the initial group described had
been investigated, and given 10 days treatment with
antibiotic prior to operation.   These children were
allocated to Treatment Groups A - E (Table 1) including
one group who received no antibiotic.   Treatment was
administered regularly in the patient's home before
admission to hospital and in hospital until 6 hours prior
to operation.   At operation blood samples were taken
for antibiotic-assay and the tonsil tissue homogenates
were similarly assayed in addition to their bacteriological examinations.

RESULTS

Throat Swab Examinations

478 consecutive patients were swabbed and of these
144 (30%) yielded beta-haemolytic streptococci although
the numbers were often very small on culture.
Haemophilus species were isolated from 92 (19%) and in a
further 30 (6%) both pathogens were isolated.

Examination of Tonsils in Initial Group

The results are shown in Table 2 and it can be seen
that Streptococcus pyogenes or Haemophilus spp. or both
were isolated from nearly all the specimens and in large

TABLE 1

TREATMENT GROUPS

GROUP A
Erythromycin ethyl succinate oral syrup ("Erythroped")
                    200 mgm in 5 ml q.i.d.
                    for children under 8 years

                    400 mgm in 5 ml q.i.d.
                    for children over 8 years

GROUP B
Penicillin 'V' potassium salt
                    125 mgm in 5 ml q.i.d.
                    for children under 5 years

                    250 mgm in 5 ml q.i.d.
                    for children over 5 years

GROUP C
No treatment

GROUP D
Erythromycin ethyl succinate oral syrup
                    250 mgm in 5 ml q.i.d.
                    for children under 8 years

                    500 mgm in 5 ml q.i.d.
                    for children over 8 years

GROUP E
Penicillin 'V' potassium salt
                    125 mgm in 5 ml q.i.d.
                    for children under 5 years

                    250 mgm in 5 ml q.i.d.
                    for children over 5 years

numbers.   Repeated washing of the encapsulated tissue
did not affect the number of organisms isolated from
the stripped tissue which suggests that the organisms
are situated deep within the tissue and not at the
surface.   This was confirmed by histological examination
of a number of specimens which clearly demonstrated the
focal distribution of the bacteria.   The average number
of viable Streptococcus pyogenes isolated was 10^7 per
gram and only slightly less for Haemophilus spp.

Other streptococci, such as Streptococcus viridans,
commensal Neisseria and Corynebacteria were also isolated
but in considerably smaller numbers, never more than 10^6
per gram and in a few coliform bacilli and yeasts (10^5
per gram or less).

TABLE 2

BACTERIA ISOLATED FROM 133 SAMPLES OF TONSIL TISSUE

Organism	Number	Average number (Colony count)
β-streptococci	74 (56%)	1.2×10^7/gm
Haemophilus	85 (64%)	0.7×10^7/gm
Both	30 (23%)	

Other pathogens
  Staph.pyogenes
  Neisseria
  Pneumococcus
	19	

Examination of Tonsil Tissue after Antibiotic

(Treatment Groups A,B,D,E).   The results of examination
of tonsils from children in Treatment Groups A to E are
shown in Table 3.   Those of Group C receiving no antibiotic confirm the results of the Initial Group described
above and are in sharp contrast to those of the other
Groups receiving antibiotic.

Although none of the tonsil tissue specimens
examined was sterile there was apparent elimination of
haemolytic streptococci and Haemophilus in the majority.
Streptococci were isolated from fewer samples from those
receiving erythromycin or penicillin than Haemophilus,
and in considerably smaller numbers.   Haemophilus spp.
were isolated from fewer samples from those who had
received erythromycin than penicillin and the average
number of organisms was smaller.   The effect of higher
dosage of erythromycin used in Treatment Group D was not
significantly different from that of the lower dose
(Treatment Group A).

Antibiotic Sensitivity

(Table 4).   All the strains of Streptococcus pyogenes
and other haemolytic streptococci isolated both before
and after treatment were sensitive to less than 0.5 ug
per ml of penicillin and to less than 2.5 ug per ml of
erythromycin.   The Haemophilus spp. isolated included
Haemophilus influenzae, Haem.parainfluenzae and Haem.
haemolyticus and a number of non-identifiable strains.
Generally these organisms were more resistant to
penicillin but about a third were sensitive to 0.5 ug per
ml of penicillin - mainly strains of Haem.parainfluenzae
and some Haem.haemolyticus.   All the Haemophilus spp.

TABLE 3

RESULTS OF TREATMENT

No.of patients receiving		Number no orgs.	No.with Haem.	Av. no. /gm	No.with strept.	Av. no. /gm
Erythromycin (Gp.A)	20	12	4	10^6	4	8×10^4
Penicillin (Gp.B)	20	12	7	10^7	5	3×10^4
No antibiotic (Gp.C)	19	0	15	$>10^7$	15	10^7
Initial series	133	0	85	10^7	74	10^7
Erythromycin (Gp.D)	19	10	5	2×10^5	4	$<10^5$
Penicillin (Gp.E)	22	14	8	10^6	3	$<10^5$

were sensitive to 25 ug per ml of erythromycin but a considerable proportion required between 2.5 and 25 ug per ml for inhibition.

Antibiotic Assay

It was possible only to sample the blood of patients under anaesthetic prior to operation and this was approximately 6 hours after the last dose of antibiotic. The mean values and range of levels found in the blood and tonsil tissue are shown in Table 5 and it can be seen that these do not attain the higher M.I.C's of the organisms found in the tissue.

DISCUSSION

The results of these investigations show clearly that throat swabbing, even when carefully carried out and with rapid bacteriological examination is not a reliable measure of the presence of organisms such as Streptococcus and Haemophilus in the deeper tissue of the tonsils, and give little indication of the actual number of viable organisms present.

Ample bacteriological evidence has been presented to support the decision to remove diseased tonsils if it is agreed that the numbers of potential pathogens isolated from the tissue constitute an undesirable focus of infection. Ninety-eight per cent of the samples of tissue removed at tonsillectomy yielded around 10^7

TABLE 4

ANTIBIOTIC SENSITIVITY

Organisms Isolated Before Treatment

	Number of strains	Penicillin 0.5 ug/ml	Erythromycin 2.5	12.5	25
Streptococcus pyogenes	122	122	122	-	-
Haemophilus spp.	98	30	58	81	98

Organisms Isolated After Treatment

Streptococcus pyogenes	16	16	16	-	-
Haemophilus spp.	24	10	14	18	24

TABLE 5

CONCENTRATIONS OF ANTIBIOTIC IN SERA AND TONSILS
ug/ml

		Erythromycin Group A	Group B	Penicillin Groups B and E
Sera	Mean	0.8	1.2	0.8
	Range	0.15-3.2	0.4-4.8	0.2-4.0
Tonsils	Mean	2.2	3.2	1.3
	Range	0.4-5.0	0.8-7.8	0.25-3.8

bacteria per gram which could be the source of toxin harmful to the patient and antigen to sensitise his immunological tissue.

It has been shown conclusively that systemic antibiotic such as erythromycin or penicillin can control the growth of these bacteria in the tonsils although eradication is not certain in the dosages used over a period of 10 days. Streptococcus is apparently more easily suppressed than Haemophilus by such short term treatment with antibiotics and this is probably related to the greater susceptibility of these organisms to both antibiotics as measured by their in vitro M.I.C's. However susceptible Streptococcus pyogenes survived in a number of patients in whom the penicillin tissue concentrations must have exceeded the M.I.C's for considerable periods during treatment. Haemophilus spp are more resistant to penicillin and a proportion of strains are relatively resistant to erythromycin, and this may be the main reason for failure to eliminate these organisms with either antibiotic. It is possible however that uniform penetration of antibiotic through the inflamed, hypertrophied and sometimes fibrous tissue is insufficient to ensure that all the microflora is subjected to adequate concentrations no matter what dose is given. Certainly the results with higher doses of erythromycin are disappointing and by themselves do not justify the use of larger amounts of the drug.

ACKNOWLEDGEMENTS

I have to thank Drs. J.F. Birrell, FRCS, and J. McCallum, FRCS, for access to patients and material and the nursing staff of the Unit concerned. Drs. J.D.M. Gould and S.E. Criswell gave valuable help and Dr. Derrick Jackson advice. The support of laboratory assistants and the provision of antibiotics used by Abbott Laboratories, Queenborough, Kent is gratefully acknowledged.

SINUSITIS IN PAEDIATRICS

Dr G. Herz and Dr J. Gfeller

Specialists in Paediatrics

Basel and Dübendorf / Switzerland

Purpose of Trial

The purpose of this trial was as follows:

1. To discuss the diagnosis of sinusitis in childhood from the viewpoint of the practising paediatrician.

2. To assess the results of the treatment of sinusitis in childhood with a selected antibiotic, doxycycline.

3. To determine how rapidly children treated with doxycycline show subjective and objective improvement.

4. To determine the tolerance of this antibiotic in day-to-day practice.

Method

Patients admitted to this trial were cases diagnosed as suffering from sinusitis in our two separately-run practices. The diagnosis was in all cases made on the basis of the history, the clinical picture, and radiography, and any necessary laboratory investigations were carried out. The course of the disease, and objective improvement or cure, were observed not merely clinically, but also with the help of X-Rays, B.S.R. and haematological investigations. We also determined how rapidly subjective improvement occurred in the treated children.

For methodological reasons a single antibiotic - doxycycline - was used for the treatment of sinusitis, and treatment was supplemented by antipyretics, antitussives and nose- and ear-drops. Doxycycline was given in the recommended doses: 4 mg/kg body weight on the first day, followed by 2 mg/kg body weight daily thereafter. The dose in the patients aged 14 - 17 was 200 mg on the first day, followed by 100 mg daily thereafter. The antibiotic was administered once daily in the form of syrup or capsules, with or just after a meal. Children aged less than 6 were not admitted to the trial on account of the possibility of enamel hypoplasia and tooth staining.

RESULTS

Table 1

Age Distribution - 106 Children

Age in years	Number of children	%
6 7 8	12 17 } 40 = 11	37.7 %
9 10 11 12	9 21 } 45 = 11 4	42.5 %
13 14 15 16 17	4 6 5 } 21 = 3 3	19.8 %
Total	106	

Table 2

Diagnosis - 106 Children

Maxillary Sinusitis	60	56.6 %
Ethmoidal Sinusitis	6	5.7 %
Maxillary + ethmoidal sinusitis	26	24.5 %
Maxillary + frontal sinusitis⟩ Ethmoidal + frontal sinusitis⟩	3	2.8 %
Pan-sinusitis	11	10.4 %
Total	106	100 %

Table 3

History in 106 Children

1.	Cough	76
2.	Headache	66
3.	Pyrexia	58
4.	Rhinitis	41
5.	Inappetence	14
6.	Sore throat	10
7.	Fatigue	5
8.	Abdominal pain (3x) Vomiting (2x)	5

Table 4

Clinical Findings in 106 Children with Sinusitis

1.	Pharyngitis	88
2.	Retropharyngeal drip	60
3.	Tenderness over sinus points	45
4.	Associated otitis media	37
5.	Deterioration in general condition	34
6.	Tender enlarged angular lymph-nodes	31
7.	Bronchitis	25
8.	Rhinitis	23

Table 5

Duration of treatment with Doxycycline - 106 Children

In days	Number	%
10 - 14	18	17 %
15 - 21	72	68 %
more than 21	16	15 %
Total	106	100 %

Table 6

Results of treatment - 106 Children

Assessment:

Cured	77	=	72.6 %	Total success rate:
Improved	23	=	21.7 %	
Failed	6	=	5.7 %	94.3 %

Table 7

Subjective Improvement - 106 Children.

RAPID:	In days	No of children	
in 4 - 7 days	4 - 5	18	
	6 - 7	47	
	Total	65	98
MODERATE:			
in 8 - 28 days	8 - 10	20 } 33	
	12 - 14	13	
	16 - 21	7	
	28	1	
	Total	41	

Table 8

Objective Improvement or Normalisation of Roentgenogram

106 Children

RAPID:	In days	No of patients	%
within 2 - 3 weeks	7 - 10 11 - 14	19 } 60 = 41	56.6 %
	15 - 21	20	
	Total	80 =	75.5 %
MODERATE:			
within 4 - 5 weeks	22 - 28 29 - 35	13 5	
	Total	18 =	17 %
SLOW:			
within 5 weeks		2 =	1.9 %
FAILURES:		6 =	5.7 %
	Total	106 =	100 %

The tolerance of the antibiotic used in this trial was extremely good in nearly all the children and adolescents. In only one case did a child vomit the first dose, and another child complained of transient gastric upset.

Discussion

Sinusitis is one of the commonest diseases which confront the paediatrician in his practice. Children are often brought with non-specific complaints, and only a thorough history and objective examination can make the correct diagnosis, which is then confirmed radiologically. The frequency of sinusitis in childhood does not surprise the paediatrician: we must anticipate involvement of the paranasal sinuses in any catarrhal inflammatory condition of the

nasopharynx (8), since the immunological and proliferative processes of the nasopharynx favour the implication of the sinus mucosa.

The diagnosis of sinusitis in this study was confirmed radiologically in each case, and the results of treatment were assessed
not only clinically, but also by X-Ray at appropriate intervals.
Patients with a history of allergy or with vasomotor rhinitis were
excluded from this trial.

Table 3 shows details from the medical history. Cough and
irritating cough were complained of surprisingly frequently - in
76 cases. The parents of 22 children reported that irritating cough
was most marked at night. Headache, which was complained of by 66
of our patients, is also one of the commonest symptoms of children
with sinusitis. Our summary shows that pyrexia was present in 58
cases, but that this important sign was absent in nearly half the
patients. We regard rhinitis as an important symptom, and in many
cases this was the presenting symptom in an otherwise unremarkable
history. To summarise, we can from our experience describe the
tetrad of cough - especially irritating cough at night, headache,
often localised in the frontal region, rhinitis and pyrexia as the
most important points in the history which would lead to a suspicion of sinusitis. Vague abdominal pains, which are said to be the
commonest symptom of maxillary sinusitis in childhood, e.g., in the
study by Bjönnes and Gugler (4) they are said to occur in 24 % of
cases, were only occasionally complained of in our series. Our
observations can be compared with the interesting details of the
medical history concerning the symptomatology of sino-bronchitis
given by Schmid: cough in 47 % of cases, rhinitis in 39 %, headache
in 24 %, a rise in temperature in 41 %, loss of appetite in 21 %,
vomiting in 9 %, fatigue in 7 %, and abdominal pain in 2 % (13).

Clinically, retropharyngeal drip (60 cases) was particularly
common, in addition to the most common finding of pharyngitis
(88 cases). Typical tenderness to pressure was found in 45 cases,
but we had expected to find this sign more frequently. Otitis and
bronchitis are not characteristic for the diagnosis of sinusitis,
but on the other hand, the bronchitis which commonly co-exists
(in 25 of our cases) clearly indicates that many cases of sinusitis
are in fact cases of sino-bronchitis or the descending respiratory
tract syndrome.

The results of the B.S.R. determinations and white cell counts
were interesting. It was striking that the B.S.R. was increased in
only about half of the patients, and then for the most part only
moderately so. Values of more than 30 mm in the first hour were

found in about 9 % of cases. In only barely 32 % of the children
was there a definite leucocytosis (more than 10,000 leucocytes).
Hence, normal values for the B.S.R. and white blood count should
not mislead the clinician in the differential diagnosis of sinusitis.
Only radiology can provide a definite confirmation of the diagnosis
of sinusitis. However, normalisation of the B.S.R. and white cell
count provide useful criteria of the healing process. In addition,
we determined the platelet count in our patients, and even when
the antibiotic was used for long periods, found no reduction in
this to below the normal range.

Sinusitis was commonest in the 9-12 year old group, i.e., in
42.5 % of our series. The older age-groups and adolescents were
less common, in about 19.8 % of cases. The proportion of children
aged 6 - 8 was relatively high, at 37.7 %. Schmid regards the 7-12
year old group as being at particular risk, particularly in relation to chronicity and complications (13).

If we consider the individual diagnostic groups, it is seen
that maxillary sinusitis, with an incidence of 56.5 %, and a combination of maxillary and ethmoidal sinusitis, with an incidence
of 24.5 %, were commonest. Pan-sinusitis was present in about 10 %
of cases in our series. Frontal sinusitis was rare, and this is in
accord with the late aeration of the frontal sinuses.

Duration of Treatment

On the basis of general experience, we regard 2 - 3 weeks as
appropriate in most children. The purpose of treatment must be to
ensure complete cure and to prevent chronicity or relapse. In some
cases good results can be achieved with shorter periods of treatment, while other, stubborn cases of sinusitis require more than
three weeks' treatment. Schmid recommends as a basic rule that
antibiotic therapy should be continued for 3 - 4 weeks, and warns
against premature discontinuance of the antibiotic "since otherwise relapse will inevitably occur within a short time" (13).

Results of Treatment

Where our course of treatment was carried out, success was
achieved in the majority of patients, i.e., in 94.3 % of cases.
No serious septic complications, such as brain abscess, meningitis,
osteomyelitis, etc., occured in any case, neither were irrigation
or operation required.

Several authors have used doxycycline successfully in the treatment of sinusitis (1, 2, 3, 5, 9, 11).

Axelsson and Brorson explain the good results of treatment with doxycycline on the grounds of its high degree of penetration into the sinuses (2). Other authors have also demonstrated adequate concentrations of doxycycline in sinus secretions (2, 6, 7, 10, 12). Axelsson et al (3) believe, on the basis of the results of treatment of 97 adults with doxycycline, that irrigations can be avoided with the use of this antibiotic.

We deliberately eschewed microbiological investigation in our series, since we regard the causal significance of pathogens in nasal or throat swabs as dubious in cases of sinusitis. Conservative treatment was successful, and it was furthermore impossible for this reason to carry out cultures of sinus pus to determine the causative organisms. Several cases of failure to respond to treatment suggest that these were probably those with insensitive organisms.

In selecting the antibiotic for this trial we decided on doxycycline because references in the literature show the high concentrations achieved by doxycycline in the sinus mucosa and sinus secretions (2, 6, 7, 10, 12), and because we ourselves, in a previous trial (9), were able to confirm the excellent clinical results reported by other authors in the treatment of infections of the respiratory tract, including sinusitis, with doxycycline.

One of the purposes of this trial was to determine how rapidly doxycycline acts, on the basis of the criteria described above.

Rapid subjective improvement in 65 patients (61.3 %), and rapid objective improvement in 80 (75.5 %) are evidence that doxycycline is a rapidly effective antibiotic.

The tolerance of doxycycline was very good in nearly all patients. Mild signs of gastro-intestinal intolerance occurred in two cases.

This is without doubt a most satisfying result, and one of particular significance in paediatrics. A further advantage for the paediatrician is the simplicity of dosage, with a single daily dose.

Summary

The authors discuss the problem of the diagnosis of sinusitis in children from the viewpoint of the practising paediatrician, on the basis of 106 children and adolescents aged between 6 and 17 years, and suffering from sinusitis. Maxillary sinusitis (56.5 %) and a combination of maxillary and ethmoidal sinusitis (24.5 %) were commonest, and pan-sinusitis occurred in about 10 % of cases.

The commonest complaints in the history were cough, headache, pyrexia and rhinitis. The commonest clinical findings were pharyngitis, retropharyngeal drip, tenderness to pressure over the sinus points, otitis media, a deterioration in the general condition, enlarged tender angular lymph-nodes, bronchitis and rhinitis.

The results of treatment of sinusitis in childhood with the antibiotic used here, doxycycline, are assessed. A successful result was obtained in 94.3 % of cases: cure in 77 patients (72.6 %) and marked improvement in 23 (21.7 %). There were six failures (5.7 %). In the majoritiy of children - 72 cases (68 %), the duration of treatment was 15 - 21 days. It was 10 - 14 days in 18 children (17 %) and more than three weeks in 16 children (15 %).

Rapid subjective improvement was seen in 65 cases (61.3 %), and rapid objective improvement in 80 (75.5 %).

The tolerance of doxycycline was very good in nearly all patients. Mild symptoms of gastro-intestinal intolerance were seen in two cases.

Literature

1. AGBIM, O.G. : A Comparative Trial of Doxycycline and Ampicillin in the Treatment of Acute Sinusitis.
    Chemotherapy 21 (Suppl. 1), 68-75, 1975

2. AXELSSON, A., BRORSON, J.-E.: Concentration of Antibiotics in Sinus Secretions.
    Ann. Otol. 82, 44-48, 1973

3. AXELSSON, A., CHIDEKEL, N., GREBELIUS, N., JENSEN, C., SINGER F.:
    Treatment of Acute Maxillary Sinusitis
    Ann. Otol., Rhin. Laryngol., 82, 2, 186-191, 1973

4. BJOENNESS, H., GUGLER, E. : Zur Behandlung der Sinusitis im
                                Kindesalter.
                        Therapeutische Umschau, 30, 6, 452-456, 1973

5. BOSKOVIC, D. : Erfahrungen mit Vibramycin in der H.N.O.-Heil-
                    kunde.
                    Zeitschrift für Therapie, 7, 475-478, 1971

6. ENEROTH, C.M., LUNDBERG, C., WRETLIND, B. : Antibiotic Con-
                    centrations in Maxillary Sinus Secretions and
                    in the Sinus Mucosa.
                    Chemotherapy 21 (Suppl. 1) : 1-7, 1975

7. GNARPE, H., LUNDBERG, CH. : L-Phase Organisms in Maxillary
                                Sinus Secretions.
                        Scand. J. Infect. Dis. 3: 257-259, 1971

8. HARNACK, G.A. von : Kinderheilkunde.
                        Springer Verlag Berlin, Heidelberg, 1971

9. HERZ, G., GFELLER, J. : Vibramycin in Paediatrics.
                        Chemotherapy 21 (Suppl. 1), 58-67, 1975

10. LISS, R.H., NORMAN, J.C. : Visualization of Doxycycline in Lung
                    Tissue and Sinus Secretions by Fluorescent
                    Techniques.
                    Chemotherapy 21 (Suppl. 1) : 27-35, 1975

11. LUMIO, J.S. : Doxycycline Hydrochloride (Vibramycin) in Oto-
                    rhinolaryngological Infections.
                    Chemotherapy 12 : 101-106, 1967

12. LUNDBERG, CH., GULLERS, K., MALMBORG, A.-S. : Antibiotics in
                    Sinus Secretions.
                    The Lancet, 107-108, July 13, 1968

13. SCHMID, F. : Die Sinobronchitis.
                    Pädiat. Prax., 555-564, 1972

SULFAMETOPYRAZINE (SMP) IN THE CHEMOPROPHYLAXIS OF EXACERBATIONS OF CHRONIC BRONCHITIS

Darke, C.S.   Launchbury, A.P.

Consultant Physician   Pharmaceutical Adviser
Northern General Hospital   Pharmitalia (UK) Ltd.
Sheffield   Barnet, Herts.

INTRODUCTION

The sputum of chronic bronchitics frequently becomes muco-purulent or purulent with the onset of infection; such episodes are particularly frequent during the winter months. Given the fact that there is a natural fear of recurrent infections in the minds of very many bronchitic subjects and the danger that repeated infections will lead to a reduction of the respiratory reserves, it is understandable that many workers have tried to reduce the frequency and severity of exacerbations of chronic bronchitis with the aid of chemoprophylaxis. Others have endeavoured, by intermittent therapy, to provide prompt treatment of infections but this method of control suffers from the disadvantage that it may provide an opportunity for infection to become established before drugs are administered. The studies involving continuous antibacterial cover, indicate that worthwhile protection may be conferred in this way. For example, the use of tetracyclines for continuous chemoprophylaxis of chronic bronchitis was studied by two groups of workers for full five-year periods; Calder et al (1968) and Johnston et al (1969) both found that the drug was effective in reducing the frequency and severity of exacerbations. Pines (1967) had similar success with a long-acting sulphonamide and later demonstrated that co-trimoxazole could also be effective when used in this manner (Pines 1973). The position has been reviewed by the Committee on Therapy of the American Thoracic Society which concluded that patients who have frequent and/or prolonged exacerbations benefit from continuous prophylactic administration of antimicrobials (American Thoracic Society, 1971).

However, one of the difficulties with regimes studied to date
has been that difficulty is encountered in ensuring that patients
take their drugs regularly and as prescribed. Investigations on
the conscientiousness with which prescribed medication is taken,
have shown that the reliability of tablet taking is inversely
related to the frequency of the dosage (Gatley, 1968), the number
of preparations the patient is taking and to the age of the
patient (Blackwell, 1973). The purpose of this paper is to
demonstrate that once-weekly medication with a chemotherapeutic
agent with a long half-life is tolerable and acceptable over a
long period and apparently taken conscientiously. The acceptability of the regimen was evidenced by the small number of
defaulters. The drug chosen for the study was sulfametopyrazine
which is a long-acting sulphonamide with pharmacokinetic properties which commend it for the chemoprophylaxis of chronic
bronchitis. Its long half-life of about 65 hours enables it to be
administered at weekly intervals as a 2g. water-dispersible tablet
(Kelfizine W). High blood levels are obtained varying from about
130 mcg. per ml. on the first day to about 25 mcg. per ml. on the
7th day after administration (Donno et al, 1967, Devriendt et al
1970, Krüger-Thiemer et al, 1969). Sulfametopyrazine penetrates
well into body fluids and secretions including saliva (Colombo,
1963), tonsillar tissue (Cis, 1970) and, of particular importance
in the present context, sputum (Giura and Menghini, 1971). In
sputum the concentration of sulfametopyrazine is consistently
about 20% of the plasma level. It has the broad spectrum of
activity characteristic of sulphonamides which typically includes
Streptococcus pneumoniae and Haemophilus influenzae.

MATERIALS AND METHODS

The trial was carried out in general practice with the
collaboration of 583 practices throughout the United Kingdom and
most parts of the Republic of Ireland. All the observations were
limited to the winter months between October 1973 and March 1974.
Care was taken to include areas representative of urban, industrial
and rural conditions. Each practitioner was asked to endeavour to
contribute about 15 bronchitic subjects to the study. While no
specific control group was studied in parallel with those receiving
sulfametopyrazine, a measure of control was achieved by randomly
extracting a group of 1120 patients and comparing the frequency of
exacerbations during the trial winter with those suffered by these
patients during the previous winter when they received no continuous
cover with sulfametopyrazine. To enable this work to be done, the
participating practitioners were asked to record the number of
exacerbations suffered the previous winter on entry of each
patient to the trial.

Most patients admitted to the trial had documentary evidence

of chronic bronchitis with or without associated emphysema or asthma.
Patients with a history of right heart failure or actual evidence
of oedema were accepted but patients with pulmonary tuberculosis
or lung cancer were excluded. Either sex was admissible but the
study did not include children (81% of patients in fact were over
the age of 45). On entry into the study, the purpose of which was
explained in full to the patient, the amount / character of sputum,
antibiotic requirements and periods off work or confinement to house
or bed, were recorded. It was not possible to make routine measurements of ventilatory capacity since the appropriate apparatus was
not universally available in the practices participating. Concurrent therapy was recorded and continued during the study at the
practitioner's discretion. In many instances, the sputum was
rendered mucoid before entry into the trial by administration of a
broad spectrum antibiotic. The trial protocol permitted each
practitioner to treat exacerbations occurring during the survey
period with antibiotics as appropriate but required continued
administration of sulfametopyrazine at the same weekly intervals
throughout.

RESULTS

A total of 6521 patients were included in the study, 72% of
them being male. As can be seen from Table 1, roughly two thirds
of the patients were severely disabled in that they had complicating disease:

TABLE 1: Associated Chest Conditions

Emphysema	1710	Emphysema + Cardiac Failure	442
Asthma	1083	Asthma + Cardiac Failure	87
Cardiac Failure	370		
Emphysema + Asthma	595	Emphysema + Asthma + Cardiac Failure	175

As will be seen from Table 2, 81% of the patients entered
into the trial were aged 45 and over, the largest single group
being in the 55-64 year age range:

TABLE 2: Ages of Patients

Up to 34 yrs.	437	55-64 yrs.	2,142
35-44 yrs.	426	65 yrs. and over	1,994
45-54 yrs.	1,171		

Table 3 shows that the treatment periods varied considerably depending on when the patients first presented to their practitioner; approximately two thirds of the subjects (4014) received the drug for more than three months:

TABLE 3: Numbers of Patients in Various Treatment Periods

Up to 1 month	479	4-5 months	1,196
1-2 months	629	5-6 months	1,012
2-3 months	955	6+ months	641
3-4 months	1,165		

Out of the total population of 6521 patients, 4129 (63.4%) required no antibiotics during the period of the study (Table 4):

TABLE 4: Analysis of Results: Antibiotic Requirements

No antibiotics required	4,129	(63.4%)
1-2 courses required	1,168	(17.9%)
More than two courses	280	(4.3%)
Records incomplete for	944	(14.4%)

The difference between this group and the others who derived less benefit is highly significant ($P < 0.001$). A further 1168 (17.9%) required only one or two courses of antibiotics. Thus nearly two thirds of the total trial population suffered no significant bacterial infection throughout the period. Another 20% only had one or two exacerbations in contrast to the previous winter when an average of 4-5 exacerbations were recorded per patient.

As will be seen from Table 5, nearly 50% of patients in the study had mucopurulent or purulent sputum on admission:

TABLE 5: Initial Sputum States

Mucoid	2,486	(38.1%)	
Mucopurulent	873	(13.7%))	
Purulent	2,204	(33.8%))	47.5%
Not recorded	938	(14.4%)	

At the end of the study period (Table 6), a significant ($P < 0.001$) number of patients experienced a reduction in the quantity of sputum (3279 patients, 50.3%):

TABLE 6: Analysis of Results: Trends of Sputum States

	Better	Same	Worse
Purulence	2,956	2,284	219
Quantity	3,279	2,005	185

The data for the presence or degree of purulence shown on Table 6 can be further broken down. Under the headings 'Better' and 'Worse', the 3175 patients are divided as shown in Table 7:

TABLE 7: Details of Shifts of Sputum States During Trial Period

"Better"		"Worse"	
Purulent - mucopurulent	353	Mucopurulent to purulent	13
Purulent - mucoid	2,013	Mucoid to purulent	117
Mucopurulent - mucoid	590	Mucoid to mucopurulent	89
Totals:	2,956		219

Thus a change from some degree of purulence to a mucoid sputum was seen in 2,603 patients (47.4% of the 5,459 patients for whom sputum data were recorded). Omitting the patients recorded as "unchanged" as to purulence or otherwise of sputum, this percentage becomes 82%, i.e. of those showing a change with regard to sputum purulence, 82% showed a shift to diminished purulence or to a mucoid sputum. This 82% is composed of 63.4% (2,013) who showed change from purulent to mucoid and only 18.6% (590) who changed from mucopurulent to mucoid. These figures are highly significant ($P<0.001$).

The randomly-extracted group of 1120 patients, used as a retrospective control, was analysed with reference to the numbers of exacerbations each individual had suffered during the trial period as compared with the number recorded, before entry to the trial, during the previous winter period 1972/73 when no sulfametopyrazine was prescribed prophylactically. It was found that during the winter 1972/73 when patients received no sulfametopyrazine, the average frequency of exacerbations was 4.2 per patient; this contrasts with the average frequency of 0.4 per patient during the trial period 1973/74 when sulfametopyrazine was received continuously. Table 8 tabulates the distribution of exacerbation frequency within this group for the two winters, and it is notable that during the 1973/74 period, there is a substantial shift to the zero to two frequency range.

Side-effects were relatively few in number occurring in only 2.5% of patients in the trial and in all instances were very mild;

TABLE 8: Comparison of Two Winters in Randomly-Extracted Group of
1120 Patients

1972-3 Without Sulfametopyrazine		1973-4 With Sulfametopyrazine	
Patients	Exacerbations	Patients	Exacerbations
13	0	782	0
56	1	154	1
203	2	61	2
173	3	21	3
304	4	16	4
151	5	3	5
200	6-30	2	8-9

Table 9 shows that these unwanted effects were divided almost
equally between rashes and gastrointestinal upsets. No serious
drug reaction such as the Stevens-Johnson syndrome occurred:

TABLE 9: Side-Effects

Rash	87	(1.3%)
Others, comprising:	78	(1.2%)
Nausea	54	
Vomiting	9	
'Sick'	4	
'Dizzy'	6	
Headache	1	
'Couldn't say'	3	
'Couldn't take tablets'	1	

DISCUSSION

Virus infections of the respiratory tract are known to be
relatively common initiators of exacerbations of chronic bronchitis
(Stenhouse et al, 1967, Fisher et al, 1969, Lambert & Stern, 1972,
Carilli et al, 1974, Horn and Yealland, 1974), and it is very
probable that these occurred throughout both winter periods 1972/3
and 1973/4. However, sputum purulence is attributable to secondary
bacterial infection and prevention of this phase with sulphonamides
or other antimicrobials is generally thought to be highly beneficial.
It is believed that the ten-fold reduction in frequency of infections
requiring antibiotic therapy demonstrated in this study, could be
attributable to the suppression of the secondary bacterial invasion
by the sulphonamide used. The results could hardly be attributed to
the mildness of the weather, since the two previous winters were
comparably mild.

Subjective assessment of response to treatment is fraught with difficulties and liable to be biased in favour of a new approach in any uncontrolled trial. Nevertheless, it is worth recording that in this instance the participating physicians were firmly of the opinion that the drug had benefited their patients in about two thirds of the whole group. Furthermore, this opinion was endorsed by many patients who were worried when the drug was stopped and asked to receive it during the following winter.

Both Streptococcus pneumoniae and Haemophilus influenzae may develop resistance to certain antibiotics (May 1972), though it has been shown that this likelihood is reduced particularly in the case of H. influenzae if drugs are given continuously rather than intermittently (ibid). While further studies are being carried out to determine whether resistance develops significantly in response to long-term sulfametopyrazine administration, the results to date suggest that it does not.

The inference from this large general practitioner study is that the weekly administration of 2g. of sulfametopyrazine is safe and effective in reducing the antibiotic requirements of chronic bronchitics with minimal side-effects.

ACKNOWLEDGEMENT

Thanks are expressed to Mr. P. Parker for his help in performing the detailed statistical analysis of the case data.

REFERENCES

American Thoracic Society, Committee on Therapy,"Chemotherapy of Chronic Bronchitis", American Review of Respiratory Disease, (1971), 104, 776-7

Blackwell, B., (1973), New Engl. J. Med., 289, 249

Calder, M.A., et al (1968), Brit. J. Dis. Chest, 62, 93-99

Carilli, A.D., et al (1964), New Engl. J. Med., 270, 123-7

Cis, C., (1970), Annali di Laringologia, Otologia, Rinologia, Faringologia, Fasc. 6, 448-58

Colombo, E. (1963), Rivista Italiana di Stomatologia, 18, 1158-72

Devriendt, A., et al (1970), Europ. J. Clin. Pharmacol., 3, 36-42

Donno, L., et al (1967), Il Farmaco (Ed. Prat), No. 8, 444-53

Fisher, M., et al (1969), Brit. Med. J., 4, 187-92

Giura, R., and Menghini, P. (1971), Giornale Italiano di Chemioterapia, 18, 19-22

Horn, M.E.C., and Yealland, S. J. (1974), Arch. Dis. Child, 49, 516-9

Johnston, R.N., et al (1969), Brit. Med. J., 4, 265-9

Krüger-Thiemer, E., et al (1969), Chemotherapy, 14, 273-302

Lambert, H.P., and Stern, H., (1972), Brit. Med. J., 3, 323-7

May, J.R. (1972), "The Chemotherapy of Chronic Bronchitis and Allied Disorders" The English Universities Press Ltd., pages 74-84

Pines, A. (1967), Brit. Med. J., 3, 202-4

Pines, A., (1973), The Practitioner, 210, 556-8

Stenhouse, A.C., (1967), Brit. Med. J., 3, 461-3

CHEMOTHERAPY OF CHRONIC BRONCHITIS IN CHILDREN

Suzuko Uehara,[*][**] Itaru Terashima,[*] Yoshiko Muramatsu,[*]
Keishi Kishimoto[*] and Seiji Kubo[*]
[*] Department of Pediatrics, School of Medicine
Chiba University, Chiba, Japan
[**] Training Institute for Nurse Teacher
Chiba University, Chiba, Japan

Summary. Dominant pathogens in the washed sputum and the
effects of antibiotics were studied in 40 children with chronic
bronchitis during 1964-1974. H. influenzae, especially of type
b, was found in 38 cases, associated with pneumococcus in 21 and
S. aureus in 2. Administration of appropriate antibiotics, such
as ampicillin, proved effective in eliminating or reducing the
organisms as well as clinically. However, relapses occurred
after discontinuance of antibiotics. Although large doses of
ampicillin delayed the recurrence of the pathogens, superinfections were more likely to occur during the treatment. In spite
of the treatment with antibiotics, only eight cases out of 21
children with chronic bronchitis had considerable clinical
improvement from two years' observation.

It has been found out through our ten years' observation on
the lower respiratory disorders in children that bacterial infection is most frequently encountered in chronic bronchitis.
Chronic bronchitis is relatively common with adults, however,
it has been infrequent in childhood and its definition still
remains to be established. Criteria of chronic bronchitis in
our clinic is prolonged moist cough for more than six months.
The purpose of this study is to elucidate the dominant pathogens
in chronic bronchitis in children and to make clear the effects
of antibiotics on this disease. The subjects studied were 40
children with chronic bronchitis of the ages from four to fifteen
during the period from 1964 to 1974.

The procedure for sputum examination was the same as that
described in the preceeding report.(Uehara, 1970) In an attempt
to improve culture reliability, the sputum was subjected to

Table 1. Dominant Pathogens in Washed Sputum
Chronic Bronchitis 40 cases

H. influenzae + D. pneumoniae   21(52.5%) Serotypes of H. influenzae
H. influenzae   17(42.5%)
S. aureus   2(5.0%)   type b 29(80.6%)
                                             type a   5(13.9%)
        Superinfection with GNR: other than type a & b
                                                    1(2.8%)
                Pseudomonas   4   non-typable
                Klebsiella   2   1(2.8%)
                E. coli   1
                Cloaca   1   36 cases examined

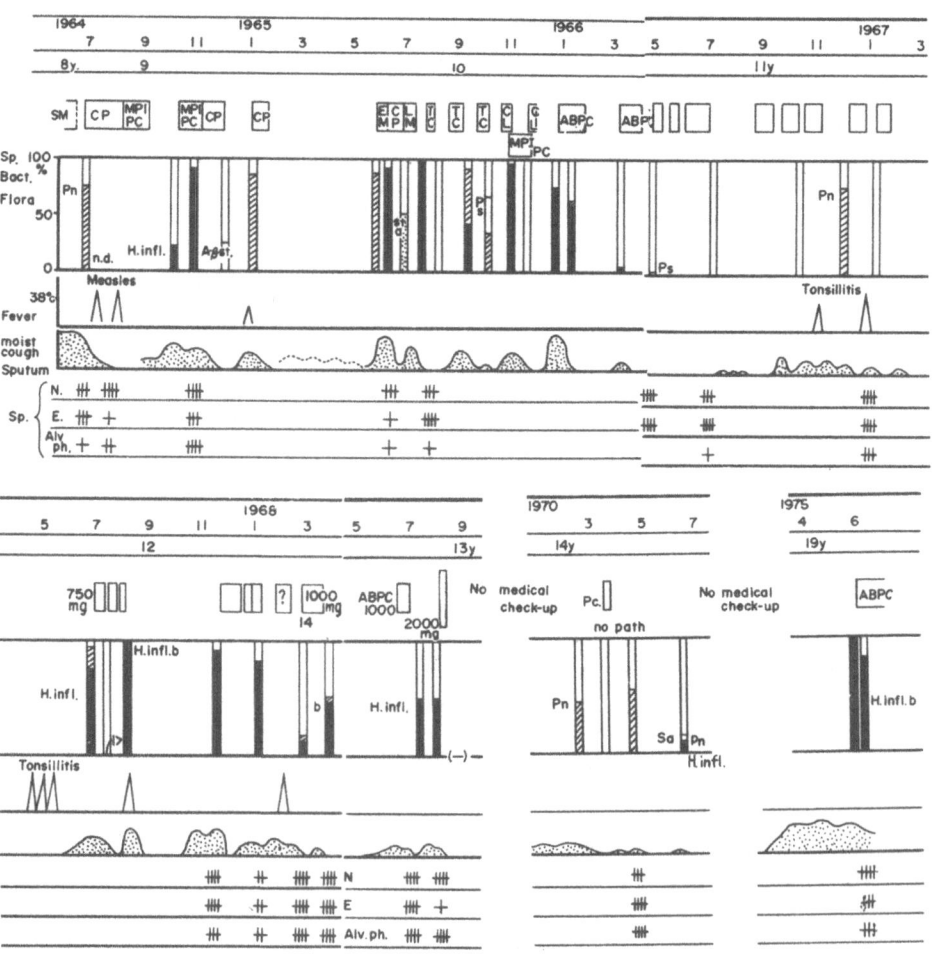

Fig.1. Clinical course of chronic bronchitis (Y.J. f)

repeated washings with sterile saline. The presence of alveolar
phagocytes was considered as an important indication of "bronchial secretion". Dominant pathogen was defined as the strain that
constitutes more than 50% of the washed sputum flora counted as
colonies.

Table 1 summarizes dominant pathogens in washed sputum
obtained from the 40 cases of children with chronic bronchitis.
H. influenzae was isolated in 95.0% of the patients. Simultaneously or alternatively with H. influenzae, pneumococcus was found
in 52.5%. However, H. influenzae seemed to be more closely
related to the disease. There were two cases of S. aureus
included. The strains of H. influenzae isolated from 34 cases
were typable: 29 belonged to type b and five to type a. It has
been noticed that the majority of the strains isolated from children were typable, although those from adults have been reported
mostly to be non-typable.

Case Report (Fig. 1)   The patient was an eight year-old
girl. Before she attended our clinic in July 1964, She was
diagnosed and treated as pulmonary tuberculosis because of persisting productive cough. In our clinic the diagnosis was
chronic bronchitis. H. influenzae and pneumococcus were isolated
from the sputum. The pathogens disappeared after chloramphenicol
and tetracycline treatment with clinical improvement. However,
the pathogenic organisms reappeared many times in spite of the
treatment. Then, ampicillin was selected as an alternative drug
after that. H. influenzae was eliminated for a year and a half,
and treatment was discontinued for six months. Then, the clinical and bacteriological relapse occurred. Administration of a
large dose of ampicillin resulted in a relatively good course with
little cough. She did not respond to our annual inquiry for five
years. She visited us with a complaint of productive severe
cough in June 1975. She was nineteen years old. She had purulent sputum which contained a large number of neutrophils yield-
ing heavy growth of H. influenzae, which we interpret as a sign
of acute exacerbation of the disease. This is a rare case in
which chronic bronchitis occurring in childhood has been followed
into adulthood. Such study will throw light in the relationship
between chronic bronchitis of children and of adults.

Table 2 shows the effects of antibiotics regarding the
disapperance of H. influenzae and pneumococcus in the sputum.
Any agent succeeded in eliminating pneumococcus. As regards
H. influenzae, ampicillin, chloramphenicols and tetracyclines
were effective except for three cases. Disappearance of the
organism was confirmed within two days in the earliest in the
consecutive examination. Amoxycillin given in a dose half of
that for ampicillin, proved effective in only two trials out of
five. A discrepancy was found between the sensitivity of

Table 2. Effects of Antibiotics on Pathogens in Washed Sputum

1) Disappearance of Pathogens   Chronic Bronchitis

Antibiotics / Pathogens	PC	ABPC	AMPC	CP	TP	TC	DOTC MINO	EM	ABPC*
H.influenzae							6		
dominant	1	27	5	9	5	7	2 4	4	15
disappeared	0	25	1	8	4	7	1 3	0	15
significantly reduced		1	1	1	1		4		
% effective	0 %	96.3%	40.0%	100.0%	100.0%	100.0%	66.7%	0 %	100.0%
slightly reduced or unchanged	1	1	3	0	0	0	1 1	4	0
D.pneumoniae									
dominant	2	4	2	2	1	1	0	2	0
disappeared	1	4	2	2	1	1	0	2	0
significantly reduced	1								
% effective		100.0%							
slightly reduced or unchanged	0	0	0	0	0	0	0	0	0

No. of Episodes

ABPC 30 mg/kg/day   CP 30mg/kg/day   TC 25mg/kg/day   ABPC* 60-80mg/kg/day

AMPC 15mg/kg/day   TP 20mg/kg/day   DOTC,MINO 2-4mg/kg/day EM 25mg/kg/day

2) Reappearance of Pathogens

	H. influenzae		D. pneumoniae	
after Chemotherapy (ordinary doses)				
disappeared reappeared within 30 days	49		13	
(dominant)	26	53.1%	7	53.9%
The same pathogen	22	44.7%	3	23.1%
(dominant)	(17	34.7%)	(3	23.1%)
different pathogens	D.pneumoniae	3	H.influenzae	4
	S.aureus	1		
after ABPC (large doses)				
disappeared reappeared within 30 days	15			
	2	13.3%		
(dominant)	(1	6.7%)		
after 30 days	5	33.3%		
(dominant)	(4	26.7%)		

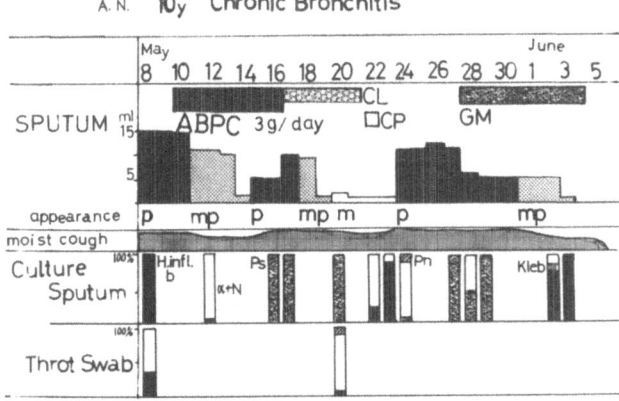

Fig.2. Case A.N.(f) Chronic Bronchtis
          treated with a large dose of ampicillin

	H.influenzae			D.pneumoniae			Staph. aureus		
No.	Sp.	Np.	Th.	Sp.	Np.	Th.	Sp.	Np.	Th.
1									
2									
3									
4									
5									
6									
7									
8									
9									
10									
11									
12									
13									
14									
15									
16									
17									
18									
19									
20									
21									
22									
23									
24									
25									
26									
27									
28									
29									
30									
31									
32									
33									
34									
35									
36									
37									
38									
39									
40									

dominant   □ non-dominant

Fig.3. Bacteriological findings
        of chronic bronchitis. 40 cases.

TABLE 4

Clinical Course of Chronic Bronchitis in Children

two years' observation   21 cases

Course	Moist Cough & Sputum	Dominant Pathogens in Sputum	Relapses	Antibiotics	No.of Cases	
very good	disappeared	negative	(-)	not necessary	1	8
good	markedly reduced	transiently positive	(-)	not necessary	7	
moderately good	reduced	transiently positive	(+)	occasionally necessary	12	13
poor	persistent	positive	(++)	necessary	1	

H. influenzae to erythromycin and its clinical effects.

     The important problem in the chemotherapy of chronic
bronchitis is how to prevent the recurrence of pathogens in the
sputum and at the same time how to minimize the superinfections
with gram-negative rods and other organisms. H. influenzae or
pneumococcus reappeared in 44.9% or 23.1% of the episodes,
respectively, within 30 days after chemotherapy was discontinued.
Staphylococcus aureus and β-streptococcus also appeared at times,
but disappeared in a short period of time. On the other hand,
substitution of pathogens such as pseudomonas, E. coli and
Klebsiella are sometimes found in sputum during the treatment
with broad-spectrum antibiotics.

     In order to eradicate H. influenzae large doses of
ampicillin were administered orally for about five days in a
modified dosage based on Dr. May's recommendation for 15
episodes.(May, 1964)   60-80 mg/kg/day was considered suitable
for children. There was a clinical responce within a few days
with disappearance of the organism. However, reappearance in
dominance of the organism occurred after 24 days, three months,
three months, six months and seven months, respectively. As far
as elimination of H. influenzae is concerned, this treatment

seemed to be more satisfactory. However, it should be stressed
that there is more danger of superinfections with pseudomonas
(Fig. 2) and other gram-negative rods. Therefore, patients
should be hospitalized during the treatment with succesive
bacterial examinations. If moist cough and sputum increase again
and appearance of the sputum turns to purulent after some
clinical improvement, superinfection should be suspected. In
such case treatment with the drug should be immediately discontinued and alternative antibiotics should be selected.

Among possible underlying disorders of chronic bronchitis,
oto-rhino-laryngeal diseases, especially chronic sinusitis,
found in 72.2% of the cases, should be considered. Figure 3
shows bacterial flora of the sputum, nasopharyx and throat in
the cases with chronic bronchitis. H. influenzae was found to be
dominant in 26 cases in both sputum and nasopharynx, pneumococcus
in 14 and staphylococcus in one. H. influenzae remained in the
nasopharynx, even when the pathogen had disappeared in the
sputum after chemotherapy. Serotypes of H. influenzae isolated
from the nasopharynx were identical with those from the sputum in
69.2% of the cases and its existence were related to having
sinusitis.

Taking allergic factors into consideration, we are using the
bacterial vaccine in 20 cases after chemotherapy.

According to two years' observation on 21 cases with chronic
bronchitis, only eight cases had considerable clinical improvement, while the others had clinical exacerbations with
H. influenzae and/or pneumococcus in the sputum.(Tab.4.)

References

1) May, J.R. and Delves D.M.(1964), Thorax, 19, 298-305
2) Uehara, S., Muramatsu, Y., Terashima, I., Nomoto, Y. and
   Kubo, S.(1970), Progress in Antimicrobial and Anticancer
   Chemotherapy, Tokyo Univ. Press, p.789-793

PHARMACOLOGICAL AND CLINICAL STUDIES WITH CEPHACETRILE AS A TREATMENT FOR LOWER RESPIRATORY TRACT INFECTIONS

A.L. THOMAS* AND D.S. REEVES

DEPARTMENT OF MEDICAL MICROBIOLOGY

SOUTHMEAD HOSPITAL, WESTBURY-ON-TRYM, BRISTOL BS10 5NB

Cephacetrile is a new derivative of 7-amino-cephalosporanic acid available in injectable form for intramuscular or intravenous administration and is not thought to be nephrotoxic (Opitz et al, 1970). This trial was designed to study the drug when used to treat patients with lower respiratory tract infections.

MATERIALS AND METHODS

Twenty three patients in the general medical and surgical wards of our hospital who were thought to have lower respiratory tract infections were treated. As sputum reports could not be expected for at least 48 hours treatment was begun immediately on clinical grounds. A general clinical assessment was made and the patient seen daily during the treatment period, the final clinical assessment was made one month later at follow-up. Clinical improvement was judged on changes in their subjective feeling of well being, skin colour, dyspnoea and other physical signs. All patients had general supportive treatment including physiotherapy. White blood count, ESR, temperature and chest X-ray before and after treatment were done but were unhelpful in assessing therapy. Liver and renal function tests were also performed. Sputum cultures were taken before and at the end of treatment. The mean inhibitory concentration of Haemophilus influenzae isolated, together with serum and plasma levels of the drug were measured using standard methods. 1 gram of cephacetrile in 2 mls of 2% lidocaine was given by intramuscular injection into the thigh each 12 hours for an average of

* Present address :- K.R.U.F. Institute of Renal Disease,
  Royal Infirmary, Cardiff CF2 1SZ, Wales.

Table 1 – Patients Admitted to Trial

Clinical State: Poor   5
                   Moderate   15
                   Good   3
                                                   Total   23

Male/Female   16/7

Average age (years)   61.6

Congestive cardiac failure   7

Previous Chronic respiratory disease :
                        Chronic bronchitis   11
                        Bronchiectasis   1

7 days.   There were 16 males and 7 females.   Their initial features are shown in Table 1 and their diagnoses in Table 2.

RESULTS

Clinical assessment.   Sixteen patients were clinical successes
(69%) in that they showed clinical improvement which was maintained
up to their follow up visit.   Three patients were considered to be
partial successes in that they made a satisfactory response in the
treatment period but on follow-up were found to have needed further
antibiotic treatment.   There were 4 clinical failures, all over 60
years of age, in poor general condition and, like the partial
successes, had histories of chronic bronchitis.   It became clear
that patients with a history of chronic chest disease did not do as
well as those with no previous disease.   The post operative group
of patients did particularly well (see Table 3).

Table 2 – Respiratory Infections Treated with Cephacetrile

Diagnosis	Number
Acute exacerbations of Chronic Bronchitis	7
Lobar Pneumonia	5
Postoperative Chest Infection	5
Bronchopneumonia	4
Bronchiectasis	1
2^0 to Congestive Cardiac Failure	1
Total	23

Table 3 — Clinical Results of Chronic Chest Disease and Post
        Operative Groups Treated with Cephacetrile

Group	No.	Success	Partial Success	Failure
Chronic Chest	12	5	3	4
Post Operative	5	5	-	-

Microbiology. Twelve patients had at least one pathogen
reported from the pre-treatment sputum. Haemophilus influenzae
was the most frequently reported organism and it was eliminated in
3 out of the 7 cases. Patients growing Haemophilus influenzae
resistant to cephacetrile were not taken off cephacetrile provided
that they continued to improve clinically. All strains of H.
parainfluenzae, Strep. pneumoniae and Esch. coli were eliminated,
m.i.c.'s of Haemophilus influenzae at the time of the trial were
in the range 4 - 16 ug/ml.

Toxicology. There were no adverse effects attributable to
cephacetrile on any of the toxicological parameters studied. One
patient showed a rise in blood urea nitrogen from 30 mg/100 ml to
63 mg/100 ml but the serum creatinine did not rise.

Tolerability and side-effects. There were no gastro-intestinal
side effects or skin rashes. One female patient did complain of
pain at the injection site and injections were stopped for that
reason.

Pharmacology. Serum levels in 18 patients showed a mean 1
hour level of 28.9 ug/ml falling to a mean of 2.16 ug/ml at 8 hours.
These serum levels are similar to those found by other workers (Wise
et al, 1974). Urinary excretion was variable, the mean urine concentration was 117 ug/ml. As might be expected serum levels remained higher in patients with low creatinine clearances.

DISCUSSION

When assessing the efficacy of a drug in acute respiratory
infections it is the final clinical result which is of importance
to the clinician, cephacetrile showed a satisfactory result in 83%
of the patients which is similar to studies with other agents
(Bayley et al, 1970; Galbraith, 1967). No advantage could be
seen over other antibiotics particularly as the drug has to be given
by intramuscular injection. A dose interval of 4 - 6 hours is
recommended to maintain serum levels above the m.i.c.'s for Haemophilus species. Patients with chronic respiratory disease did
badly probably because of the relatively poor activity of all
cephalosporins against the predominant pathogen Haemophilus

<u>influenzae.</u>   This may be related to the higher ratio of peak serum
levels/m.i.c. achieved by more well tried drugs such as ampicillin
and chloramphenicol (Williams and Andrews 1974).   However cephacetrile certainly would be useful in post-operative patients, particularly if they were penicillin sensitive and where parentral
therapy is often mandatory.   It is encouraging that there were no
undersirable effects of the drug and particularly no evidence of
nephrotoxicity.

ACKNOWLEDGEMENTS

     We should like to thank Mr. M.J. Bywater and Mr. H.A. Holt for
technical assistance.   Dr. V.B. Whitmarsh of CIBA Laboratories for
advice and supply of cephacetrile and the physicians and surgeons
of Southmead Hospital for allowing us to study their patients.

REFERENCES

1. BAYLEY, A.J. (1970). British Journal of Diseases of the Chest.
       64, 232.
2. GALBRAITH, H.J.B. (1967). Postgraduate Medical Journal, 43
       (Suppl.) 58.

3. OPITZ, A., KNOOP, H., KRAFT, D., OFFERMANN, G., SCHAFFER, K.,
       AND HERRATH, D. v.   Advances in Antimicrobial and Anti-
       neoplastic Chemotherapy, vol. 9, p.1345 (Urban and Schwar-
       zenberg, Munich 1972).
4. WILLIAMS, J.D., ANDREWS, J. (1974). British Medical Journal,
       1, 134.
5. WISE, R., REEVES, D.S., HEPBURN, P.R. (1974). Chemotherapy
       20: 177.

THE ACTIVITY OF MINOCYCLINE AGAINST TETRACYCLINE RESISTANT PATHOGENS IN THE RESPIRATORY TRACT

J.D. Williams, W. Farrell and M. Wood*

Department of Medical Microbiology, The London Hospital
Medical College, London E1 2AD.
*Medical Unit, The London Hospital, London E1

INTRODUCTION

Following its discovery, tetracycline was for several years one of the main antibiotics used in the treatment of infections of the upper and lower respiratory tract. More recently its use has been declining, partly due to the introduction of other agents such as ampicillin and co-trimoxazole, and partly due to the emergency of tetracycline resistant strains of β-haemolytic streptococci (Robertson, 1965, 1968; Fallon, 1973), Streptococcus pneumoniae (Percival et al, 1961) and Haemophilus influenzae (Williams and Andrews, 1974).

Because of the activity of minocycline against tetracycline resistant staphylococci (Steigbigel et al, 1968a) and gram-negative bacilli (Simmons, 1974), we have investigated minocycline with a view to its potential use in respiratory infections. In view of the variability of absorption of minocycline reported by Alestig and Lindberg (1974) we carried out a cross-over study of tetracycline and minocycline absorption in healthy volunteers.

METHODS

A total of 25 strains of group A streptococci, 39 strains of pneumococci and 51 strains of Haemophilus species was isolated from a variety of upper respiratory sites. The sensitivities of the organisms to tetracycline and minocycline were determined by incorporating each antibiotic into DST agar (Oxoid) containing either 5% horse blood for group A streptococci and pneumococci, or 0.5% lysed horse blood with 10 µg/ml NAD for Haemophilus, to

give a range of final concentration of 0.06 to 128 µg/ml. The
minimum inhibitory concentration (M.I.C.) was read after overnight
incubation at 37°C.

For the pharmacology experiments each subject was given
250 mg tetracycline ('Achromycin', Lederle) and one week later
200 mg minocycline (Lederle). The doses were given orally
after an overnight fast. Blood samples were then taken at intervals for a period of 24 hours. The total amount of urine excreted
in the 24 hours following drug administration was also collected.

Serum and urine levels of minocycline and tetracycline were
determined by the method recommended by Cyanamid International
(Technical publication RL 02387 and RLA 10239).

RESULTS

a)   The results of the M.I.C.s of minocycline and tetracycline
are shown in Table 1.

TABLE 1

M.I.C.s OF TETRACYCLINE AND MINOCYCLINE FOR STRAINS OF GROUP A STREPTOCOCCI, PNEUMOCOCCI AND HAEMOPHILUS

Organism	No.of strains	Tetracycline M.I.C. µg/ml	Minocycline M.I.C. µg/ml
Group A streptococci	10	64	4 - 32
	5	32	4 - 8
	2	16	4
	8	0.25 - 1.0	0.25 - 1.0
Pneumococci	1	64	2
	5	32	1 - 8
	7	16	1 - 2
	1	8	0.5
	2	4	1 - 2
	23	0.25 - 1.0	0.06 - 0.05
Haemophilus	1	64	2
	2	32	1 - 2
	13	8 - 16	0.25 - 1.0
	1	4	1.0
	2	2	0.25
	32	0.25 - 1.0	0.125- 1.0

1.   Group A streptococci

Of the 25 strains investigated 17 (68%) were not inhibited
by 8 µg tetracycline per ml and were considered resistant.   The
remaining 8 strains were fully sensitive to 1 µg tetracycline per
ml.   The tetracycline sensitive strains required similar M.I.C.s
of minocycline but there was a reduction in the M.I.C. of all
tetracycline resistant strains with minocycline.   However the
M.I.C. of minocycline for the resistant strains was never lower
than 4 µg/ml.

2.   Pneumococci

A total of 39 strains was tested, of which 16 (41%) were
judged resistant to tetracycline having an M.I.C. of 4 ug/ml or
more.   These 16 tetracycline resistant strains required lower
M.I.C.s of minocycline, 13 of them being inhibited by 2 µg
minocycline per ml.   The remaining 23 tetracycline sensitive
pneumococci also had a reduced M.I.C. with minocycline compared
with tetracycline.

3.   Haemophilus species

The M.I.C. of tetracycline for 51 haemophilus strains, the
majority of which were H.influenzae, showed that 16 (31%) were
not inhibited by 4 µg tetracycline per ml.   Thirty two (63%) had
M.I.C.s of 0.25 - 1.0 µg tetracycline/ml.   The action of minocycline on tetracycline resistant Haemophilus was marked.   These
strains had on average an eightfold reduction in the M.I.C. of
minocycline as compared with tetracycline.

b)   Pharmacology

1.   Serum

The serum concentration of each antibiotic in the 6 subjects
is shown in Fig. 1.

Minocycline reached peak values in the serum of 2.70 to 3.70
(mean 3.10) µg/ml and tetracycline 1.40 to 3.25 (mean 2.64) µg/ml.
For the dosage administered the half-life of minocycline was
longer when measured by graphical extrapolations, varying between
12 and 22 hours (mean 17 hours) than that of tetracycline which
ranged from 3 - 11 (mean 7.3) hours.

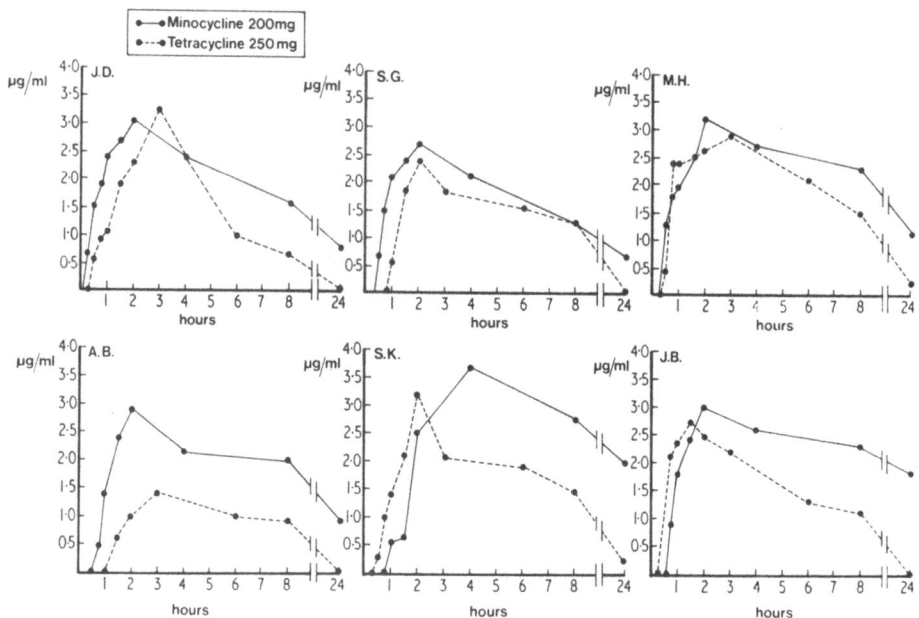

Fig.1 Antibiotic concentrations in serum of 6 subjects after
       administration of 200 mg minocycline and 250 mg tetracycline

2.   Urine

        The amounts of the antibiotic excreted in the urine during
the 24 hours following administration were 35 to 53% (mean 46%)
of the given dose for tetracycline and 3.5 to 5.9% (mean 4.8%)
of the administered minocycline.

                              DISCUSSION

        The use of tetracycline in upper respiratory tract infections
has been declining due to the recognition of tetracycline resistant organisms. A recent survey shows that in the U.K. tetracycline resistance among haemolytic streptococci of group A is
approximately 30% (Kensit et al, 1975). Although the M.I.C.s of
minocycline for haemolytic streptococci are almost one-quarter of
those of tetracycline the reduction is not sufficient to bring
tetracycline resistant strains within the range of minocycline.
The 17 resistant strains tested all required 4 µg or more of
minocycline per ml to inhibit growth. The blood levels of minocycline we obtained correlate well with those of Steigbigel et al
(1968b) and Cartwright et al (1975), i.e. with peak serum levels
of 2.7 to 3.7 (mean 3.1) g per ml. The half-life ranged from
12 to 22 (mean 17) and the mean 0 - 24 hour and 0 - α integral

concentration was 43.9 and 71.1 μg/hr/ml^{-1} respectively.

The activity of minocycline against those pathogens usually
associated with the lower respiratory tract (<u>Strep.pneumoniae</u>
and <u>Haemophilus influenzae</u>) are however of considerable clinical
interest and are reported in detail elsewhere (Wood et al, 1975).
The fall in M.I.C. of minocycline compared to tetracycline was
sufficient to bring most tetracycline resistant pneumococci into
the therapeutic range - 2 μg per ml or less. All the tetracycline
resistant strains of <u>Haemophilus influenzae</u> had M.I.C.s of minocycline below 2 μg per ml. The efficacy of minocycline in the
treatment of lower respiratory tract infections with tetracycline
resistant organisms can only be established by clinical trial.
The outcome of such trials is awaited with interest.

REFERENCES

Alestig, K., Lingberg, J. (1974) Studies on the absorption and
    excretion of minocycline and a comparison with doxycycline.
    Infection, <u>2</u>, 137.

Cartwright, A.L., Hatfield, H.L., Yeadon, A., London, E. (1975)
    A comparison of the bioavailability of minocycline capsules
    and film-coated tablets. J. Antimicrobial Chemotherapy, <u>1</u>,
    (3) (In press).

Fallon, R.J. (1973) Tetracycline resistant -haemolytic strepto-
    cocci. B.M.J., <u>4</u>, 300-301.

Kensit, K., Farrell, W. (1975) Survey of tetracycline resistance
    of pneumococci and group A streptococci in the United Kingdom.
    Proc. 9th International Congress of Chemotherapy (In press)

Percival, A., Armstrong, E.C., Turner, G.C. (1969) Increased inci-
    dence of tetracycline resistant pneumococci in Liverpool in
    1969. Lancet, <u>1</u>, 998-1000.

Robertson, M.H. (1965) -haemolytic streptococci in South West
    Essex with particular reference to tetracycline resistance
    B.M.J., <u>2</u>, 569-571.

Robertson, M.H. (1968) Tetracycline resistant streptococci in South
    West Essex: a continuing survey. B.M.J., <u>3</u>, 349-350.

Simmons, N.A. (1974) Comparative activity of minocycline and tetra-
    cycline. B.M.J., <u>1</u>, 158-159.

Steigbigel, N.H., Reed, C.W., Finland, M. (1968a) Susceptibility of
    common pathogenic bacteria to seven tetracycline antibiotics
    in vitro. Am.J.Med.Sci., (255), 179-195.

Steigbigel, N.H., Reed, C.W., Finland, M. (1968b) Absorption and
    excretion of five tetracycline analogues in normal young
    men.   Am.J.Med.Sci. (255), 296-312.

Williams, J.D., Andrews, J. (1974) Sensitivity of Haemophilus
    influenzae to antibiotics. B.M.J., 1, 134-137.

Wood, M.J., Farrell, W., Kattan, S., Williams, J.D. (1975)
    Activity of minocycline against respiratory pathogens.
    J.Antimicrobial Chemotherapy, 1 (3) (In press)

AMOXICILLIN IN THE TREATMENT OF RESPIRATORY DISEASES IN CHILDREN

Z. Jedličková *, M. Šimková , A. Rubín,
M. Hejzlar and M. Rýc
* Postgraduate Medical and Pharmaceutical Institute

Prague 10, Ruská 85, Czechoslavakia

SUMMARY

In diseases caused by agnets such as Streptococcus pneumoniae in the pathogenic phase, nonpenicillinase-producing staphylococci, Haemophilus influenzae, Streptococcus beta haemolyticus group A, E. coli, Proteus mirabilis, in respiratory diseases, the expedient administration of amoxicillin (Amoxil Beecham) was not only confirmed in vitro but also clinically. Compared with ampicillin it is of advantage to administer amoxicillin 3 times per day. Amoxicillin application allows an extension of the night rest of the child and reduces practically ampicillin doses to half. Side-effects were observed in one case only. The children tolerate medicine very well, expecially syrup; apparently its taste agrees with them.

The character of the bacterial cell damage after amoxicillin incubation in vitro was demonstrated by electron microscope. Short-term incubation of Streptococcus pneumoniae cells in a 0.5 mcg/ml amoxicillin concentration was proved to induce a significant damage of bacterial cells. Analogue changes in Haemophilus influenzae wre obtained after long incubation. In Klebsiella ozaenae cells, on the other hand, higher doses of anoxicillin (5 mcg/ml) were necessary.

Anoxicillin, chemically alpha-amino-para-hydroxybenzyl-penicillin (orginally called BRL 2333, commercial name Amoxil) is the structural analogue of ampicillin. According to literary data (Acred et al. 1971, Geddes and Williams 1974, Suttherland et al. 1972) amoxicillin has better parameters: it is better absorbed from the digestive tract (Bodey and Nance 1972), forms a 2-3 times higher serum level at comparable doses (Croydon and Sutherland 1971, Neu 1974, Rolinson 1974, Shiota 1974) and is better tolerated at oral application (Fiedelman 1974, Fujii et al. 1974, Sabto et al. 1973). The efficacy of amoxicillin, ampicillin and other antibiotics in vitro was separately studied and therapeutic effect of the preparation was tested in respiratory diseases in children.

MATERIAL AND METHODS

Prior to application, the effectiveness of the preparation was verified in vitro in several bacterial agents cultivated in respiratory and other infections, by qualitative was well as quantitative method, in order to determine the actual conditions of sensitivity of these agents in Czechoslovakia.

Microbial agents cultivated from pharyngeal and nasal swabs were tested for sensitivity with regard to chemopreparations-amoxicillin included - to be used for treatment. For test with gram-negative rods they were: ampicillin, carbenicillin, co-trimaxazole, nitrofuranes, nalidixic, acid, chloramphenicol, tetracyclin, colistin, gentamicin, kanamycin, streptomycin. Gram-positive ocooi were tested for sensitivity to amoxicillin, penicillin, oxacillin, ampicillin, carbenicillin, co-trimoxazole, cephalosporin, erythromycin, lincomycin, spiramycin, chloramphenicol, tetracyclin, gentamicin and kanamycin. Swabs were taken before the preparation was applied, during treatment and after the symptoms had disappeared.

The preparation was administered in 44 children- 24 boys and 20 girls _ with the following diagnoses:

Pneumonia	31 children
Bronchitis acuta	6 children
Bronchitis spastica	3 children
Pansinusitis	1 child
Lymphadenitis submandibularis	1 child
Disease of the urinary tract	1 child

In the evaluation of the effect, the clinical status of the child was decisive. The presence of microbial flora on the tonsils and in the nose, blood count, GPT, urea, urinary sediment and chest X-ray changes were studied.

Amoxil was administered in syrup od capsulles form to patients aged from 12 days to 18 years and was only applied in acute cases. It was either administered as the sole antibiotic or together with other medicaments. In small children the preparation was administered in form of syrup, in older children in capsulles. Doses varied from 30 - 50 mcg/kg per day.

Table 1

IN VITRO ACTIVITY OF AMOXICILLIN

ORGANISMS	NUMBER	MIC mg/ml RANGE	MEAN MIC	ZONE DIAMETER m m
STREPTOCOCCUS PNEUMONIAE	44	0,005 – 0,12	0,05	16 – 22
—॥— PYOGENES GROUP A	65	0,01 – 0,12	0,05	34 – 44
HAEMOPHILUS INFLUENZAE	29	0,05 – 0,75	0,50	16 – 22
NEISSERIA GONORRHOEAE	30	0,005 – 0,25	0,06	
SALMONELLA SPP.	41	0,25 – 8	2	16 – 28
ESCHERICHIA COLI	53	0,5 –>128	16	12 – 28
ENTEROBACTER AEROG.	7	64 –>128		< 12 – 19
SHIGELLA SONNEI	50	0,5 –>128	16	
PROTEUS MIRABILIS	105	0,5 –>128	8	< 12 – 30
—॥— RETTGERI	20	16 –>128		< 12 – 27
KLE BSIELLA OZAENAE	12	4 – 64	64	< 12 – 19

NOTE: ABOUT 70-80% OF TESTED STRAINS

Table 2

CHILDREN ACCORDING TO THE AGE AND AMOXIL ACTION

AGE	BOYS	+	±	O	A	GIRLS	+	±	O	A	TOTAL
UP TO 1 MONTH	1	1				3	2		1		4
2 MONTHS						1	1				1
3-6 —॥—	2	2				1	1				3
7-12 —॥—	4	3	1			1	1				5
1-2 YEARS	1		1			2		2			3
3-5 —॥—	5	4		1		5	5				10
6-7 —॥—	6	4		1	1	3	3				9
8-12 —॥—	4	2	2			4	2	2			8
13-18 —॥—	1	1									1
TOTAL	24	17	4	2	1	20	15	4	1		44

+	VERY GOOD EFFECT
±	LESSER —॥—
O	NO —॥—
A	ALLERGY

The effect of this antibiotic in vitro was studied by
electron microscope in 3 bacterial species (Streptococcus penum-
oniae 4/49, Haemophilus influenzae 1/58 and Klebsiella ozaenae
11/67).   Cultures grown on Brian Heart Infusion Broth were incubated
with amoxicillin in a 0.5 mcg/ml concentration (Streptococcus
pneumoniae and Haemophilus influenzae) and 5 mcg/ml concentration
(Klebsiella ozaenae) for 1,2 and 4 hours.   After this the suspensions
were fixed with 5 p.c. water solution of formaldehyde purified
by repeated washing by distilled water and applied to carbon
coated formvar membranes.   After having been chromium-shadowed,
preparations were evaluated by electron microscope Philips EM 300-
operating by 80 kv.

RESULTS

Preliminary results of sensitivity test for various microbial
agents are indicated in Table 1.

All cultivated microorganisms were tested for sensitivity
with regard to amoxicillin:

	Number of strains	
	Sensitivity	Resistance
Streptococcus pneumoniae in pathogenic phase	27	2
Haemophilus influenzae	2	-
Streptococcus beta haeomolyticus group A	7	-
Staphylococcus aureus	3	5
Coliform microorganisms	2	11
Enterobacter spp.	-	6

The temperature decrease occurred on the first day, at the
lastest on the second day, excepting a single case when the
temperature decreased after 72 hours.   The clinical symptoms
disappeared in 6 days on average.   The total treatment lasted 7-
14 days.   The blood count corresponded to the clinical course,
in one case the transaminases increased slightly during administration being, however, again within normal limits when the
treatment was finished.   But this increase might have been induced
by the toxic effect of the bacterial agens.   In children with
pneumonia and infection of the urinary tract in agenesis of the
right kidney, the inflammatory changes persisted in the urinary
sediments event after pneumoniahad dissappeared.   On termination
of therapy the X-ray picture was in all children without inflammatory
foci, in some cases hilar shadows remained.

In the total of 44 children (Table 2) Amoxil was of good effect in 32 children (i.e. 72.7%), of lesser effect in 8 children (18.2%), being of no effect in 3 children (6.8%)½ Because cutaneous allergy was ascertained in one child, its treatment had to be discontinued on the third day of administration. The reaction was of massive form (from small morphons to maculopapular pimples persisting for four days). - Amoxil showed no effect in one newborn girl with pneumonia bilateralis; later Staphylococcus aureus, E. coli, Enterobacter spp., resistant to amoxicillin, were determined. - Amoxil administration to a boy aged 2 1/2 years with pansinusitis, where Streptococcus pneumoniae sensible to this drug had been determined in the swab, was also of no effect at all. - The last case with no effect was a 6 years old by with pneumonia, otitis media bilateralis susp. and gammaglobulinaemia.

Electron microscopical examinations proved that Streptococcus pneumoniae cells were damaged in 0.5 mcg/ml Amoxil concentration (Fig. 1) in vitro, only within a 1 hour incubation. The damage causes a defect of bacterial cell reproduction and leads to the growth of considerably prolonged cell forms. Haemophilus influenzae, after being incubated in a 0.5 mcg/ml amoxicillin concentration, shows similar changes only within a 4 hours incubation. A 6 hours incubation causes already a complete lysis of bacterial cells (Fig.2). In Klebsiella ozaenae cells, 5 mcg/ml amoxicillin concentration causes visible damages within a 2 hours incubation; the character of damage is analogous to that of Streptococcus pneumoniae (Fig.3).

REFERENCES

Acred, P., Hunter, P.S., Mizen, L. and Rolinson, G.N. (1971), Antimicr. Agents a. Chemotherapy-1970, Am. Soc. Microbiol. 416.

Bodey, G.P. and Nance, J. (1972), Antimicr. Agents a. Chemotherapy 1.358.

Croydon, E.A.P. and Sutherland, R. (1971), Antimicr. Agents a. Chemotherapy - 1970, 427.

Fiedelman, W. (1974), Current Ther. REasearch 16, 1287.

Fujii, R., Nakazawa, S., Yoshoika, H., Nishimura, T. and Kobayashi, Y. (1971), Exc. Med. Series No 326, S 107

Geddes, A.M. and Williams, J.D. (1974). Exc. Med. Series No 326, S 116.

Handsfield, H.H., Clark, H., Wallace, J.F., Holmes, K.K., and
Turck, M. (1973), Antimicr. Agents a.Chemotherapy 3, 262.

Nakazawa, S. (1974), Exc. Med. Series No 326, S 1.

Neu, H.C., (1974), J. Inf. Dis. 129, Suppl. S 123.

Neu, H.C., (1974), J. Inf. Dis. 129, Suppl. S 272.

Rolinson, G.N (1974)., Exc. Med. No 326. S 1.

Sabto. J., Carson, P. and Morban, T. (1973),
Med. J. Austr. 2, 537.

Shiota, K, (1974), Exc. Med. No 326, S 135.

Sutherland, R., Croydon, E.A.P., and Rolinson, G.N. (1972),
Brit. Med. J. 3,13.

Williams, J.D. and Andrews. J. (1974).
Brit. Med. J.1, 134.

Wise, P.J. and Neu, H.C. (1974)
J. Inf. Dis. 129, suppl. S 266.

THE ANTIMICROBIAL SENSITIVITIES OF URINARY PATHOGENS, 1971-1974

R. N. Grüneberg M.D. M.R.C.Path.

University College Hospital

London W.C.1

INTRODUCTION

It is sometimes necessary to start treatment of urinary tract infection before the results of laboratory investigations are available. Under such circumstances, up to date information on the antimicrobial sensitivities of urinary pathogens is needed to guide the clinician. This paper reports the findings in one laboratory in London in the years 1971-1974.

METHODS

Urine samples are derived from various sources:
1. Patients in the wards or attending outpatient clinics at the following hospitals: St. Pancras Hospital, The Hospital for Tropical Diseases, and the National Temperance Hospital. No attempt has been made to differentiate between inpatient and outpatient derived strains, all being classified as "Hospital Strains".
2. Patients attending General Practitioners in the district whose specimens are sent to the laboratory. Organisms from these specimens are referred to as "General Practice Strains".

The laboratory methods used are the same for all urine samples. A urine sample is regarded as showing significant bacteriuria if it is shown to contain more than 100,000 organisms of a single type per ml. of urine, using a surface viable counting technique on cysteine-lactose electrolyte-deficient medium (C.L.E.D.). Anti-bacterial sensitivities are determined using Stokes' method (1968) in which the zone size given by the test strain is compared on every plate with that given by a known sensitive control organism.

TABLE 1

ORGANISMS ISOLATED FROM GENERAL PRACTICE U.T.I. IN 1971-4

	1971		1972		1973		1974	
Esch.coli	340	78.5%	308	73.6%	390	76.0%	451	77.1%
Proteus mirabilis	40	9.2%	42	10.0%	40	7.8%	38	6.5%
Klebsiella-Enterobacter spp.	10	2.3%	14	3.3%	22	4.3%	27	4.6%
Enterococci	10	2.3%	16	3.8%	12	2.8%	17	2.9%
Staphylococci	22	5.1%	24	5.7%	34	6.6%	41	7.0%
Pseudomonas aeruginosa	4		4		3		2	
All other organisms	7		10		12		9	
Total	433	100%	418	100%	513	100%	585	100%

TABLE 2

ORGANISMS ISOLATED FROM HOSPITAL U.T.I. IN 1971-4

	1971		1972		1973		1974	
Esch.coli	306	55.4%	456	55.4%	312	52.3%	382	58.3%
Proteus mirabilis	63	11.4%	108	13.3%	92	15.4%	68	10.4%
Klebsiella Enterobacter spp.	93	16.8%	126	15.3%	98	16.4%	91	13.9%
Enterococci	22	4.0%	28	3.4%	29	4.8%	35	5.3%
Staphylococci	18	3.3%	24	2.9%	18	3.0%	21	3.2%
Pseudomonas aeruginosa	15	2.7%	43	5.2%	14	2.3%	25	3.8%
Candida spp.	11	2.0%	4	0.5%	8	1.3%	11	1.7%
All other organisms	24		33		25		22	
Total	552	100%	822	100%	596	100%	655	100%

TABLE 3

PROPORTIONS OF ALL URINARY PATHOGENS FULLY SENSITIVE TO
VARIOUS ANTIMICROBIALS IN GENERAL PRACTICE, 1971-4

% of strains fully sensitive (ranking)

Drug	1971 (433 strains)	1972 (418 strains)	1973 (513 strains)	1974 (585 strains)
Ampicillin	88.2 (4)	84.4 (6)	82.4 (7)	81.2 (7)
Cotrimoxazole	96.6 (1)	96.4 (1)	94.9 (1)	93.2 (1)
Cephaloridine	87.5 (5)	85.1 (4)	86.6 (5)	83.1 (6)
Colistin sulphamethate	85.0 (7)	82.3 (7)	86.8 (4)	87.9 (4)
Nalidixic acid	90.7 (3)	87.6 (3)	88.2 (3)	86.0 (5)
Nitrofurantoin	85.6 (6)	85.1 (4)	85.5 (6)	88.4 (3)
Sulphonamide	76.4 (8)	73.2 (8)	75.6 (8)	73.7 (8)
Tetracycline	72.5 (9)	69.6 (9)	73.3 (9)	73.6 (9)
Trimethoprim	94.0 (2)	94.4 (2)	90.0 (2)	89.5 (2)

TABLE 4

PROPORTIONS OF ALL URINARY PATHOGENS FULLY SENSITIVE TO
VARIOUS ANTIMICROBIALS IN HOSPITAL PRACTICE, 1971-4

% of strains fully sensitive (Ranking)

Drug	1971 (552 strains)	1972 (822 strains)	1973 (596 strains)	1974 (655 strains)
Ampicillin	66.1 (7)	64.2 (7)	66.6 (8)	61.2 (7)
Cotrimoxazole	83.9 (2)	81.7 (2)	82.2 (1)	76.2 (3)
Cephaloridine	69.9 (6)	68.1 (6)	68.7 (5)	63.2 (6)
Colistin sulphamethate	76.8 (4)	78.6 (4)	74.1 (3)	78.0 (2)
Nalidixic acid	84.8 (1)	82.6 (1)	81.6 (2)	80.6 (1)
Nitrofurantoin	70.3 (5)	71.8 (5)	68.3 (6)	72.7 (4)
Sulphonamide	61.9 (8)	62.2 (8)	67.7 (7)	57.4 (8)
Tetracycline	55.8 (9)	56.1 (9)	53.4 (9)	48.6 (9)
Trimethoprim	79.9 (3)	80.7 (3)	73.9 (4)	71.5 (5)

TABLE 5

THE PERCENTAGE OF URINARY ESCH. COLI FROM GENERAL
PRACTICE U.T.I., 1971-4, FULLY SENSITIVE TO
VARIOUS ANTIMICROBIALS

Drug	1971 (340 strains)	1972 (308 strains)	1973 (390 strains)	1974 (451 strains)
Nitrofurantoin	97.6	97.0	96.9	98.3
Sulphonamide	77.3	75.3	75.1	74.3
Ampicillin	91.4	88.9	87.4	85.6
Trimethoprim	98.5	99.6	97.9	97.9
Colistin sulphate	100.0	99.6	100.0	100.0
Nalidixic acid	99.1	99.0	98.4	97.8
Tetracycline	81.2	81.2	79.3	80.0
Cephaloridine	91.2	88.7	87.7	85.6
Cotrimoxazole	99.2	99.6	99.0	98.9

TABLE 6

THE PERCENTAGE OF URINARY ESCH.COLI FROM HOSPITAL
U.T.I., 1971-4, FULLY SENSITIVE TO
VARIOUS ANTIMICROBIALS

Drug	1971 (306 strains)	1972 (456 strains)	1973 (312 strains)	1974 (382) strains)
Nitrofurantoin	95.7	97.7	96.5	97.8
Sulphonamide	69.6	68.9	78.6	66.4
Ampicillin	84.4	81.3	82.4	74.3
Trimethoprim	96.8	96.8	97.2	91.7
Colistin sulphate	100.0	100.0	99.7	100.0
Nalidixic acid	98.1	98.4	100.0	97.1
Tetracycline	75.8	78.3	76.9	67.8
Cephaloridine	86.6	81.9	83.0	74.3
Cotrimoxazole	97.0	95.2	98.1	93.4

RESULTS

The types of organisms isolated from infected urines from General Practice in the years 1971 - 1974 are presented in Table 1. Similar results from Hospital Practice are shown in Table 2. The proportions of all urinary pathogens fully sensitive to various antimicrobials in General Practice are shown in Table 3 which also ranks the antimicrobials in order of in vitro effectiveness for each year. Table 4 represents the similar observations for the urinary pathogens from Hospital Practice. Tables 5 and 6 show the percentages of all urinary Esch. coli sensitive to various antimicrobials from 1971-1974 in General Practice and in Hospital Practice respectively.

DISCUSSION

The organisms isolated from urinary infections in General Practice and in Hospital are shown in Table 1 and 2 respectively. From each source the types of organisms varied little from year to year, and the proportions of each are typical of general experience. There are substantial differences in the infecting flora in General Practice compared with that in Hospital. Thus, the usually antibiotic sensitive Esch. coli was responsible for 73-78% of General Practice infections but only 52-58% of Hospital U.T.I. This difference in the species distribution could be the underlying cause of the difference in antibiotic sensitivity of the infecting urinary flora in the two situations. An analysis of the degree of antibiotic resistance of Esch. coli causing U.T.I. in General Practice is presented in Table 5 and a similar analysis of Esch. coli causing U.T.I. in Hospital Practice is shown in Table 6. It can be seen by comparing Tables 5 and 6 that there are still differences in antibiotic sensitivity in the two situations when organisms of the same species are compared, but that the major cause of the differences in sensitivity is variation in species distribution. Thus in 1974 85.6% of Esch. coli causing U.T.I. in General Practice were sensitive to Ampicillin compared with 74.3% sensitive in Hospital. Comparing all urinary pathogens in 1974, 81.2% of General Practice strains were sensitive to Ampicillin whereas only 61.2% of Hospital Strains were sensitive.

Inspection of Tables 3 and 4 shows that urinary pathogens, whether in General Practice or in Hospital, are in general very anti-biotic sensitive. Urinary Esch. coli are even more sensitive to antimicrobials than are the generality of urinary organisms, despite their potentiality for the accumulation of plasmid-mediated resistances (R Factors). In General Practice the provisional

treatment of a clinically diagnosed U.T.I. with any of the antimicrobials tested (Table 3) could readily be justified. Some of
these choices are more apparent than real; trimethoprim is not used
independently of sulphonamide, and cephaloridine requires parenteral
administration which is not often convenient in General Practice.
Colistin is not used as a routine treatment for U.T.I. A choice
made solely on the basis of breadth of antimicrobial spectrum in
General Practice in 1974 would rank the drugs in decreasing order
of preference thus: co-trimoxazole, nitrofurantoin, nalidixic acid,
a cephalosporin, ampicillin, a sulphonamide, a tetracycline. The
treatment choice would not be made solely on these grounds, of
course, since considerations such as frequency of administration,
nature and frequency of side effects, acceptability to the patient
and cost must be taken into account.

In Hospital Practice the choice of urinary antimicrobial agents
(Table 4) is wider, since parenteral treatment can be undertaken,
although oral therapy is usually preferred. The choice of initial
treatment before laboratory results are available, if based solely
on the antimicrobial spectrum in 1974 (Table 4) would be, in
decreasing order of preference: nalidixic acid, colistin sulphate,
co-trimoxazole, nitrofurantoin, a cephalosporin, ampicillin, a
sulphonamide, a tetracycline. It should be repeated that the
choice would not be made solely on these grounds.

In view of the concern felt in the medical profession about
the possibility of deterioration in the efficacy of antimicrobial
agents in the face of plasmid-mediated resistances (R Factors), it
is interesting to note (Tables 3, 4, 5 and 6) the relatively small
changes in the sensitivities observed in the four years 1971 - 1974.
Among General Practice urinary pathogens of all kinds only ampicillin has shown a marked decline, from 88.2% to 81.2% of all strains
fully sensitive. When urinary Esch. coli from General Practice are
considered alone (Table 5) it can be seen that the decline of
ampicillin sensitivity is again shown from 91.4% to 85.6%, but that
it is mirrored by a similar decline of sensitivity to cephalosporin
from 91.2% to 85.6%. In Hospital Practice (Table 6) the urinary
Esch. coli show similar decreases of sensitivity between 1971 and
1974 in the case of ampicillin (from 84.4% to 74.3%), cephalosporin
(from 86.6% to 74.3%), and tetracycline (from 75.8% to 67.8%).
Resistance to these three agents, ampicillin, cephalosporin; and
tetracycline may all be plasmid-mediated. In general (Tables 5 and
6) the susceptibility of urinary pathogens to antimicrobial agents,
resistance to which is not plasmid-mediated, (nitrofurantoin, nalidixic acid), has been maintained with little change. In General
Practice there has been no significant change in the proportion of
urinary Esch. coli fully sensitive to trimethoprim and therefore
also sensitive to co-trimoxazole (Table 5).

It has been shown (Fleming, Datta and Grüneberg, 1972) that

resistance to trimethoprim can be plasmid-mediated, but this has not been reflected in the General Practice urinary flora. Inspection of Table 6, however, shows a decline in the senstivity of urinary Esch. coli in this hospital (where R Factor mediating trimethoprim resistance was first recognised) from 96.8% to 91.7% between 1971 and 1974. This experience is not general since most hospitals do not at present have the R Factor concerned (Jobanputra and Datta, 1974). Experience in this hospital shows, so far, that antibiotic prescribing policies limiting the use of sulphonamide, ampicillin and co-trimoxazole are capable of eradicating R Factor mediated trimethoprim resistance from the hospital flora (Grüneberg et al, 1975).

It appears, therefore, that tnere is a slow change in the pattern of susceptibility of urinary pathogens to various antimicrobial agents, that this change may be more marked in the case of drugs the resistance to which is R Factor mediated but that this situation can be modified by appropriate action. Urinary pathogens are still generally sensitive to most antibiotics and in nearly all cases there is a wide choice of chemotherapeutic agents.

REFERENCES

Stokes, E.J. (1968)
Clinical Bacteriology, 3rd Edition, London: Arnold p.179

Fleming, M.P., Datta, N. and Grüneberg, R.N. (1972)
Trimethoprim resistance determined by R Factors.
British Medical Journal, 1, 726

Grüneberg, R.N., Leakey, A., Bendall, M. J. and Smellie, J. M. (1975)
The bowel flora in urinary tract infection: the effect of chemotherapy with special reference to co-trimoxazole.
Kidney International. (in the Press)

Jobanputra, R. S. and Datta, N. (1974)
Trimethoprim R Factors in enterobacteria from clinical specimens.
Journal of Medical Microbiology, 7, 169.

A CLINICAL METHOD OF ASSESSING THE EFFECT OF

CHEMOTHERAPY IN EXACERBATED CHRONIC PYELONEPHRITIS

H.Gelinov, A.Astrug, L.Todorova

Clinic of Nephrology

Medical Academy, Sofia, Bulgaria

Any clinical method for evaluation of the therapeutic qualities of a new antimicrobial drug used for the treatment of exacerbated chronic pyelonephritis, in addition to the fundamental requirement for exact knowledge of the causative agent and its susceptibility to the tested drug, prompts selection of the most appropriate clinical form of pyelonephritis and of the most convincing parameters for assessment and categorization of the therapeutic effect. With the present work we set ourselves the task, by following up the parameters adopted by us for evaluation of the therapeutic effect, to emphasize their significance, incidence and in the treatment of exacerbated chronic pyelonephritis. Our patients were treated with gentamycin.

Material and Method

For a 3-year period, from April 1971 through May 1974, a total of 112 patients (39 men and 73 women) with a mean age of 54.7 years received gentamycin treatment. Of these 98 had exacerbated chronic pyelonephritis, 7 acute pyelonephritis and 7 urosepsis. Forty-nine patients (43.6 per cent) had varying degree of azotemia and 62 (55.4 per cent - a variety of accompanying diseases. In all patients daily records of the temperature were taken and the constitutional symptoms followed up. Complete urinalysis with bacterial counts was performed before treatment and on the 2nd, 3rd, 5th and 10th day of treatment. The laboratory control included erythrocyte,

leucocyte and differential counts, ESR, blood urea, serum creatinine, creatinine clearance, floculation tests,
serum bilirubin, and electrolyte balance - at the onset
and at the end of treatment. Eventual damage to the 8th
cranial nerve was carefully searched for (22 patients
were subjected to thorough otoneurologic examination).
Fifteen patients, six of them with nitrogen retention,
had the serum gentamycin levels measured; in another
group of 15 patients gentamycin clearance was performed.
The minimal inhibiting concentration (MIC) was determined in 11 patients.

     The daily dose of intramuscular gentamycin was 80-
180 mg (average 1.2 mg/kg), duration of treatment - 5-20
days (average 10.8 days). In azotemic patients the
single dose was reduced, in accordance with the creatinine clearance values.

     The effect of gentamycin treatment was evaluated by
the following six parameters: bacteriuria, leucocyturia,
fever, leucocytosis, ESR and constitutional symptoms
(lumbar pain and micturition disturbances). The results
were classified in a 3-grade scale: 'very good' - disappearance of bacteriuria and leucocyturia and abatement
of other symptoms; 'good' - disappearance of bacteriuria,
reduction of leucocyturia and abatement of at least two
of the other symptoms; 'no effect' - persistence of bacteriuria and leucocyturia, regardless of whether the
other symptoms have been controlled or not.

                         Results

     We shall announce only the results which are direct-
ly related to the subject of the present report. As is
seen in the Table, 96 of the 112 patients (85.7 per cent)
were favourably affected: in 39 patients (34.8 per cent)
the therapeutic effect was very good, and in 57 (50.9 per

Number of cases	Sex		effect of treatement	
	Male	Fe-Male	very good and good	without any effect
112	39	73	96 (85.7%)	16 (14.3%)

cent)- good.   Treatment was ineffective in 16 patients.
All failures were in patients who had varying degree of
renal failure and accompanying diseases.   The presence
or absence of effect on the individual symptoms, expressed in absolute numbers and in percentage, is seen in Fig.
1; the relation between renal function and therapeutic
effect is shown in Fig.2.

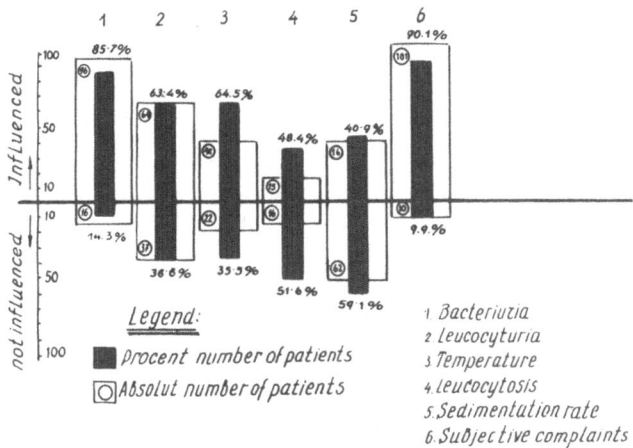

Figure 1

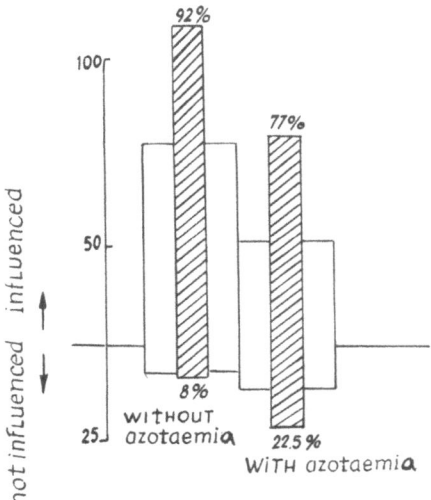

Figure 2

Discussion

In the event of favourable therapeutic index the clinical trial of a new renal-urinary chemotherapeutic agent raises the following basic questions: 1. Dose-interval-route of administration; 2. selection of patients; 3. choice, follow-up and assessment of the parameters permitting objective evaluation of the therapeutic effect. With gentamycin, the clinical experience gained so far has answered the first question. As to the selection of patients, data available in the literature and the results of our studies show that the most appropriate clinical form for testing a new renal-urinary chemotherapeutic agent is the nonobstructive (hematogenous) form of pyelonephritis with preserved renal function and absence of acute or chronic accompanying diseases. The requirements for maximal removal of all impeding factors are best observed in this clinical form. Only 32 of our patients met the afore-mentioned requirements. They all highly benefited from gentamycin treatment.

As for the third basic question - choice, follow up and evaluation of the parameters - the afore-mentioned six parameters have long since been established in the literature. The first two - bacteriuria and leucocyturia - are specific, the remaining four - nonspecific. Proceeding from the results obtained in our patients, a diagnostically worth assessment of these parameters not only by the 'specificity-nonspecificity' symptom, but also by the symptoms: 'subjectiveness-objectiveness', 'effectiveness of treatment' and 'incidence'. We suggest that the parameters be arranged in the following order, according to their diagnostic significance: objectiveness -subjectiveness, specificity-nonspecificity, effectiveness of treatment and incidence. This sequence, related to our patients, is shown in Fig.1. It becomes clear why the subjective symptoms, though most common and best affected by treatment, actually occupy the last place, or why fever, effectiveness of treatment and incidence are diagnostically superior to ESR. For the lack of space we are not able to afford further discussions. Finally, we want to point out that with strict observance of the requirements of this clinical method and in eventual control studies with a known drug under conditions of random selection or individual mode of administration, it seems most justifiable from a therapeutic point of view to attempt treatment of abacterial forms of exacerbated chronic pyelonephritis.

GEOGRAPHICAL VARIATION IN URINARY INFECTIONS IN GENERAL PRACTICE:

A COMBINED STUDY IN HOLLAND AND ENGLAND

G.A. Takken, Wijk-aan-Zee, Holland and
Valerie M. Moss and W. Brumfitt
The Royal Free Hospital

Pond Street, Hampstead, London NW3 2QG

During the last decade there has been a great deal of interest in the geographical differences in the incidence of various diseases, for example, multiple sclerosis. In the case of infectious disease this problem has also aroused great interest in the varying sensitivity of the causitive organisms. Urinary infection is a worldwide problem and attention has already been focussed on the different serotypes of <u>Escherichia coli</u> responsible for infection in domiciliary practice when material is obtained from different locations, and reports on the sensitivity of the organisms isolated have shown a great variation (see for example McAllister 1974, Senewiratne et al 1973). Whether this is due to true differences or technical problems remains to be seen. Other obvious points of interest would be the influence of climatic and seasonal variations as well as factors such as diet. In order to investigate these problems we decided to organise parallel studies in two general practices in Holland and in England, as an initial pilot study. We were concerned about the differences in bacteriological techniques and consequently it was decided that by using the dip-slide and the filter paper strip method it would be possible to transport the bacteriological specimens to a central laboratory. In this case the department chosen was at The Royal Free Hospital, London. We hoped that by doing this we would ensure uniformity in technique and therefore results. We report here the findings of the first nine months of a study carried out in a single-handed practice of about 2,000 patients situated in Wijk-aan-Zee, Holland, and in Hertfordshire where we have also been able to undertake a screening programme in a group practice of 16,000 patients. This study is now half completed but the data is not yet ready for analysis.

In the Dutch study, all patients who presented with definite

symptoms of urinary infection were included. When the patient
arrived a full history was taken using a specially designed proforma.
The patient was examined clinically and blood specimens were taken
for haematological and biochemical tests which were carried out at
Red Cross Hospital, Be
vervek. The urine specimens were examined
clinically and microscopically in the doctor's office but the dip-
slides and filter paper strip tests were done on two consecutive
urine specimens (collected by the clean-catch technique after
appropriate swabbing using sterile distilled water). The dip-slides
were found to be a suitable medium for the filter paper strip
inoculation and this simplified transportation. Initially, transport
was by air-freight but this proved costly and relatively inefficient
and we have now changed to the efficient and more economical method of
using ordinary postal services. The interval before arrival is from
2 to 4 days during which time the organisms have incubated at ambient
temperature. By inspection of the specimens on arrival we have been
unable to confirm findings of Arneil et al (1970) that incubation at
room temperature is adequate for the development and analysis of the
number of colonies on the dip-slide. Therefore the specimens were
incubated on arrival at the Royal Free, but it has become apparent
that incubation before dispatch of the specimens might well prove to
be more appropriate.

    The present communication is concerned with the preliminary
results from the first nine months of the study in The Nederlands.
Fifty-eight patients attended with a history of urinary infection,
but for a variety of reasons (such as pregnancy and lack of collaboration) the number who were prepared to be fully investigated
amounted to 41. The patients were mainly female (38) and 3 males.
Of the female patients, 22 were married, 14 were single and 2 were
widowed. The age group is at first sight unusual in that 23 were
between 17-30, only 8 were in the range 31-50, but 10 were over 50.
In fact, examination of the age distribution of the patients in the
practice concerned indicated that this agreed with actual age
distribution. Of considerable interest is the finding that the
history showed no fewer than 29 female patients had a previous history
of urinary infection and of these 25 had a clear history of what they
described as "cystitis", 8 had suffered from acute pyelonephritis, 6
had had gynaecological operations and 2 were known to have a calculus.
Only 12 patients had no previous history of urinary infection.
Regarding the frequency of infection judged by symptoms and pyuria 58
patients presented over a period of nine months - which is equal to
38 per 1,000 per year. The 15 with accompanying significant bacteriuria represented an annual incidence of 10 per thousand, which is in
agreement with several previous studies (Fry et al 1962, Loudon and
Greenhalgh 1962, Mond et al 1965).

    We were very interested to compare the results of microscopy
carried out in the doctor's office (on the basis of finding more than
5 cells per high powered field)with the presence of a significant

bacteriuria (10^5 organisms per ml). All 41 patients had a significant pyuria but only 15 (37%) had a significant bacteriuria.

It is clearly important to decide on the merits of the dip-slide and filter paper strip techniques. Both tests were positive in 15 patients, and according to our protocol only these were taken to have significant bacteriuria. However, one dip-slide was positive and the strip negative, and one strip was positive and the dip-slide negative. There were two patients with counts of 10^4 per ml or more but these were also excluded because they were less than 10^5 per ml. Bacteria found in significant bacteriuria conformed to the usual pattern, bearing in mind that there were two patients with calculus and 6 had had gynaecological operations. Organisms isolated from first specimens were 11 <u>E.coli</u>, 2 <u>Micrococcus</u> spp. (as judged by novobiocin resistance), 1 <u>Klebsiella pneumoniae</u> and 1 <u>Proteus vulgaris</u>. With regard to <u>E.coli</u> none of the first isolates was resistant to trimethoprim or nitrofurantoin but one was resistant to sulphonamide.

We were interested to observe the results of treatment. The drugs tested were co-trimoxazole and nitrofurantoin, given in a double blind trial using a random number list. Co-trimoxazole was given in the usual dose of two tablets every 12 hours for 7 days and nitrofurantoin in a dose 100 mg twice daily. Interestingly, all 15 patients with significant bacteriuria were cured but, of course, the number is small. All the 41 patients with typical symptomatology and pyuria were treated and the cure rate in this larger group was 33 (88%) with 8 failures. Of those that failed, 5 were treated with co-trimoxazole and 3 with nitrofurantoin. These differences are not significant.

The side effects were rather frequent but a number were mild and it was only necessary to discontinue treatment in 3 patients. The nature of the side effects is shown in the Table which were those to be expected with treatment given. Two patients given nitrofurantoin had vomiting in addition to the nausea. Vomiting was not found in patients given co-trimoxazole.

SIDE EFFECTS IN 41 PATIENTS
(7 days treatment)

Co-trimoxazole (2 tablets 12 hourly)	9
Nitrofurantoin (100 mg 12 hourly)	5

Haematology and biochemistry carried out on all 41 patients before and after chemotherapy did not show any evidence of toxicity.

In previous studies on urinary infection the question of

seasonal variation has been discussed but no conclusions reached.
Although in the present study the numbers are small, consideration
of the patients with significant bacteriuria shows two obvious
clusters. Patients 8 to 13 inclusive presented in the period 22
August to 14 October 1974 and a second cluster of 4 patients
presented between 24 March and 14 April 1975. Thus, 10 of the 15
patients with significant bacteriuria were seen during 10 weeks of
the 9 month study.

The present study will continue until 100 patients have been
investigated and the results compared with the study at present in
progress in England, which it is hoped will yield 200 - 300 patients
with urinary infections.

Acknowledgements

We are grateful to Mr J.J. Kuneman and Dr J. Cooper of The
Wellcome Foundation for their invaluable help.

REFERENCES

Arneil, G.C., McAllister, T.A. & Kay, P. 1970 Lancet 1, 119.
Fry, J., Dillane, J.B., Joiner, C.L. & Williams, J.D. 1962
    Lancet 1, 1318.
Loudon, I.S.L. & Greenhalgh, G.P. 1962 Lancet 2, 1246.
McAllister, T.A. 1974 J.Internat.Med.Res.2, 400.
Mond, N.C., Percival, A., Williams, J.D. & Brumfitt, W. 1965
    Lancet 1, 514.
Senewiratne, B., Senewiratne, K. & Hettiarachchi, J. 1973
    Lancet 3, 222.

SULFAMETOPYRAZINE AS TREATMENT FOR BACTERIURIA IN PREGNANCY, AND EFFECTS ON BOWEL FLORA

D.S. REEVES

DEPARTMENT OF MEDICAL MICROBIOLOGY

SOUTHMEAD HOSPITAL, BRISTOL, BS10 5NB, ENGLAND

Sulfametopyrazine (2-sulfanilinamido-3-methoxypyrazine; SMP) is an ultra long-acting sulphonamide. It is the only sulphonamide available in the U.K. with which therapeutically adequate blood levels of drug are maintained for up to a week following a single dose. In patients with asymptomatic infections as bacteriuria in pregnancy this represents an advantage since it is possible for a patient to forget to take some or all of the doses in a multi-dose regime in the absence of symptoms. The importance of treating bacteriuria in pregnancy while the infection remains asymptomatic is well established. The use of a single dose of SMP (2 grams) as treatment for such patients has been already reported (Reeves, 1975), where the development of a two-dose regime of SMP is also described. Reported here are the comparative results of treating bacteriuria in pregnancy with SMP (2 grams), SMP (2+2 grams), or sulphadimidine (SD, in full dosage).

Break-through infections with sulphonamide resistant organisms occur during long-term therapy with sulphonamide and are attributed to alteration of bowel flora to resistance (Winberg et al, 1973). There was a possibility that the low total dose comprising a course of SMP might have less effect on bowel flora. A study of faecal flora before and after treatment was therefore undertaken.

METHODS

Clinical Protocol

Women attending ante-natal clinics at Southmead Hospital for

the first time were screened for significant ($>10^5$ bacteria/ml)
bacteriuria. Patients with bacteriuria attended a special clinic
where they were documented, a confirming urine specimen taken, and
treatment given.   2 weeks later the patients attended for follow-
up when changes in symptomatology, any side-effects were recorded,
and a further urine specimen taken.   Check specimens of urine for
bacteriuria were taken at about 4-weekly intervals for the rest of
pregnancy.

A treatment was given by random code as follows: (i) SMP 2
grams taken in the clinic; (ii) SMP 2 grams taken in the clinic
and 2 grams 4 days later; (iii) SD 1 gram 6-hourly for 7 days.

A cure was defined as absence of the original infecting
organism in a follow-up specimen.   The presence of a new bacterial
species (or a different type of the same species) was considered to
be a re-infection and thus not a failure of treatment.

The minimal inhibitory concentrations (MIC's) of sulphonamide
for the urinary isolates was determined by an agar plate dilution
technique.   The medium was Oxoid D.S.T. agar with 2% lysed horse-
blood, and the inoculum was $1 - 1.5 \times 10^3$/ml.

Investigation of Faecal Flora

Patients coming to the clinic for the first time were instruc-
ted how to bring a sample of faeces with them.   They also brought
a sample to any post-treatment follow-up visit.   Patients with a
history of antibiotic therapy within the past 3 months were excluded
from this study.

As controls, similar pairs of faeces samples were taken from
5 patients treated with nitrofuratoin, and 5 with hexamine hippurate.   Neither is thought to have an action on bowel flora and
this was more ethical than leaving patients untreated.

A piece of a faeces sample was emulsified in saline and spread
on a MaConkey agar plate. After incubation 10 colonies of entero-
bacteria were taken at random for storage and subsequent m.i.c.
determination to sulphonamide in batches by a standard agar plate
dilution method.   As a means of assessing changes in faecal flora
the m.i.c. of sulphonamide for each of the 10 colonies was allocated
a code:-

m.i.c. (mg/l)	Code	m.i.c. (mg/l)	Code
10	1	100	4
25	2	200	5
50	3	200	6

Table 1: Infecting Organisms Divided by Treatments

Treatment	Esch. coli	Proteus mirabilis	Klebsiella spp.	Other	Totals
SMP 2g	44	1	3	1	49
SMP 2+2g	37	1	–	2	40
SD	38	1	1	–	40

The number of organisms of each code in a specimen was multiplied by that code, and the sum of the products was taken as a measure of the overall sulphonamide resistance of the 10 colonies taken.

RESULTS

Outcome of Treatment

The infecting organisms are showing in Table 1. The results of treatment divided by sensitivity of the infecting organism are in Table 2 where it can be seen that there is a strong relationship between resistant organisms and failure of treatment. The

Table 2: Results of Treatment Related to MIC of Sulphonamide of Infecting Organisms.

Treatment	Result	MIC (mg/1 SMP)			Totals
		<50	100–200	>200	
SMP 2g	C2C6	23	5	2	30
	C2	4	0	0	4
	C2F6	2	1	0	3
	F2	5	3	4	12
SMP 2+2g	C2C6	22	3	2	27
	C2	3	0	0	3
	C2F6	3	0	0	3
	F2	3	0	4	7
SD	C2C6	13	4	0	17
	C2	0	6	0	6
	C2F6	2	0	0	2
	F2	8	1	6	15

C2C6 – Original infecting organism absent from urine at 2 and 6 weeks follow-up.

C2 – Original infecting organism absent from urine at 2 weeks follow-up but not tested at 6 weeks.

C2F6 – Original infecting organism absent from urine at 2 weeks follow-up but present at 6 weeks.

F2 – Original infecting organism present in urine at 2 weeks follow-up.

Table 3: Cure Rates and Side Effects of the Three Regimes of
          Sulphonamides.

Treatment	Cure rate: follow-up at		Side Effects		
	2 weeks	6 weeks	Absent	Present	Not Assessable
SMP 2g	37/49(83%)	30/45(67%)	41	6(13%)	7
SMP 2+2g	33/40(83%)	27/37(73%)	38	4(10%)	5
SD	25/40(62%)	17/34(50%)	27	13(33%)	6

cure rates are in Table 3 together with the incidence of side-
effects.

Effect on Faecal Flora

The results for patients given nitrofurantoin or hexamine
hippurate (i.e. where no change would be expected to be induced by
therapy) are in Table 4. As in no case was there a change of resistance code greater than 10, a change greater than 10 was taken
as significant in subsequent analyses. The results on the 46
individual pairs of faeces during the sulphonamide therapies are
not shown for reasons of space. The mean codes before and after
therapy together with the number of significant changes are in
Table 5.

With all three regimes of sulphonamide there was an increased
bacterial resistance to the treatment apparent in the faeces.

Table 4: Effect of Nitrofurantoin or Hexamine Hippurate on Sulpho-
          namide Resistance of Faecal Flora.

Treatment	Sulphonamide resistance code in individual patients		
	Before Therapy	After Therapy	Change
Nitrofurantoin	6	10	+ 4
(50 mg t.d.s.)	11	10	− 1
	10	10	0
	28	20	− 8
	53	43	− 10
mean	21.6	18.6	− 3
Hexamine	24	31	+ 7
hippurate	20	20	0
(Hiprex, 1	22	14	− 8
tablet t.d.s.)	23	15	− 8
	42	40	− 2
mean	26.2	24.0	−2.2

Table 5:   Mean Sulphonamide Resistance Codes and Changes in Codes
for the 3 Sulphonamide Therapies and the Control Therapies.

Treatment	No. of pairs of faeces	Mean Codes Before therapy	Mean Codes After therapy	Mean Codes Change	No. of significant changes in codes Upwards	No. of significant changes in codes Downwards
Nitrofur-antoin	5	21.6	18.6	-3	None - by definition	
Hexamine hippurate	5	26.2	24.0	-2.2		
SMP 2 gram	16	27.1	40.8	+13.7	7	1
SMP 2+2 gram	14	28.5	42.4	+13.9	7	2
SD	16	24.0	29.8	+5.8	5	1

DISCUSSION

There has been only a single previously published report on
the use of SMP as treatment for bacteriuria in pregnancy. The cure-
rate using a 2 gram dose was 62% (Williams and Smith, 1970) which
is very similar to that described here. It was hoped that using a
larger dose of SMP would improve this cure-rate and this is in fact
borne out, although the difference (67% and 73% for SMP 2 and SMP
2+2 grams respectively) is not statistically significant. A rate
of 73% is however similar to many previously reported treatments
for bacteriuria in pregnancy (see Williams et al, 1968). The low
cure-rate given by sulphadimidine is disconcerting since this regime was included to act as a "yardstick" against which those with
SMP could be compared. Previous experience with sulphadimidine
(Williams et al, 1965 and 1968) showed cure-rates of 73% and 78%,
with few side-effects. The large number of side-effects reported
here may be responsible for a low cure-rate since it is likely the
patients stopped their medication.

Previous reports of the use of an ultra long-acting sulphonamide in bacteriuria in pregnancy are few. We used sulphadoxine
(not marketed in U.K.) and found cure-rates of 79% and 52% in London
and Birmingham respectively (Williams et al, 1968). The highest
cure-rates have been reported using co-trimoxazole (87% of 86
patients; Williams et al, 1969) but this combination is not now
advised for use in pregnancy. While SMP would appear to be no more
efficacious in curing bacteriuria in pregnancy than other agents,
side-effects were infrequent. The two rashes that occurred were
not more severe nor longer lasting than is usual with sulphonamides
of a shorter half-life.

It is disappointing that the low total dose give less as much
effect on faecal flora as a full course of sulphadimidine. This

may be attributable to entero-hepatic circulation the existance of
which Devriendt et al (1970) postulated on pharmacokinetic grounds.

REFERENCES

Devriendt, A., Jansen, F.H., and Weemaes, I. (1970). European
Journal of Clinical Pharmacology 3: 36-42.

Williams, J.D., Brumfitt, W., Condie, A.P., and Reeves, D.S.
(1969). Postgraduate Medical Journal. 45, November suppl. 71-5.

Williams, J.D., Brumfitt, W., Leigh, D.A. and Percival, A. (1965).
Lancet i; 831-4.

Williams, J.D., Condie, A.P., Franklin, I.N.S., Leigh, D.A.,
Reeves, D.S., and Brumfitt, W. (1968). Ed. O'Grady and Brumfitt,
W., London. pp 160-169.

Williams, J.D., and Smith, E.K. (1970). British Medical Journal,
651-3.

Winberg, J., Bergstrom, T., Lincoln, K., Lidin-Janson, G. (1973).
Clinical Nephrology, 1, 143.

Reeves, D.S. (1975). Journal of Antimicrobial Chemotherapy, 1,
171-186.

A COMPARATIVE STUDY OF TICARCILLIN AND GENTAMICIN IN THE TREATMENT OF COMPLICATED URINARY TRACT INFECTIONS

Paul O. Madsen and Torben B. Kjaer

From the Urology Section, Veterans Administration Hospital and the Department of Surgery, University of Wisconsin School of Medicine, Madison, Wisconsin 53706

SUMMARY

Ticarcillin is a semisynthetic penicillin for parenteral use with an antibacterial spectrum similar to that of carbenicillin but better in vitro activity against Pseudomonas aeruginosa.

The two antibiotics ticarcillin and gentamicin were compared in a prospective randomized study of 80 elderly male patients with complicated urinary tract infections due to hyperplasia of the prostate, cancer of the prostate, urethral strictures, and stones. The two groups of patients were comparable as to infecting microorganisms and underlying urinary tract pathology. No patients had indwelling catheters. All microorganisms isolated were sensitive to the two antibiotics by the disc sensitivity test. Ticarcillin was diluted in 0.5% lidocaine to reduce pain on injection. Both antibiotics were well tolerated but the patients receiving gentamicin showed a statistically but not clinically significant increase in the blood urea nitrogen and serum creatinine values following treatment, suggesting slight renal toxicity. Both antibiotics were effective in eradicating the infections with no significant difference between the two groups in cure rate as defined by a negative urine culture one week following discontinuation of the treatment.

Ticarcillin (BRL 2288, α-carboxy-3-thienylmethylpenicillin, disodium salt) is a semisynthetic penicillin with an antibacterial spectrum similar to that of carbenicillin. When compared to carbenicillin, it is of particular interest because ticarcillin is significantly more active in vitro against Pseudomonas aeruginosa, slightly more active against E. coli and it is active against certain proteus species (Beecham-Massengill Pharmaceuticals, 1974). Ticarcillin is not absorbed after oral administration.

Table 1

Distribution of Bacteria Isolated from the Urine
in the Two Patient Groups

Organism	Treatment Group	
	Ticarcillin (n = 40)	Gentamicin (n = 40)
Escherichia	20	20
Klebsiella-Enterobacter	2	4
Proteus	9	13
Pseudomonas	9	6

The present study was carried out to compare the safety and
efficacy of ticarcillin and to compare it to gentamicin in the treatment of complicated urinary tract infections in an elderly male
patient population.

MATERIALS AND METHODS

Eighty elderly male patients (average age 72 years) with complicated urinary tract infections due to obstruction of the lower
urinary tract, from benign hyperplasia or cancer of the prostate or
urethral strictures were treated with ticarcillin intramuscularly 1
g every 8 hours for 7 days or gentamicin 80 mg intramuscularly every
8 hours for 7 days in a prospective, randomized study. Ticarcillin
was diluted in 0.5% lidocaine to reduce pain on injection.

All patients had relatively normal renal function as expressed
by a serum creatinine $\leq$ 1.5 mg% and/or a blood urea nitrogen of $\leq$
25 mg%. The two patient groups were comparable as to the infecting
microorganisms (Table 1) and to the pathology of the urinary tract.
No patients had indwelling catheters. All of the microorganisms
isolated from the urine were susceptible to gentamicin and ticarcillin by the disc sensitivity method (Bauer et al., 1966).

Urine cultures with colony count were carried out before treatment, on the third and seventh day of treatment and 1 week following
discontinuation of treatment.

Complete blood count, blood urea nitrogen, serum creatinine,
serum alkaline phosphatase, lactic dehydrogenase (LDH) and serum
glutamic oxaloacetic acid (SGOT) were determined within 48 hours before initiation of treatment and again on the last day of treatment.

These therapeutic results were defined according to the urine

Table 2

Results of Treatment of Complicated Urinary Tract Infections with
Ticarcillin and Gentamicin in 80 Patients (All Figures in %)

		Negative Culture	Relapse or Persistence	Reinfection or Superinfection
Third Day of Therapy	Ticarcillin	87	8	5
	Gentamicin	90	2	8
End of Therapy	Ticarcillin	92	3	5
	Gentamicin	94	3	3
One Week Follow-up	Ticarcillin	54	36	10
	Gentamicin	70	20	10

cultures: cure: negative culture at 1 week following treatment;
persistence: more than 10^5 colonies/ml of the original bacteria
during treatment; relapse: negative cultures during therapy and
more than 10^5 colonies/ml of the original organism at follow-up;
reinfection: more than 10^5 colonies/ml different from the original
bacteria at follow-up; and superinfection: more than 10^5 colonies/
ml different from the original bacteria during therapy. Microorganisms were identified by routine bacteriological methods without
specific typing.

RESULTS

Both antibiotics were well tolerated by all patients without
any detectable clinical side effects. The bacteriological results
are listed in Table 2. In our patient material, the therapeutic
results would be expected to be poor. Both antibiotics however,
cleared up practically all urine cultures and in both patient groups
more than half the patients were cured as defined by having a negative urine culture 1 week following discontinuation of the treatment.
The effect of the two drugs on the renal function is outlined in
Table 3. It can be seen that there is a statistically but not clinically significant increase in the serum creatinine and blood urea
nitrogen values following gentamicin treatment whereas no such
change was noted in the patients treated with ticarcillin. These
results support the opinion that penicillin derivatives have less
nephrotoxicity than the aminoglycoside antibiotics. There were no
significant differences in complete blood count values and alkaline
phosphatase values before and after treatment. There was in both
groups a statistically but not clinically significant increase in
LDH and SGOT values before and after treatment (paired t-test).

It can be concluded that ticarcillin appears to be as effective

Table 3

Blood Urea Nitrogen (BUN) and Serum Creatinine Values Pre and Post
Treatment with Ticarcillin and Gentamicin in 80 Patients

Treatment		BUN (mg%)		Serum Creatinine (mg %)	
		Pre R_x	Post R_x	Pre R_x	Post R_x
Ticarcillin	Mean ± 1 SD	18.7 ± 7.1	19.7 ± 9.5	1.21 ± 0.45	1.22 ± 0.45
	Paired t-test	Not significant		Not significant	
Gentamicin	Mean ± 1 SD	18.1 ± 6.9	21.4 ± 11.4	1.15 ± 0.33	1.24 ± 0.45
	Paired t-test	$p < 0.02$		$p < 0.05$	

as gentamicin in the treatment of complicated urinary tract infections due to susceptible bacteria in an elderly male patient population. Ticarcillin also appears to have less of a nephrotoxic effect
than gentamicin.

REFERENCES

1. Bauer, A. W., W. M. Kirby, J. C. Sherris, and M. Turck. 1966.
    Antibiotic susceptibility testing by a standardized single disk
    method. American Journal of Clinical Pathology, 45:493–496.

2. Beecham-Massengill Pharmaceuticals, Bristol, Tennessee. Clini-
    cal Investigation Prospectus. 1974.

STUDIES ON ANTITUBERCULOSIS ACTIVITY OF AMIKACIN

Yuzo Kawamori and Natsuo Nishizawa

Senboku National Hospital

Sakai, Osaka, Japan

Amikacin is a derivative of kanamycin, which was semisynthesized by Dr. Kawaguchi of Bristol-Banyu Research Institute in Japan.

Because this is a derivative of kanamycin A as shown in Figure 1, it is expected that amikacin has an antituberculosis activity.

Table 1 shows the growth inhibiting effect against tubercle bacilli of amikacin in vitro. Among 26 strains isolated from the sputum of pulmonary tuberculosis patients, 10 were sensitive to 0.2 mcg per ml of amikacin or kanamycin in Dubos' liquid media, and other 4 strains were sensitive to 0.5 mcg per ml of both drugs but resistant to 0.2 mcg per ml. Seven strains which were resistant to 20 mcg per ml of kanamycin were resistant to the same concentration of amikacin, as well.

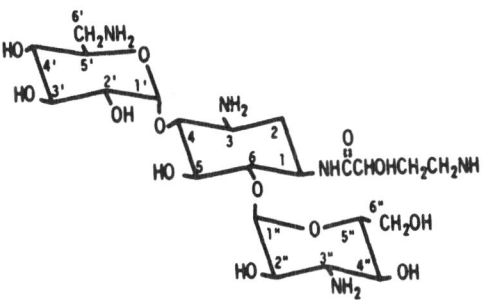

Figure 1. Chemical Structure of Amikacin (AMK)

Table 1. MIC of AMK and KM against TB-B in Dubos' liquid media

MIC (mcg/ml)		No. of strains
AMK	K M	
0.2	0.2	10
0.5	0.5	4
0.2	0.5	1
0.5	2.0	3
> 20	> 20	7
5	> 20	1

And the remaining 5 strains were more sensitive to amikacin than
to kanamycin, that is, one was sensitive to 0.2 mcg per ml of amikacin and to 0.5 mcg per ml of kanamycin, 3 strains were sensitive
to 0.5 mcg per ml of amikacin and sensitive to 2 mcg per ml of
kanamycin, and one strain resistant to 10 mcg per ml of kanamycin
was sensitive to 5 mcg per ml of amikacin. On the slant of egg
media, minimal inhibiting concentration of amikacin was higher
than that in the Dubos' liquid media, just as that of kanamycin,
showing 25 mcg per ml of MIC for sensitive strains to amikacin
and kanamycin. From the results, we are sure that amikacin has an
antituberculosis activity at the same grade as, or somewhat higher
than kanamycin A.

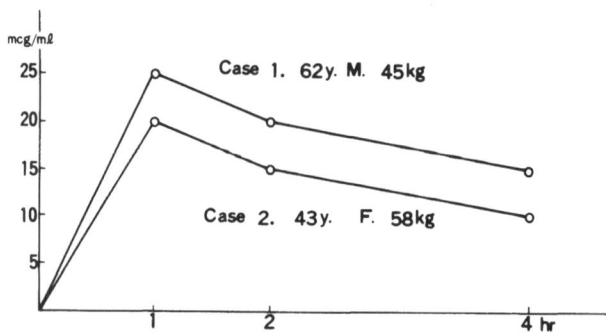

Figure 2. Serum levels of AMK following i.m. injection of 200mg.

Table 2. Serum levels of AMK and KM 4 hours after i.m. injection

Drug	Dose	No. of tested cases	Serum levels (mcg/mℓ)
AMK	200 mg	2	8.0 ~ 9.5
	400 500 mg	6	10.2 ~ 17.0
KM	500 mg	3	6.0 ~ 8.4
	1 g	5	10.8 ~ 22.0

The serum levels of amikacin after intramuscular injection were estimated comparing to that of kanamycin. The concentrations of both drugs were tested by the disc-agar-plate method with B.subtilis as indicating organism, and the solution of amikacin in pH 7.0 phosphate buffer was used as the standard curve. Two patients of pulmonary tuberculosis having normal renal and hepatic functions were injected with 200 mg of amikacin, and the serum were obtained after 1, 2 and 4 hours. As shown in Figure 2, 22 or 25 mcg per ml after one hour, 15 or 20 mcg per ml after two hours and 10 or 15 mcg per ml after four hours were given. This pattern of serum levels is similar as that of kanamycin.

Summarized results of estimation of serum levels 4 hours after the administrations of amikacin and kanamycin are shown in Table 2. Most of them were tested cross over in 8 patients. It was observed that the injection of 400 or 500 mg of amikacin could keep about the same levels in serum after 4 hours as those of 1 g of kanamycin.

The sera 4 hours after administration of both drugs were also tested for antimycobacterial activity by the method originally reported by Dr. Dye. The sera were diluted two fold in series with Dubos' liquid media and inoculated with ten days culture in the same media of three strains of tubercle bacilli. After two weeks, the end point of dilution, in which the growth were completely inhibited, were estimated. As shown in Table 3, the sera obtained 4 hours after injection of 400 or 500 mg of amikacin could inhibit completely the growth of strains sensitive to 0.2 mcg per ml of both drugs at the 16 to 32 fold dilutions just as those after administration of 1 g of kanamycin.And against a strain sensitive to 5 mcg per ml of amikacin but resistant to 10 mcg per ml of kanamycin, the sera obtained after injection of 500 mg of amikacin did inhibit their growth at 4 to 8 fold dilution, while those after injection of 1 g of kanamycin could not inhibit it even at a 4 fold dilution.

Table 3. Antimycobacterial activity of serum 4 hours after
         i.m. injection of AMK or KM

MIC against test strain (mcg/ml)		Drug	Dose (mg)	Endpoint of dilution for complete inhibition
A M K	K M			
0.2 (2 strains)	0.2	AMK	200	8 x
			400	16 x
			500	16 – 32 x
		KM	500	4 – 8 x
			1,000	16 – 32 x
5	20	AMK	500	4 – 8 x
		KM	500	∠ 4 x
			1,000	∠ 4 x

Dr. Akiyoshi of the Tokyo Medical and Dental University had
reported the experimental studies on ototoxicity of amikacin and
shown that the ototoxicity of amikacin was in the same grade of
that of kanamycin when both drugs were given in the same dose.
From the results of our own studies and Dr. Akiyoshi's experiments
it was supposed that the administration of 500 mg of amikacin
would keep the same grade of clinical effects against tuberculosis
patients as that of 1 g of kanamycin with less side effect than
that of the latter. Dr. Yamamoto and others including ourselves
studied the clinical observations concerning the daily administration of 500 mg of amikacin for three months, followed by a three
times a week injection of the same dose for another three months.
The cases were selected among pulmonary tuberculosis with cavities
and positive sputum, who had been treated already with antituberculosis drugs of the first line. Among 103 cases included in the
trial, 74 cases were given the drug for 6 months, while the others
are still continueing. Table 4 shows the percentages of negative
conversion of the culture which were divided into three groups
according to the numbers of the accompanying sensitive drugs.

Table 4. Culture negative conversion (KM-sensitive cases)

Accompanying Sensitive drugs	Months treated					
	1	2	3	4	5	6
0	25 %	25 %	25 %	25 %	25 %	33 %
1	64	80	88	77	77	80
2 or more	69	83	95	97	96	96

Table 5. Side effects   Withdrawn cases in parentheses

Total cases	103
Cases with side effects	14 (5)
Tinnitus	4
Tinnitus with hearing disturbance	6 (3)
Hypoaesthesia around the mouth	2
Headache	2 (2)

While the rate of negative conversion in the cases treated accompanying without other antituberculosis drug or with resistant drugs was only 25 %, the negative conversion in the cases with one sensitive accompanying drug were observed in 80 % at 2 months or later of treatment, showing higher rate than expected. In the cases treated with two or more of accompanying drugs, over 90 % of conversion were detected.

The side effects during the administration of amikacin are shown in Table 5, that is, in 14 cases adverse symptoms including tinnitus, hearing disturbance and headache were observed, while it was necessary to withdraw the drug in 5 cases of the trial. However, as these cases with side effects had been treated with streptomycin, kanamycin or other aminoglycoside antibiotics for more than 6 months, more precise observation should be performed for the original treatment cases.

From the results of the above mentioned experimental and clinical studies on amikacin, we consider that the drug would be more effectively than kanamycin for the cases of pulmonary tuberculosis that are indicated for kanamycin treatment.

IN VITRO, PHARMACOLOGICAL AND CLINICAL STUDIES WITH AMIKACIN

Manuel Valdivieso, M.D., Gerald P. Bodey, M.D., Ronald
Feld, M.D., Victorio Rodriguez, M.D. and Peter B. Schwartz,
M.D.

Department of Developmental Therapeutics, Department of
Gynecology, The University of Texas System Cancer Center,
M.D. Anderson Hospital and Tumor Institute, Houston, Texas
U.S.A.

ABSTRACT

Amikacin, a new aminoglycoside antibiotic, was found to have
broad spectrum in vitro activity against most gram-negative bacilli.
Amikacin was also effective against 74% of 26 isolates of gram-negative bacilli known to be resistant to gentamicin. Pharmacological
studies in humans demonstrated that adequate serum concentrations of
amikacin could be safely reached and maintained by continuous infusions. Using these two schedules, amikacin cured 64% of 155 episodes
of identified infections occurring in cancer patients. The majority
of infections were pneumonia and septicemia. The most commonly
identified pathogens were E. coli, organisms of the Klebsiella-
Enterobacter-Serratia group and P. aeruginosa. The cure rate for
infections produced by these organisms was 79%. Included were 5 of
8 infections produced by organisms resistant to gentamicin. The
results with continuous infusions of amikacin in patients with
severe neutropenia were as good as the results with intermittent
infusions in patients with adequate neutrophil counts. Optimum results were obtained in neutropenic patients when a serum concentration
of approximately 15 µg/ml was maintained.

INTRODUCTION

Patients with cancer are frequently affected by infections produced by gram-negative bacilli. Results of therapy for these
infections are still suboptimal particularly during periods of severe

neutropenia. Consequently, they remain the most common immediate
cause of death in cancer patients (3,4,5). The recent emergence of
pathogenic organisms which are resistant to multiple antibiotics,
including gentamicin, has complicated the problem. Thus, the need
for continuing studies of promising new antibiotics is of importance.

Amikacin is a new aminoglycoside antibiotic which is chemically
related to kanamycin (6). Amikacin is of special interest because
of its broad spectrum of activity in vitro against most gram-negative bacilli, including some organisms which are resistant to other
aminoglycoside antibiotics (2). A review of our experience with
amikacin indicates that this is a very effective antibiotic for the
treatment of gram-negative bacilli infections in cancer patients.

MATERIALS AND METHODS

The sequential in vitro, pharmacologic and therapeutic studies
with amikacin were begun in the Department of Developmental Therapeutics of the University of Texas M.D. Anderson Hospital and Tumor
Institute in 1972. The in vitro activity of this antibiotic was
studied in 466 clinical isolates of gram-negative bacilli (2). All
organisms were cultured from blood specimens obtained from patients
previously admitted to this institution. Susceptibility tests were
conducted by use of the broth dilution technique.

. The therapeutic efficacy of amikacin was investigated during
216 febrile episodes occurring in 178 cancer patients. All patients
were presumed or proven to have infection caused by gram-negative
bacilli and had a temperature of 101 or greater. Half of the
patients received amikacin after 48 to 72 hours of unsuccessful
therapy with a combination of cephalosporin and carbenicillin.

After appropriate cultures and other indicated tests, amikacin
was administered intravenously, either intermittently, or by continuous infusion. Patients with adequate neutrophils ($>1000/mm^3$)
received the drug by the intermittent schedule: 150 mg/M^2 administered in 50 ml of 5% dextrose solution over a 30 minute period
every 6 hours. Patients with neutropenia (<1000 neutrophils/mm^3)
received the continuous schedule. The first 14 neutropenic patients
received a loading dose of 100 mg/M^2 followed by a total daily dose
of 600 mg/M^2. All subsequent patients received a loading dose of
150 mg/M^2 followed by a total daily dose of 800 mg/M^2. An infusion
pump was used to administer the continuous infusions (IVAC TH500,
IVAC Corp., San Diego, California).

Pharmacologic studies were performed in 16 patients who were
receiving amikacin as therapy for infection. There were 6 patients
receiving the intermittent schedule and 10 patients receiving the

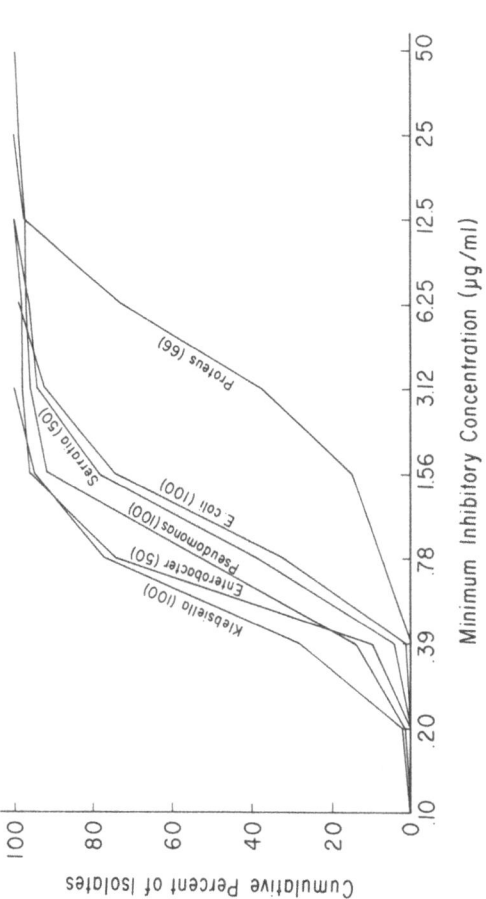

FIGURE 1.   In vitro activity of amikacin against gram-negative bacilli.   Numbers in paranthesis indicate number of isolates tested.

continuous schedule. Serum specimens were obtained before drug administration and at 0.25, 0.5, 1, 2, 4 and 6 hours thereafter. The concentrations of amikacin in blood specimens were determined by an agar well method with Bacillus subtilis ATCC 6633 as the test organism.

Serum concentrations of amikacin were determined daily in patients receiving therapy by continuous infusion and the dose of the drug was adjusted to try to maintain a serum concentration of 15 µg/ml. Therapy for all patients was continued for a minimum of 7 days or for 5 days after they became afebrile. Complete blood count, blood urea nitrogen, serum creatinine and liver function studies were obtained initially and weekly during therapy. Audiograms (Beltone audiometer, Beltone Electronics Company, Chicago, Illinois) were performed prior to, twice weekly, during and 1 to 3 days after discontinuation of therapy in 45 episodes. Consent forms were obtained according to institutional policies. The majority of organisms causing infection were tested in vitro for susceptibility to amikacin.

Patients were considered to have an identified infection if they had characteristic clinical and laboratory evidence of infection. Patients who were febrile but without characteristic evidence of infection were considered to have fever of unknown origin. Patients were considered to have been cured if they became afebrile and all clinical and laboratory signs of infection disappeared. Patients were considered to have developed superinfection when another infection caused by a different organism occurred during treatment of the original infection.

RESULTS

The in vitro activity of amikacin against gram-negative bacilli is shown in Figure 1. At a conentration of 3.12 µg/ml, amikacin inhibited over 90% of isolates of all gram-negative bacilli, except Proteus species. This antibiotic inhibited over 90% of Pseudomonas aeruginosa isolates at a concentration of 1.56 µg/ml. Nineteen of 26 (74%) isolates of gram-negative bacilli known to be resistant to gentamicin sulfate were sensitive to amikacin (Table 1). Included were 5 of 10 isolates of Pseudomonas aeruginosa and all 10 isolates of Serratia marcescens.

Results of pharmacological studies performed in patients receiving amikacin as therapy for infection is presented in Figure 2. On day 3, patients who were receiving the intermittent schedule had an initial mean serum concentration of 2.5 µg/ml. The highest mean serum concentration was obtained at the end of the infusion and was 18.3 µg/ml. The mean serum concentration at 6 hours (before

TABLE 1. Minimal Inhibitory Concentration to Amikacin of Gram-negative Bacilli Resistant to Gentamicin

ORGANISM	# ISOLATES	MIC TO AMIKACIN (μg/ml)			
		1.5 or less	3.12	6.25-12.5	>12.5
Pseudomonas	10	2	1	2	5
Serratia marcescens	10	8	2	0	0
Enterobacter sp.	3	3	0	0	0
Klebsiella sp.	2	1	0	0	1
Escherichia coli	1	0	0	0	1
TOTAL	26	14	3	2	7

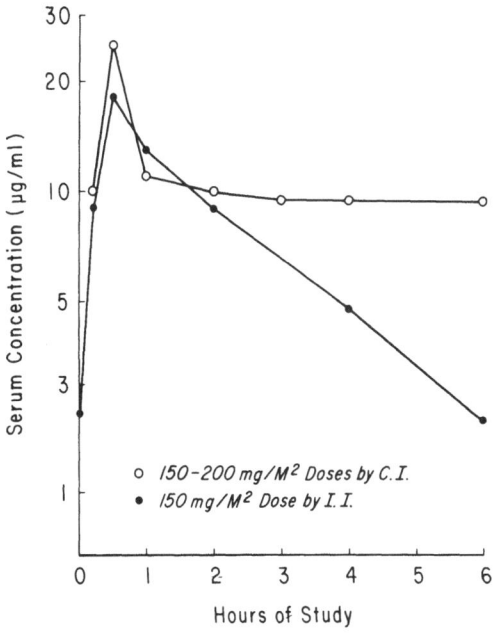

FIGURE 2. Studies were performed in patients receiving amikacin as therapy for infection. Six patients were receiving inter-mittent infusions (I.I.) and 10 patients were receiving continuous infusions (C.I.). Studies were conducted on day number 3 of therapy.

initiation of next infusion) was 2.4 µg/ml. The serum half-life on
day 3 was 1.7 hours. Among the patients who received a loading dose
of 150 mg/M^2 of amikacin administered intravenously over a 30 minute
period, followed immediately by a total daily dose of 800 mg/M^2 administered as a continuous infusion, the highest mean serum concentration was obtained at 30 minutes and was 24.8 µg/ml. The mean
serum concentration at 1 hour was 11 µg/ml and remained above 8 µg/ml
thereafter.

One hundred and seventy-eight cancer patients had 216 febrile
episodes and were treated with amikacin. Eighty-eight patients had
solid tumors, 78 had leukemia, 11 had lymphoma and 1 had aplastic
anemia. There were 97 males and 81 females. The median age was 48
years with a range of 14 to 87 years. Amikacin was administered by
continuous infusion during 92 febrile episodes in 67 patients.
During the remaining 124 febrile episodes in 111 patients, amikacin
was administered by the intermittent schedule.

The overall response rate for the 216 febrile episodes treated
with amikacin was 64%. Identical response rate was observed among
the 155 episodes of documented infections and the 61 episodes in
which infection was suspected but not proven. The most common
types of documented infection were penumonia and septicemia;
although infections of soft tissue and urinary tract were also
common (Table 2). The highest response to amikacin occurred among
patients with urinary tract infections (96%). The lowest response
was obtained among patients with pneumonia (53%). The response
rate was slightly though not significantly higher (p=.29) for
patients with pneumonia who received continuous infusions of amikacin
(62%) as opposed to those who received amikacin intermittently (47%).
Similar differences were observed among soft tissue infections where
the overall response was 54% and the response obtained by continuous
infusion of amikacin was higher (70% vs 44%).

TABLE 2. Response to Amikacin by Type of Infection and Schedule of
          Therapy

INFECTION	TOTAL		CONTINUOUS		INTERMITTENT	
	NUMBER	%RESPONSE	NUMBER	%RESPONSE	NUMBER	%RESPONSE
Pneumonia	53	53	21	62	32	47
Septicemia	43	67	23	65	20	70
Soft Tissue	28	54	10	70	18	44
Urinary tract	24	96	4	100	20	95
Others	7	57	1	0	6	67
TOTAL	155	64	59	66	96	63

TABLE 3. Response to Amikacin by Infecting Organism and Method of Therapy

ORGANISM	TOTAL		CONTINUOUS		INTERMITTENT	
	NUMBER	%RESPONSE	NUMBER	%RESPONSE	NUMBER	%RESPONSE
E. coli	31	81	9	78	22	82
Klebsiella-Enterobacter-Serratia group	29	79	14	88	15	73
Ps. aeruginosa	11	82	3	100	8	75
Other*	10	70	--	--	10	70
Gram-positive cocci	8	75	2	100	6	67
Multiple organism	27	41	11	27	16	50
Unknown organisms	39	46	20	60	19	32
Single gram-negative bacillus	81	79	26	85	55	76

*4 cases due to Proteus sp., 2 cases due to Citrobacter sp. and 1 case each due to Acinetobacter sp., Aeromonas sp., Hemophilus influenza and Salmonella enteriditis.

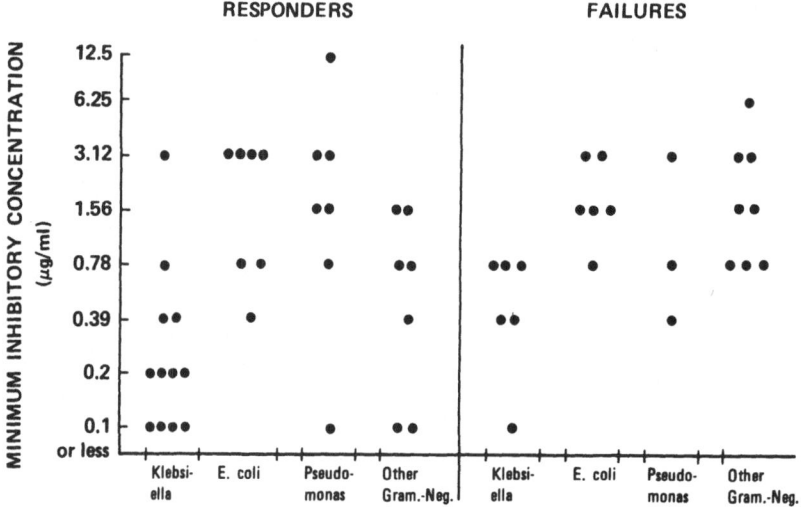

FIGURE 3. Clinical response to amikacin therapy related to in vitro
sensitivity of infecting organisms. Studies were performed
on 56 of the gram-negative bacilli causing infections.

TABLE 4. Responses to Gentamicin, Tobramycin and Amikacin in Relation to Changes in Neutrophil Counts

NEUTROPHILS/mm³	GENTAMICIN		TOBRAMYCIN		AMIKACIN	
	#	%	#	%	#	%
<100	23	22	25	24	27	63
101-1000	26	62	15	60	30	70
>1000	51	57	42	69	98	62
Decreased	45	40	31	35	42	50
Increased	55	50	51	65	113	69
TOTAL	100	50	82	54	155	64

- number of infections   % - percent response

TABLE 5. Response and Toxicity Related to Serum Concentration of
Amikacin

SERUM CONCENTRATION (µg/ml)	EPISODES OF IDENTIFIED INFECTION	% RESPONSE	TOTAL EPISODES	% TOXICITY*
<10	16	63	32	3
10-15	21	76	34	12
15-20	5	80	7	29
>20	9	78	10	50

*Audio or nephrotoxicity

The etiologic agent could be identified during 116 of the 155
episodes of documented infection (Table 3). The majority of infections in which an organism could not be identified were cases of
pneumonia and cellulitis. The most frequently identified pathogens
were E. coli, organisms of the Klebsiella-Enterobacter-Serratia
group and P. aeruginosa. There were no differences in the response
rate among these organisms. The response to amikacin of infections
produced by single gram-negative bacilli was slightly higher for
patients who received the continuous infusion therapy (85% vs 76%).
The poorest results were observed in the treatment of infections
produced by unknown organisms or by multiple organisms.

In vitro sensitivity studies using the broth dilution
technique were performed on 56 of the 79 gram-negative bacilli
causing infections (Figure 3). With exception of 2 organisms, all
were sensitive to 3.12 µg/ml or less of amikacin. The doses of
amikacin administered were sufficient to maintain serum concentrations above this level. However, 23 of the 56 organisms which
caused infections failed to respond. The response rate was only
49% among the 37 infections caused by organisms with an MIC greater
than 0.39 µg/ml. However, the response rate was 79% among the 19
infections caused by organisms with MIC of 0.39 µg/ml or less.
Therefore, response to amikacin was related to the in vitro sensitivity of the infecting organisms. Five of 8 infections produced
by gram-negative bacilli resistant to gentamicin in vitro responded
to amikacin.

The relationship between the response to amikacin and the
number of circulating neutrophils during the period of infection;
as well as a comparison with our previous experience with gentamicin
and tobramycin is presented in Table 4. There was no correlation
between the initial neutrophil count and response to amikacin
therapy. However, the response rate was higher for patients who
responded to their infection with an increment in their neutrophil
count (69%) than for those patients whose neutrophil count decreased
during their infection (50%). Similar results were obtained previously with gentamicin and tobramycin (1,10). The major difference
was that patients with initial severe neutropenia ($<100/mm^3$) responded better to amikacin (63%) than to gentamicin (22%) and
tobramycin (24%). This difference was statistically significant
(p=.001).

Daily serum concentrations were determined during 83 febrile
episodes in neutropenic patients who received amikacin by continuous infusion (Table 5). During 51 of these episodes the patients
had identified infections. The response was higher for the 35
infections in which the patient's serum concentration was maintained
at greater than 10 µg/ml (79% vs 63%). There was no apparent advantage in maintaining a serum concentration greater than 20 µg/ml.
In fact, toxicity was unacceptably high at this level.

TABLE 6. Nephrotoxicity During Amikacin Therapy

RENAL FUNCTION		TOTAL		CONTINUOUS		INTERMITTENT	
INITIAL	SUBSEQUENT	#	%	#	%	#	%
Normal	Normal	167	87	81	94	86	81
Normal	Abnormal	25	13	5	6	20	19
Abnormal	Worsened	13	54	6	100	7	39
Abnormal	Improved	11	46	0	0	11	61

- episodes   % - percent

Seven episodes of superinfection occurred in patients receiving
amikacin. Four episodes occurred in patients receiving treatment
for septicemia. The remaining 3 episodes of superinfection occurred
in patients who were treated for pneumonia. Septicemia was the most
common superinfection and occurred in 5 patients. The remaining 2
superinfections were a surgical wound infection and a urinary tract
infection. All of the superinfections were caused by gram-positive
organisms or anaerobic bacteria. Two superinfections were caused by
multiple organisms.

The major side effect observed during amikacin therapy was
azotemia (Table 6). The patient's renal function was normal prior
to the onset of therapy in 192 episodes and subsequently became
abnormal in 13%. The patient's renal function was abnormal initially in the remaining 24 episodes and worsened subsequently in
54%. Among patients who had normal renal function initially,
azotemia occurred more frequently with intermittent therapy than
with continuous therapy despite higher doses (19% vs 6%). This
difference was statistically significant (p=0.01). The duration of
azotemia could not be completely evaluated since the majority of
patients who developed azotemia died from their infection. However,
in approximately 40% of the patients, azotemia was transient.
Toxicity to the eighth cranial nerve was observed in 6 patients.
Five of these patients received amikacin by continuous infusion.
With exception of a patient who developed reversible acute labyrin-
thitis, the remaining 5 patients developed irreversible hearing loss.
Hearing loss was usually bilateral and characterized by high tone
deafness. Serial audiograms were performed during 45 episodes and
only detected abnormalities in patients who complained of hearing
loss. Audiotoxicity, like nephrotoxicity, was more frequent in
patients whose serum concentration of amikacin was maintained at
more than 15 µg/ml.

DISCUSSION

The results of this study indicate that amikacin is an effective
new aminoglycoside antibiotic for the therapy of infections caused
by gram-negative bacilli. The broad spectrum of in vitro activity

against most isolates of Enterobacteriacea and Pseudomonas aerugionsa, its superiority over tobramycin and gentamicin sulfate in vitro, especially against E. coli and Klebsiella-Enterobacter-Serratia group, as well as its impressive activity against gram-negative bacilli which were resistant to gentamicin sulfate indicate the potential value of amikacin for the treatment of infections caused by these organisms.

The pharmacological studies of amikacin in humans have shown that adequate serum concentrations of this antibiotic can be safely reached and maintained by the continuous administration of amikacin. To maintain an adequate serum concentration of antibiotics constantly is of major importance in the therapy of infections occurring in patients with impaired host defense mechanism (9).

The overall response rate of 64% among cancer patients with identified infections was encouraging and somewhat superior to our previous experience with gentamicin and tobramycin (1,10). Amikacin was most effective in the therapy of infections of the urinary tract (96%) and in cases of septicemia (67%). The cure rate in cases of pneumonia, though low, was significant. Gram-negative bacillary pneumonia generally responds poorly to antibiotic therapy and in similar groups of patients, the mortality rate has ranged from 88% to 100% (7,8). Higher tissue concentration of amikacin could account for the higher response observed among patients with pneumonia who received amikacin by continuous infusion (62%) than among those patients who received amikacin by the intermittent schedule (47%). Some of the cases of pneumonia which failed to respond may have been caused by fungi or protozoa which would not be expected to respond to amikacin. Lack of sputum production due to impaired inflammatory response prevented us from identifying the etiologic agent in these cases.

Amikacin was effective in the treatment of the majority of infections produced by single gram-negative bacillus (79%). Amikacin was only partially effective (41%) against infections produced by multiple organisms. However, these types of infections have been characterized by the low response rate to most treatments, resulting in a high mortality rate. The efficacy of amikacin in the therapy of some infections produced gram-negative bacilli resistant in vitro to gentamicin sulfate was of major importance.

The decision to administer amikacin by continuous infusion to neutropenic patients was based on our previous experience with gentamicin and tobramycin (1,10). The response to these aminoglycoside antibiotics was clearly related to the patient's neutrophil counts during the period of infection. However, gentamicin and tobramycin were administered by the intermittent schedule which resulted in intervals between doses when the serum concentration fell below the concentration required to inhibit the infecting organism. This could be of major importance to the neutropenic patient who is unable to provide adequate phagocytic cells to assist in controlling his infection. Thus, an attempt was made in this study to maintain an adequate serum concentration of amikacin constantly for neutropenic patients. The 63% cure rate obtained among patients with an initial neutrophil count of less than 100 neutrophils/mm^3 compared favorably with the 25% cure rate previously found with intermittent schedules of gentamicin and tobramycin. The results with continuous infusion therapy in patients with severe neutropenia were as good as the results with intermittent amikacin therapy in patients with adequate neutrophil counts.

Nephrotoxicity and audiotoxicity were the major side effects encountered. The overall incidence of nephrotoxicity was lower than our previous experience with gentamicin and comparable to what we observed with tobramycin. However, nephrotoxicity was somewhat more common among patients who received amikacin by the intermittent schedule even when the total daily dose of amikacin in patients receiving the antibiotic by continuous infusion was higher. This observation would suggest that the peak serum concentration of amikacin might be of critical importance in the development of nephrotoxicity. The incidence of audiotoxicity, though infrequent, was more common than has previously been observed with gentamicin and tobramycin therapy.

Amikacin is an effective new aminoglycoside antibiotic for the therapy of gram-negative bacilli infections in cancer patients. Its broad spectrum of activity and its in vivo efficacy against some organisms resistant to gentamicin sulfate is of major clinical importance. Improved results were obtained in neutropenic patients by maintaining an adequate serum concentration of antibiotic constantly by a continuous infusion schedule. Optimal results were obtained when the serum concentration was maintained at approximately 15 μg/ml. A comparative study of amikacin with other aminoglycoside antibiotics is currently underway at our institution.

REFERENCES

1. Bodey, G.P., Middleman, E., Umsawasdi, T. and Rodriguez, V.: Infections in cancer patients – Results with gentamicin sulfate therapy. Cancer 29:1697-1701, 1972.

2. Bodey, G.P. and Stewart, D.: In vitro studies of BB-K8, A new aminoglycoside antibiotic. Antimicrob. Ag. and Chemother. 4:186-192, 1973.

3. Feld, R., Bodey, G.P., Rodriguez, V. and Luna, M.: Causes of death in patients with malignant lymphoma. Am. J. Med. Sci. 268:97-106, 1974.

4. Hersh, E.M., Bodey, G.P., Nies, B.A. and Freireich, E.J: The
    causes of death in acute leukemia. A study of 414 patients from
    1954-1963. J. Am. Med. Assoc. 193:105-109, 1965.

5. Inagaki, J., Rodriguez, V. and Bodey, G.P.: Causes of death in
    cancer patients. Cancer 33:568-573, 1974.

6. Kanaguchi, H., Naito, T., Nakaguna, S. and Fugisana, K.: BB-K8,
    A new semisynthetic aminoglycoside antibiotic. J. Antibiot.
    25:695-708, 1972.

7. Pennington, J.E., Reynolds, H.Y. and Carbone, P.P.: Pseudomonas
    pneumonia. A retrospective study of 36 cases. Am. J. Med.
    55:155-160, 1973.

8. Sickles, E.A., Young, V.M., Greene, W.H. and Wiernik, P.H.:
    Pneumonia in acute leukemia. Ann. Intern. Med. 79:528-534, 1973.

9. Valdivieso, M., Feld, R., Rodriguez, V. and Bodey, G.P.: Amikacin
    therapy of infections in neutropenic patients. Am. J. Med. Sci.
    (In press).

10. Valdivieso, M., Horikoshi, N., Rodriguez, V. and Bodey, G.P.:
    Therapeutic trails with tobramycin. Am. J. Med. Sci. 268:149-
    156, 1974.

CLINICAL STUDY OF BBK8 ON GENTAMICIN (GM)

RESISTANT GRAM NEGATIVE RODS (GNR)

Susumu Tomioka, Yoshio Kobayashi, Mitsuto Hasegawa

School of Medicin, Keio University

35 Shinanomachi, Shinjuku-ku, Tokyo, Japan

Summary
1. Incidence of resistant strains of GNR against B-lactam antibiotics was higher in strains isolated from urine and blood rather than from sputum, especially in those isolated from blood.
2. Also, Gentamicin resistant strains were isolated more frequently from urine and blood than from sputum.
3. Strains of Proteus, Klebsiella and Pseudomonas which are resistant to Gentamicin have been increased in past two years.
4. Gentamicin resistant strains of GNR did not show the cross resistance to Amikacin (BBK8).
5. Amikacin showed therapeutic effect on P.aeruginosa septicemia which was highly resistant to Gentamicin and on Proteus mirabillis septicemia.

Recently the increase of Gram negative rods (GNR) infections has been pointed out in various fields. GNR septicemia has remarkably increased also in and after 1972 at Keio University Hospital. Moreover, it has been often experienced that these infectious organisms were resistant to B-lactam antibiotics. Gentamicin resistant strains also appeared in the last few years. Accordingly we investigated the sensitivity distribution of GNR strains which were isolated recently at Keio University Hospital by clinical specimens and examined antibacterial activity of Amikacin on the strains resistant to Gentamicin.

MIC of Ampicillin was over 200ug/ml against 15 out of 25 strains of E.coli which were isolated from blood during 3 years from 1972 to 1974. MIC of Cephalothin was greater than 100ug/ml against 14 strains and it was 50ug/ml against 9 out of 26 strains of E.coli. Apparently sensitivity of these strains was fairly lower than that

of strains which were isolated at the same time from other than
blood. This relationship was observed also between Klebsiella and
Cephalothin. The results revealed that sensitivity of the strains
isolated from blood to B-lactam antibiotics had been strikingly low
in recent years.

Sensitivity distribution of E.coli, Klebsiella, Proteus and
Enterobacter clinically isolated from urine or sputum to B-lactam
antibiotics. Kanamycin and Gentamicin was also examined by isolated
sourse. The sensitivity of these strains was examined by disc
method. The resistance of Klebsiella and Enterobacter isolated from
urine against B-lactam antibiotics was prominently higher than that
of strains isolated from sputum. Resistance of strains isolated from
in patients was fairly higher. These organisms also showed similar
resistance against Kanamycin and Gentamicin. However, this trend
was not noticeable in E.coli at present.

With regard to isolates in 1974, the details of detection of
the Gentamicin resistant strains was examined by specimen of sputum,
urine, pus and blood and by in and out patients. The results
revealed that 15-20% of GNR isolated from urine or blood in 1974
were Gentamicin resistant strains. As shown in Table 1, the rate of
Gentamicin resistant Klebsiella isolated from urine reached to 28.6%.
Also here, we recognized that the resistance of organisms was apt to
be different depending on specimens from which strains were
clinically isolated.

Gentamicin resistant strains had been highly detected in 1974
as mentioned above, therefore, the details of detection of Gentamicin
resistant strains during last few years was investigated. Test
strains were limited to those clinically isolated from in patients
at Keio University Hospital in and after 1972. From the results
shown in Table 2, the rates of Gentamicin resistant strains in 1972
were under 2% in the strains of Proteus, Klebsiella, Pseudomonas and
E.coli each. However, as shown in this Table 2, Gentamicin resistant
strains had rapidly increased in and after 1973 when the use of
Gentamicin began to be strikingly on the increase. In 1975 the

Table 1. Incidence of Gentamicin Resistnat Strains (in %)
(1974, In-Patients)

Sources	E.coli	Klebsiella	Entero-bacter	Proteus sp.	Pseudo-monas
Sputum	2.0	1.9	1.3	4.6	3.2
Urine	5.8	28.6	17.2	17.5	18.7
Pus	3.5	6.0	4.8	6.0	4.2
Blood	18.2	18.2	13.3	——	16.7

Table 2. Incidence of Gentamicin Resistant Strains (in %)

Year	E.coli	Klebsiella	Entero-bacter	Proteus sp.	Pseudo-monas
1972	1.8	1.6	——	1.1	1.1
1973	3.8	2.6	——	5.3	2.3
1974	5.2	10.8	——	12.3	8.2
1975*	4.7	16.4	3.9	21.3	11.2

Note: Isolated from In-Patients
*Jan.-Mar.

rates of Gentamicin resistant strains had reached to 21.3% in the
strains of Proteus, 16.4% in Klebsiella and 11.2% in Pseudomonas
with a straight increase. Gentamicin resistant strains in E.coli
remained around 5% in 1974 and 1975. Regarding this tendency as an
important matter for treatment of GNR infections, further investigation of the sensitivity distribution of Gentamicin resistant
strains to Kanamycin, Tobramycin, Dibekacin, Amikacin and Colistin
was carried out by agar dilution method. Namely, all the strains
resistant to Gentamicin of E.coli, Klebsiella, Enterobacter and
Proteus except one strain of E.coli were sinsitive to Amikacin.
However, these strains were resistant to Tobramycin, Dibekacin and
Kanamycin.

As shown in Table 3, 24 strains of P.aeruginosa which were
resistant to Gentamicin were also sensitive to Amikacin except one
strain. Gentamicin resistant strains had cross resistance to Tobramycin and Dibekacin. But Pseudomonas cepacia and Flavobacterium
which were originally resistant to Gentamicin were also resistant to
Amikacin. Based on the antibacterial activity of Amikacin against

Table 3. Susceptibility of Pseudomonas aeruginosa*
to Several Aminoglycosides (1973-1974)

Organisms	Antibiotics	MIC (ug/ml)						
		3.13	6.25	12.5	25	50	100	200≤
	Gentamicin						3	21
	Tobramycin			1	5	15	2	1
P.aeruginosa	Dibekacin						2	22
	Amikacin	8	9	6				1
	Kanamycin							24

Inoculum: 1/100 x HIB culture fluid
*Gentamicin Resistant Strains

Gentamicin resistant strains, which was assumed from the above
mentioned results. Amikacin was given to 2 cases of GNR septicemia
who were not affected favorably by Gentamicin.

Case 1 is P.aeruginosa septicemia against which MIC of
Gentamicin was greater than 200ug/ml, associated with subarachnoidal
hemorrhage. BUN and creatinine levels were rather higher in the
begining, so 200mg/day of Amikacin was administered. Latter dose
level was increased to 600mg/day. Satisfactory clinical result was
obtained.

Case 2 is Proteus mirabillis septicemia associated with
Abdominal aneurysm. 800mg/day of Amikacin was given to this patient
from the begining. Clinical effect was not observed during combined
use of Amikacin and Chloramphenicol to which the pathogenic organism,
Proteus mirabillis was highly sensitive was performing. However, the
patients symptom was relieved as soon as administration of Chloramphenicol was discontinued considering the proberbility of antagonism
between Amikacin and Chloramphenicol. No side effect was observed
in cases 1 and 2.

A CLINICAL STUDY OF AMIKACIN - A NEW AMINOGLYCOSIDE ANTIBIOTIC

E.V. Haldane and C.E. van Rooyen

Dept. of Microbiology, V.G.H.

5788 University Ave., Halifax, Nova Scotia

Amikacin is a new aminoglycoside antibiotic derived from Kanamycin-A. Both these antibiotics have a potent broad antimicrobial spectrum, but in addition Amikacin possesses activity against some Enterobacteriaceae and Pseudomonas species which are resistant to one or more of the other aminoglycosides, including some gentamicin-resistant strains. Severe infections caused by gram-negative bacilli continue to pose a major clinical problem, particularly when the organism shows in vitro resistance to gentamicin. The purpose of this clinical study was to assess the effectiveness of Amikacin therapy in a selection of such seriously ill patients.

Twenty-eight patients were included in the study group. Most of the patients had a serious underlying pathological condition, to which the infection was superadded as an acute and frequently, life-threatening episode or complication.

There were 10 cases of UTI - 5 post-operative infections following transurethral prostatectomy, 1 carcinoma of bladder, 1 renal transplantation 2 weeks previously, 1 severe subarachnoid haemorrhage, 1 congestive cardiac failure, and 1 postoperative infection after nephrostomy for obstructed ureter of the patient's only kidney. Three of the patients were paraplegics and 2 patients had concurrent septicaemia and endotoxic shock. Three of the wound infections were in above-knee amputation stumps in patients with peripheral circulatory insufficiency, 2 of whom had multiple sclerosis; the fourth was in a shotgun wound of arm. The chronic osteomyelitis all resulted from complicated fractures which had occurred 1 to 8 years previously, 2 of the femur, 1 of the humerus. The 3 intra-thoracic infections were severe pneumonia, lung abscess, empyema and fistula superimposed on chronic obstructive lung disease, bronchiectasis, and crush injury, respectively. Intra-abdominal

infection followed perforated sigmoid colon, and hemicolostomy for
carcinoma.   The arterial grafts were followed by chronic abscess
formation with deep draining sinuses.   Septicaemia occurred in a
young paraplegic with recurrent UTI and in a man with chronic lymphatic leukaemia - this man had been desperately ill for 4 weeks and
was practically moribund when referred to our service.   The second
leukaemic patient had an ileo-rectal abscess and a gluteal abscess
and unremitting hectic temperature for several weeks, but repeated
negative blood cultures.   The final patient was a young man with
persistent Pseudomonas aeruginosa infection in 3rd degree burns of
one leg.   Thirteen patients were infected with a single strain of
organism, while 15 had mixed infections with 2 or more strains of
different gram-negative species.   Twenty-two patients had been
treated with various antibiotics immediately prior to Amikacin
therapy, including 18 who had received other aminoglycosides, mostly
gentamicin.   None had shown any significant clinical or bacteriological response to treatment.   Susceptibility of the organisms to
Amikacin was determined before therapy, using the Kirby-Bauer disc
method on Mueller-Hinton agar, and all these bacteria were sensitive
in vitro to Amikacin.   In several cases the minimum inhibitory concentration of Amikacin against the organism was also determined by
tube dilution technique.

The average treatment schedule was 15-20 mgm/Kg, given either
intravenously or intramuscularly in 3 divided doses/day to a maximum of 1500 mgm daily, for an average duration of 10 days.   In
some cases IV treatment was given for the first 5 days to assure a
rapid and sufficient serum concentration of drug, and then IM for
5 days when the patient's condition was improved.   There was some
variation in treatment schedule according to severity and type of
illness, a few patients having a twice daily schedule, and several
continuing treatment for 12-15 days.   Toxicity did not pose a big
problem.   Renal function, hepatic function and hemopoietic studies
were made before, during and after the end of the course of therapy.
One patient, who had a history of chronic otitis media in childhood,
showed evidence of some degree of hearing loss after 5 days treatment, and the drug was stopped.   The audiogram then returned to the
pre-drug level.   Some weeks later, a second course produced a
similar effect.   Two cases showed a slight rise of BUN and serum
creatinine after 8 and 10 days treatment, indicative of mild renal
impairment.   Both reached their peak levels in two weeks and thereafter returned to normal within a week.   No hepatic or hemopoietic
disfunction was noted.   Two cases had mild renal insufficiency,
including the transplant patient.   One of these was given 500 mgm
once daily, and the other 500 mgm only once every 48 hours.   Serum
levels were carefully monitored daily in these two patients and
their schedule of dosage adjusted accordingly, and an average serum
concentration of 12-15 mcg/ml was achieved with the foregoing
schedules.   Both patients did extremely well without showing any
evidence of toxic effects, and renal function improved and their
infection cleared.

The outcome of treatment in the various classes of patient is shown in Table 1. Of those with UTI 8 recovered completely, one was improved and 1 died. The patient who died, developed infection with Serratia marcescens following nephrostomy, and was comatose, in septicaemic shock, with renal failure when first seen by our service. On Amikacin therapy, he showed an initial response for 2-3 days, but on the 5th day had a sudden cardiac arrest and could not be resuscitated. The chronic osteomyelitis cases all recovered. Neither infected arterial grafts showed any improvement. Of the respiratory cases, the patient with long standing chronic obstructive lung disease, remained unchanged. There were 2 cases with infection in the course of chronic lymphatic leukaemia - one with Serratia marcescens septicaemia who was moribund when started on Amikacin. He showed considerable clinical improvement within 4-5 days, his blood culture became negative, and 2 weeks later he was sufficiently well to be discharged from hospital. The second case had resistant E.coli infection with abscesses and hectic temperature pattern, and unfortunately he showed no response to any antibiotic therapy, including Amikacin.

Two series of patients are of particular interest. During our study, we had 2 minor hospital epidemics which we successfully controlled with Amikacin. One occurred among elderly urological patients in a Veteran's hospital, and was caused by a resistant strain of Proteus rettgeri, which was subsequently serotyped by Dr. John Penner of Toronto and found to belong to Biogroup 5, subgroup 5A, which appears to be an intermediate group between P.rettgeri and Providentia stuartii. The antibiogram of this strain showed it to be sensitive only to Amikacin, gentamicin and nalidixic acid. The infections were causing great discomfort and distress to the patients affected and had not responded to any treatment including gentamicin, despite in vitro sensitivity, but all cleared up rapidly and completely with Amikacin. The second epidemic, due to a multi-resistant strain of Serratia marcescens, sensitive to Amikacin only, started in a neurosurgical ward among paraplegic patients with Foley catheter bladder drainage. This group included the patient with nephrostomy who died, but otherwise Amikacin proved satisfactory in treatment and in eliminating the organism.

Table 2 summarises the outcome of treatment in all 28 patients. Seventeen (61%) showed complete bacteriological and clinical recovery from their gram-negative infective illness; a further 6 (21%) were improved, i.e., the infecting organisms were greatly reduced in number with corresponding clinical improvement, and 4 of these progressed to complete cure without further antibiotic therapy; five (18%) failed to respond either clinically or bacteriologically and 2 of these patients died.

TABLE 1.   TYPES OF INFECTION AND RESULTS OF AMIKACIN THERAPY

	No. of Patients	Bacteria	Results
UTI	3	P.rettgeri	3 Cured
	3	Serratia marc.	2 Cured, 1 died
	1	P.rettgeri, P.vulgaris	Cured
	1	Serratia marc. Enterococcus	Cured
	1	P.vulgaris, Ps.aerug. Klebsiella, Ps.aerug.	Improved
	1	Serratia marc.Klebsiella P.mirabilis	Cured
Respiratory	1	Serratia marc., Ps.aerug. Klebsiella,Enterobacter	Failed
	1	Serratia marc.	Improved
	1	Ps.aerug. E.coli, Kleb.pneum.	Cured
Osteo-myelitis	1	Serratia marc. Klebsiella Aeromonas	Cured
	1	Serratia marc. Pseudo	Cured
	1	Pseud.aerug. Staph.pyog.	Cured
Wound	3	Pseud.aerug.	3 Cured
	1	P.vulgaris, P.rettgeri Enterococcus	Improved
Arterial Grafts	1	E.coli, Klebsiella	Failed
	1	E.coli, P.mirabilis Enterococcus	Failed
Abdominal	1	E.coli, P.mirabilis Pseud.aerug. Bacteroides	Improved
	1	E.coli, Enterobacter Bacteroides	Cured
Septi-caemia	1	P.mirabilis	Cured
	1(Leukaemia)	Serratia marc.	Cured
Misc.	1(Abscesses, Leukaemia)	E.coli	Failed
	1(Burns)	Pseud.aerug. Klebsiella Staph.pyog.	Improved

TABLE 2.   SUMMARY OF RESULTS OF THERAPY

No. of Patients	Type of Infection	Number with Single Isolate	Number with Mixed Infection	Result Cured	Result Improved	Result Failure
10	UTI	6	4	8	1	1
4	Wound	3	1	2	2	-
3	Osteomyelitis	-	3	3	-	-
3	Intrathoracic	1	2	1	1	1
2	Arterial Grafts	-	2	-	-	2
2	Intra-Abdominal	-	2	1	1	-
2	Septicaemia	2	-	2	-	-
1	Burns	-	1	-	1	-
Total 28 100%		13	15	17 61%	6 21%	5 18%

In conclusion - of 28 patients with gram negative infections, all serious and many resistant to other antibiotics, 75% were successfully treated with Amikacin. 7% showed partial response, and 18% were not improved.

Amikacin showed no cross-resistance with other aminoglycoside antibiotics, and appears to be a most valuable addition to the aminoglycoside family for the treatment of gram negative infections, in particular those with organisms resistant to the other previously available antibiotics.

TREATMENT OF SEVERE INFECTIONS WITH AMIKACIN

DAIKOS G.K.,KOSMIDIS J.C.,KAFETZIS D.AND GIAMARELLOU H.

First Department of Propedeutic Medicine,Athens University

School of Medicine, King Paul's Hospital,Athens,Greece

SUMMARY

Amikacin was administered to forty-four patients suffering from severe infections, often due to organisms resistant to many antibiotics, including gentamicin. Several aggravating factors were often present. The dose administered was 500 mg or 250 mg twice daily,but in patients with impaired renal function the dose was determined by frequent monitoring of serum antibiotic levels. In 28 cases (64 %) results were excellent, in 9 cases (20 %) they were good and in only 7 cases (16 %) a fair result was obtained. No ototoxicity was observed, but in two patients a mild, reversible rise in BUN and serum creatinine was found. Amikacin may replace gentamicin for the initial treatment of severe infections, especially in countries or hospitals with an increasing rate of resistance to gentamicin.

INTRODUCTION

Amikacin (BB-K8) is a semi-synthetic derivative of kanamycin (Kawaguchi et al, 1972), which is highly resistant to most amino-glycoside-inactivating enzymes (Price et al, 1972). It is very active against aminoglycoside-resistant strains (Reynolds et al, 1974, Price et al, 1974). Animal toxicity (Reiffenstein et al, 1973) and human pharmacokinetics (Clarke et al, 1974) resemble those of kana-mycin.

Bacterial resistance to gentamicin and other antibiotics consti-tutes a problem of increasing magnitude. A high proportion of the clinical isolates at the King Paul's Hospital, particularly pseudo-monads, are resistant to all commercially available aminoglycosides,

TABLE I

Age Group	No. Patients
11 - 20	1
21 - 30	5
31 - 40	2
41 - 50	2
51 - 60	7
61 - 70	16
71 - 80	10
80 +	1
Total	44

as well as to most other commercially available injectable antibiotics. Similar experience has been reported from another Greek hospital where 30% of Pseudomonas aeruginosa strains were found resistant to gentamicin (Papachristou and Kontomichalou, 1974).

Since most of these strains are sensitive to amikacin a clinical trial with this drug was conducted and the results are reported here.

MATERIALS AND METHODS

Forty-four patients (21 males and 23 females) were treated. Most of the patients were over 60 years of age (Table I). They were suffering from severe infections in the presence of several aggravating factors, such as coma, advanced neoplasia often with antineoplastic chemotherapy, renal failure, diabetes mellitus, severe cardiorespiratory disease, administration of corticosteroids, tracheostomy, indwelling bladder catheter or other foreign body at the infection site. Twenty-six patients were suffering from urinary tract infections, ten from infections of the respiratory tract and there were eight miscellaneous infections. The infecting organisms were Klebsiella spp (13 isolates) E.Coli (12 isolates), Pseudomonas spp (11 isolates) and Proteus spp (10 isolates). There was one isolate of each of the following: Staphylococcus aureus, Micrococcus spp and an atypical coliform. In six cases there were two infecting organisms, while in one case of cholangitis no pathogen was isolated, in spite of repeated blood cultures. The diagnosis was based on clinical, haematological, radiological and histological criteria. The dosage given was 250 mg or 500 mg twice daily, depending on the nature and severity of the infection, as well as on the infecting organism. In patients with renal failure, serum antibiotic concentrations were frequently measured and the dose modified accordingly. A peak level of about 20 μg/ml was aimed at. The treatment lasted from 6 to 17 days. All patients were closely observed for the occurrence of side effects and the following tests were performed before, during and after treatment: Haematocrit, haemoglobin, white blood count, differential count, SGOT, SGPT, serum alkaline phosphatase and bilirubin,

serum creatinine, blood urea nitrogen and complete urinalysis. In
six patients audiograms were performed before and after the antibiotic course. The overall result of the treatment was considered
"excellent", when the patient was clinically cured from the infection, the pathogen was eradicated and there was no relapse. A "good"
result indicated that the patient was clinically cured but that the
pathogen was not eradicated. This was usually observed in patients
with tracheostomies, fistulae, indwelling bladder catheters, etc.
The overall result was considered "fair"when clinical improvement
was noted but this was not entirely satisfactory and either the
pathogen was not eradicated or a new pathogen had appeared. A "poor"
result indicated that the treatment had obviously failed, there was
no improvement as far as the infection was concerned, the pathogen
was not eradicated and another antibiotic had to be given.

Minimum inhibitory concentration (MIC) and minimum bactericidal
concentration (MBC) of amikacin were determined for 77 consecutive
clinical isolates. MIC was measured by a microtitre technique using
tryptose phosphate broth and an inoculum of 10^6 bacteria/ml. MBC
was measured by quantitative subculture onto semisolid media. Killing of 99.9% of organisms was taken as cut-off point. Susceptibility of the infecting organisms to other antibiotics was determined
by discs using the Bauer-Kirby method.

Antibiotic concentrations were measured by an agar well method
using Bacillus subtilis as test organism (Bodey et al, 1974).

RESULTS

Antibiotic Susceptibility of Clinical Isolates

All the infecting organisms were sensitive to amikacin as a
prerequisite for inclusion in the study. Many of the organisms
were resistant to many agents, including gentamicin (Table II) and
18 strains were resistant to all commercially available injectable
antibiotics with the possible exception of colistin.

MIC's of amikacin for 77 clinical isolates are presented in
Table III. All 5 Pseudomonas spp strains were inhibited by 4 µg/ml,
but there were several amikacin resistant strains among the other
species tested.

Efficacy of Treatment

In 28 cases (64%) the overall result was excellent. In nine
(20%) it was good and there were seven (16%) fair results. In no
case was the result graded poor (Table IV). The best results were

TABLE II
DISC SENSITIVITY OF INFECTING ORGANISMS

	Total No.	Amik	Genta	Kana	CFT*	Tet	Amp	TMP/SMZ**
E. Coli	12	12	8	6	6	3/11	3	6/8
Atyp.colif	1	1	0	0	0	1	0	1
Klebsiella spp	13	13	5	5	3	3	1	3/4
Proteus spp	10	10	4	3	2/9	0/9	2	1/4
Pseudomonas spp	11	11	2	0	N.T.	1/6	N.T.	N.T.
Micrococcus spp	1	1	1	1	1	1	0	1
Staph.aureus	1	1	1	1	1	1	1	N.T.
	49	49	21	16	13/37	10/42	7/38	12/18

(header: STRAINS SENSITIVE TO)

CFT*: Cephalothin
TMP/SMZ**: Trimethoprim/Sulphamethoxazole

TABLE IV
EFFICACY OF TREATMENT

Organism	No. strains		Antibiotic concentration (µg/ml)										
			0.25	0.5	1	2	4	8	16	32	64	128	>128
E.Coli	20	MIC	1	-	1	-	2	5	3	5	1	1	1
		MBC	-	-	-	-	1	5	5	3	4	1	1
Klebsiella spp	32	MIC	6	2	3	8	2	7	2	-	-	1	1
		MBC	2	2	4	6	4	5	5	-	-	2	2
Proteus spp	13	MIC	1	-	-	-	3	2	3	2	1	1	-
		MBC	1	-	-	-	-	2	3	3	3	1	-
Pseudomonas spp	5	MIC	1	-	1	2	1	-	-	-	-	-	-
		MBC	-	-	-	1	2	2	-	-	-	-	-
Staph.aureus	7	MIC	1	-	-	1	1	1	-	2	-	-	1
		MBC	1	-	-	-	2	1	-	-	1	1	1

TABLE III
SUSCEPTIBILITY OF 77 CLINICAL ISOLATES TO AMIKACIN

	No.pts	Exc.	Good	Fair	Poor
Pyelonephritis acute	15	11	2	2	-
Pyelonephritis chronic	3	2	1	-	-
Cystitis acute	7	7	-	-	-
Prostatitis	1	1	-	-	-
Bronchopneumonia	9	4	3	2	-
Lobar pneumonia	1	-	1	-	-
Infected biliary fistula	2	-	1	1	-
Infected hydatid cyst liver	1	-	1	-	-
Cholangitis	1	1	-	-	-
Peritonitis	1	1	-	-	-
Cellulitis of vulva	1	1	-	-	-
Wound infection	2	-	-	2	-
Total	44	28	9	7	-

(header: Overall assessment)

obtained in cystitis (100% excellent). Mixed infections had a less satisfactory outcome. In all seven cases with a fair result at least one aggravating factor was present and in five of these there were at least two such factors. Results with infections due to aminogly-coside-resistant bacteria are shown in Table V.

Side Effects and Toxicity

The injections were painless. No adverse symptoms were observed with the exception of one neurotic patient who complained of blurred vision on the last day of treatment. Detailed ophthalmological examination including visual acuity and visual fields, was normal. As soon as the patient was reassured he stopped complaining.

In two patients a rise in blood urea nitrogen (BUN) and serum creatinine (SC) was observed. The first was a 30 year old man with multiple sclerosis, indwelling bladder catheter and chronic pyelonephritis. _Proteus rettgeri_ was isolated from his urine, which was sensitive to amikacin only. His pretreatment BUN was 30 mg/100ml and SC 1.7mg/100ml. He was given 250 mg amikacin twice daily for sixteen days. Immediately after completion of treatment, BUN was 44 mg/100ml and SC 3.6 mg/100ml. No concomitant therapy had been given. These changes were reversible, values returning to the pretreatment levels in two weeks. The second patient was a 58 year old lady with acute pyelonephritis due to E. Coli, complicating cardiac failure due to mitral stenosis. She was also suffering from chronic bronchitis. Her pretreatment BUN was 20 mg/100ml and SC 1.3 mg/100ml. Amikacin was given at a dose of 250 mg twice daily for 13 days. Digoxin and frusemide were administered concomitantly. On the seventh day of treatment, BUN was 24 mg/100ml and SC 1.4 mg/100ml, but immediately post-treatment, BUN was 74 mg/100ml and SC 3.1 mg/100ml. These changes were again reversible within two weeks.

In two further patients a transient rise in SGOT and a transient leukopenia were respectively observed. The contribution of their basic illnesses to these changes is unclear. There were no other instances of renal, hepatic, haematologic or other form of toxicity. In all cases where audiograms were performed, there was absolutely no difference between the pre- and post-treatment result.

TABLE V
RESULTS WITH AMINOGLYCOSIDE-RESISTANT STRAINS

Patients with strains resistant to	Total No.	Lab.result Erad.	Lab.result Pers.	Exc.	Good	Fair	Poor
Gentamicin	27	16	11	14	8	5	-
Kanamycin	33	20	13	18	8	7	-
All except amikacin	18	11	7	10	5	3	-

DISCUSSION

In this group of mostly old patients, suffering from severe infections, in the presence of various aggravating factors, amikacin proved a very effective antibiotic. Twenty-seven of the 44 patients had an infecting organism that was resistant to gentamicin. In 22 of those a satisfactory result was obtained. This is especially encouraging in view of the increasing concern about the spread of gentamicin-resistant strains. It may however be necessary to frequently monitor the renal function of patients with known or suspected renal failure, possibly avoiding diuretics. Eighth nerve toxicity was completely absent, as often documented by audiograms.

In conclusion, in our hands, amikacin was a very effective drug for the treatment of severe infections, often due to multiresistant organisms. Wherever gentamicin resistance is increasing, amikacin may be recommended as the aminoglycoside of choice for the treatment of severe infections. Further work is needed to determine its effect on the kidney, but otherwise, in our patients, it was safe, demonstrating a total lack of ototoxicity.

REFERENCES

Bodey,G.P.,Valdivieso,M.,Feld,R. and Rodriguez,V. (1974),Antimicrobial Agents and Chemotherapy, 5,508.

Clarke,J.T.,Libke,R.D.,Regamey,C. and Kirby,W.M.M.(1974),Clinical Pharmacology and Therapeutics, 15,610.

Kawaguchi,H.,Takayuki,N.,Nakagawa,S. and Fujisawa,K.(1972),Journal of Antibiotics, 25,695.

Papachristou,E. and Kontomichalou,P. (1974), Proceedings of the 6th National Symposium of Microbiology,Athens,p. 266-278.

Price,K.E.,Chisholm,D.R.,Misiek,M.,Leitner,F. and Tsai,Y.H. (1972), Journal of Antibiotics, 25,709.

Price,K.E.,Pursiano,T.A.,De Furia,M.D. and Wright,G.E. (1974), Antimicrobial Agents and Chemotherapy, 5,143.

Reiffenstein,J.C.,Holmes,S.W.,Hottendorf,G.H. and Bierwagen,M.E. (1973), Journal of Antibiotics, 26,94.

Reynolds,A.V.,Hamilton-Miller,J.M.T. and Brumfitt,W. (1974), British Medical Journal, 3,778.

CLINICAL STUDY OF AMIKACIN (BB-K8) IN URINARY TRACT

INFECTIONS BY DOUBLE-BLIND METHOD

Jyoichi KUMAZAWA, Seiichi NAKAMUTA and Shunro MOMOSE

Department of Urology, Faculty of Medicine, Kyushu
University
3-chome, Maidashi, Fukuoka, Japan

Clinical effect on urinary tract infections and appearance of
side effects following by the administration of a new aminoglycoside antibiotic, amikacin (BB-K8) were compared with a control drug,
aminodeoxykanamycin (AKM) by double-blind method. Concerning clinical efficacy and side effects no statistical significant difference
was noted in both treated patients with acute simple cystitis (amikacin 49 cases and AKM 56 cases), and patients with acute pyelonephritis (amikacin 21 cases and AKM 19 cases). Concerning urinary
tract infection after removing urethral indwelling catheter in
postoperation cases of bladder or prostate (amikacin 31 cases and
AKM 37 cases), there observed no significant difference in side effects between both groups. From the point of clinical efficacy,
however, it was observed that amikacin treated group was superior to
AKM treated group with a significant difference $(p < 0.05)$.

In the urological department of 11 hospitals, including the
Department of Urology, Kyushu University, the clinical effects of
amikacin were evaluated by comparing with a control drug, aminodeoxykanamycin (AKM) by double-blind method in three groups of patients with acute simple cystitis, acute pyelonephritis and urinary
tract infection following the operation of bladder or prostate (after removing the indwelling catheter).

The acute simple cystitis group comprised 122 patients, in 17
of whom the administration was discontinued. The remaining 105 patients completed the trial either with amikacin (49 patients) or
with AKM (56 patients). The acute pyelonephritis group comprised
54 patients, of whom 40 finished the trial either with amikacin (21
patients) or AKM (19 patients). The last group, patients with urinary tract infection, initially comprised 91 patients, of whom 68

were fully traced under the administration with BB-K8 (31 patients)
or AKM (37 patients). For all three groups, there was no significant difference in the number of patients between both treated
groups.

The clinical effects were summarized as follows: In the acute
cystitis, 49 patients treated with amikacin were evaluated as 38
excellent, 8 good and 3 poor with the percentage of effectiveness
93.9 %. 56 patients treated with AKM comprised 38 excellent, 15
good and 3 poor with the percentage of effectiveness 94.6 %. Hence,
no statistically significant difference was noted between both
treated groups. In the acute pyelonephritis 21 patients treated by
amikacin consisted of 14 excellent and 7 good with the percentage
of effectiveness 100 %. 19 patients treated by AKM comprised 11
excellent, 6 good and 2 poor with the percentage of effectiveness
89.5 %. There observed no significant difference between two
groups. Finally, in the urinary tract infection after the operation
of bladder or prostate, 31 patients treated by amikacin comprised
5 excellent, 16 good and 12 poor with the percentage of effectiveness 67.7 %. While 37 patients treated by AKM comprised 2 excellent
12 good and 23 poor with the percentage of effectiveness 37.8 %.
Thus, in the urinary tract infection, the amikacin treated group was
superior to AKM treated group with a statistically significant difference (p < 0.05).

Improvement of subjective symptoms and urine analysis was also
compared with. In the acute simple cystitis and acute pyelonephritis there observed no statistically significant difference between both treated groups, while in the urinary tract infection
after the operation of bladder or prostate, the amikacin treated
group showed favourable effectiveness in the improvement of albuminuria (p < 0.01) and the reduction of urine bacilli (p < 0.1).

In cases of acute simple cystitis and acute pyelonephritis,
the pathogen was mostly Escherichia coli. The clinical effectiveness in the single organism-and mixed organism-infections, and both
combined effectiveness were evaluated, however, no significant
difference was noted between amikacin and AKM treated groups. In
urinary tract infections after the operation of bladder or prostate,
the pathogen was mostly Pseudomonas aeruginosa. While in single
organism-infection, no statistically significant difference was observed in both groups, the amikacin treated group showed clinical
superiority to AKM treated group with statistical significance in
effectiveness in mixed organism-infection (p < 0.05) and in both combined effectiveness (p < 0.01).

The minimal inhibitory concentration (MIC) of amikacin, AKM,
gentamicin (GM), kanamycin (KM) and dibekacin (DKB) against pathogens was examined. The MIC of amikacin against Escherichia coli was
mostly ranged 1.56 to 6.25 mcg/ml, which was a little inferior to

GM and DKB, but superior to KM and nearly equal to AKM. The MIC
of amikacin against Pseudomonas aeruginosa was 1.56 to 12.5 mcg/ml,
which was comparable to that of GM and DKB, and superior to that of
KM and AKM.

As for the side effects, in the patients with acute simple
cystitis, 6 cases of pain at the injection site, 1 case each of
tinnitus and pyrexia were observed in the amikacin treated group,
while 2 cases of pain at the injection site, 1 case of gastric pain
and 2 cases of eruption which were discontinued the administration,
were seen in the AKM treated group. In the patients with acute
pyelonephritis, 5 patients treated by amikacin and 1 patient treated
by AKM complained of the pain at the injection site. In the patients with urinary tract infection after the operation of bladder
or prostate, 1 patient of AKM treated group complained of pain at
the injection site, but no significant difference was observed between two groups. The erythrocyte count, leucocyte count, blood
urea nitrogen, creatinine, glutamic oxaloacetic transaminase and
glutamic pyruvic transaminase in the peripheral blood were checked
as far as possible. No abnormal values were found after dosing in
both treated groups.

Consequently, it may be concluded that amikacin is highly effective for the treatment of acute simple cystitis and acute
pyelonephritis, with no significant difference clinically and bacteriologically in comparison with AKM. Amikacin is also fairly effective to urinary tract infection after the operation of bladder or
prostate, its clinical and bacteriological effectiveness being significantly superior to that of AKM.

References

1) Kawaguchi, H.; T. Naito, S. Nakagawa & K. Fujisawa: BB-K8, a
   new semisynthetic aminoglycoside antibiotic. J. Antibiotics
   25:695-708, 1972

2) Price, K. E.; D. R. Chisholm, M. Misiek, F. Leitner & Y. H.
   Tsai: Microbiological evaluation of BB-K8, a new semisynthetic
   aminoglycoside. J. Antibiotics 25:709-731, 1970

3) Reiffenstein, J. C.; S. W. Holmes, G. H. Hottendorf & M. E.
   Bierwagen: Ototoxicity studies with BB-K8, a new semisynthetic
   aminoglycoside antibiotic. J. Antibiotic 26:94-100, 1973

4) Cabana, B. E. & J. G. Taggart: Comparative pharmacokinetics
   of BB-K8 and kanamycin in dogs and humans. Antimicrb. Agents
   Chemother. 4:478-483, 1973

Andrews, J.
Artenstein, M.S.
Astrug, A.

Bankl, H.
Beavis, J.P.
Bedford, K.
Berben, J.A.
Bodey, G.P.
Brumfitt, W.
Bucholz, H.W.
Burch, K.

Campanella, L.
Caruso, D.
Catizone, F.
Chain, Sir E.
Cohen, J.D.
Concetti, F.
Constantinidou, M.
Controni, G.
Cox, F.

Daikos, G.K.
Darke, C.S.
Deane, C.A.
De Domenico, R.
Delamore, I.W.
Dingeldein, E.
Dontas, A.S.

Fabre, S.
Farrell, W.
Feld, R.
Ferguson, I.R.
Frottier, J.
Fisher, E.

Garcia, J.A.
Gaya, H.
Gelinov, H.
Gfeller, J.
Giamarellou, H.
Gorst, D.
Gould, J.C.
Gruneberg, R.N.

Haider, W.
Haldane, E.V.
Hale, J.H.
Hamilton,Miller,J.L.

Hasegawa, M.
Hejllar, M.
Herz, G.
Hicks, J.M.
Higby, D.J.
Hilmer, R.
Holloway, W.J.
Honetz, N.
Hooper, D.G.
Hossack, G.M.
Huang, J.T.

Imamura, K.
Ingham, H.R.
Ishiyama, S.
Ivamoto, H.
Iwai, S.
Izumi, M.

Jameson, B.
Jedlickova, Z.
Jennis, F.
Jensen, K.

Kafetzis, D.
Kawabe, T.
Kawamori, Y.
Kishimoto, K.
Kjaer, T.B.
Klastersky, J.
Kobata, S.
Kobayashi, Y.
Kolb, L.D.
Kosmidis, J.C.
Kotani, Y.
Krystof, G.
Kubo, S.

Lackner, F.
Lang, E.
Launchbury, A.P.
Lecart, C.
Ledger, W.J.
Luyx, A.

Madhavan, T.
Madsen, P.O.
Martin, F.
McRedie, K.B.
Miale, T.D.
Miller, D.L.

Mittermayer, K.
Miwa, T.
Mondai, J.
Moss, V.
Muramatsu, Y.
Murata, I.

Nakayama, I.
Niden, A.H.
Ninomiya, K.
Nishimura, T.
Nishizawa, Y.

Ohkoshi, M.
Okubadejo, O.A.
Owen, D.

Pacilio, G.
Paddock, G.M.
Parsons, R.L.
Peet, T.N.D.
Pichler, H.
Prieto, J.

Saenz, M.C.
Schwartz, P.P.
Schimpff, S.C.
Selkon, J.
Semoulin, R.
Shibata, K.
Shimizu, Y.
Shinagawa, N.
Simkova, M.
Smith, L.L.
Stone, H.H.
Storring, R.A.
Suzuki, S.
Suzuki, Y.

Reeves, D.S.
Reynolds, A.V.

Rodriguez, V.
Rodriguez, W.J.
Ross, S.
Rotter, M.
Roy, D.
Rubin, A.
Ryc, M.

Quinn, E.

Takken, G.A.
Terashima, I.
Thadepalli, H.
Thomas, A.L.
Todorova, L.
Tomioka, S.
Tooth, T.A.
Tramont, E.C.
Tsekos, G.N.
Turner, D.T.L.

Uehara, S.
Ueno, K.

Vachon, F.
Valdiviesco, M.
Van Rooyen, C.E.
Vincent, P.C.

Wahlig, H.
Watanabe, K.
Wewalka, G.
Wilkinson, P.M.
Williams, J.D.
Wise, R.
Wood, M.
Work, B.

Yasushi, U.
Yoshida, R.
Yura, J.